Concise Pocket Midwifery Dictionary

Concise Pocket Midwifery Dictionary

Second Edition

UN Panda MD

Senior Physician

New Delhi, India

JAYPEE *The Health Sciences Publisher*

New Delhi | London | Philadelphia | Panama

Jaypee Brothers Medical Publishers (P) Ltd

Headquarters

Jaypee Brothers Medical Publishers (P) Ltd
4838/24, Ansari Road, Daryaganj
New Delhi 110 002, India
Phone: +91-11-43574357
Fax: +91-11-43574314
Email: jaypee@jaypeebrothers.com

Overseas Offices

J.P. Medical Ltd
83 Victoria Street, London
SW1H 0HW (UK)
Phone: +44 20 3170 8910
Fax: +44 (0)20 3008 6180
Email: info@jpmedpub.com

Jaypee Medical Inc
The Bourse
111 South Independence Mall East
Suite 835, Philadelphia, PA 19106, USA
Phone: +1 267-519-9789
Email: jpmed.us@gmail.com

Jaypee Brothers Medical Publishers (P) Ltd
Bhotahity, Kathmandu, Nepal
Phone: +977-9741283608
Email: kathmandu@jaypeebrothers.com

Jaypee-Highlights Medical Publishers Inc
City of Knowledge, Bld. 237, Clayton
Panama City, Panama
Phone: +1 507-301-0496
Fax: +1 507-301-0499
Email: cservice@jphmedical.com

Jaypee Brothers Medical Publishers (P) Ltd
17/1-B Babar Road, Block-B, Shaymali
Mohammadpur, Dhaka-1207
Bangladesh
Mobile: +08801912003485
Email: jaypeedhaka@gmail.com

Website: www.jaypeebrothers.com
Website: www.jaypeedigital.com

Inquiries for bulk sales may be solicited at: jaypee@jaypeebrothers.com

Concise Pocket Midwifery Dictionary

First Edition: 2010
Second Edition: **2015**
ISBN 978-93-5152-584-4
Printed at Sanat Printers, Kundli

Preface to the Second Edition

Midwives play an important role in maternal and child healthcare and delivery. In developing countries, rural health essentially hinges on shoulders of an energetic, well-informed and dedicated midwife.

Revised edition of Midwifery dictionary would serve as a useful guide for midwives and rural health delivery personnel. It is basically written to impart and inform the midwife about basic terms used in medical science, particularly obstetrics and gynecology. The language and elaboration have been made simple and easy to comprehend. Several new diagrams (more than 100) and appendices (13) have been added to this new edition.

Since medicine is a constantly changing field, utmost care has been taken to maintain the authenticity and credibility of the information provided in this dictionary. However, some inadvertent human errors remain unavoidable. Therefore, all suggestions for improvement are cordially welcome.

Last but not least, I would like to thank the medical editors, Dr Anchal Kaushik and Ms Dikshika Joshi for helping me in revising this dictionary. I am also especially grateful to the entire staff of M/s Jaypee Brothers Medical Publishers (P) Ltd, New Delhi, India, for bringing out this fantastic dictionary.

UN Panda

Preface to the First Edition

Midwife plays an important role in maternal and child healthcare delivery. In developing countries, rural health essentially hinges on shoulders of an energetic, well-informed and dedicated midwife.

Midwifery dictionary is basically written to impart and inform the midwife about basic terms used in medical science, particularly obstetrics and gynecology. The language and elaboration have been simple and easy to comprehend. Common procedures, instruments and interventions have been also described in brief at appropriate places. The book is handy and easy to comprehend.

All suggestions for improvement are cordially welcome.

UN Panda

Contents

a. scan an ultrasound procedure

abacavir An anti-HIV drug

abasia inability to walk

abatement decrease in severity of symptoms or pain

ABC the mnemonic used for remembering the correct protocol, in order of priority, for cardiopulmonary resuscitation. A refers to airway, B to breathing and C to circulation

abciximab a human–murine monoclonal antibody that inhibits platelet aggregation, used in PTCA and unstable angina

abdomen that part of body lying between thorax and pelvis. ***a. acute*** intra-abdominal condition like perforation, obstruction that needs emergency surgical intervention

abdominal regions the nine regions of the abdomen artificially delineated by two horizontal and two parasagittal lines. The horizontal lines are tangent to the cartilages of the ninth ribs and iliac crests, respectively, and the parasagittal lines are drawn vertically on each side from the middle of the inguinal ligament. The regions thus formed are: (1) above—the right hypochondriac, the epigastric and the left hypochondriac; (2) in the middle—the right/left lateral or lumbar, umbilical, and (3) below—the right inguinal or iliac, the pubic or hypogastric, and the left inguinal or iliac

abdominal respiration A type of respiration caused by the contraction of the diaphragm and the elastic expansion and recoil of the abdominal walls

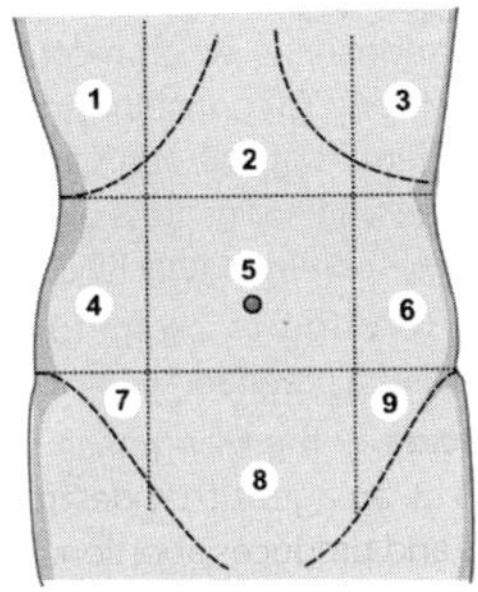

Abdominal regions

abdominoposterior in obstetrics, designating a fetus position in which the belly is forward

abducens drawing away

abduct to draw away from midline

aberration deviation from normal or usual

abetalipoproteinemia a congenital hereditary syndrome with absence of apolipoprotein B marked by acanthocytosis, ataxic neuropathy, retinitis pigmentosa, hypocholesterolemia and malabsorption

ablation removal or destruction

ablatio placentae abruptio placentae

ABO blood group blood groups containing A, B, AB, or no agglutinogen (O). AB group has no agglutinin or antibody and hence can receive blood of any group. Since O group has no agglutinogen, they can donate to any other group (universal donor)

A

ABO-incompatibility occurs in 1 in 200 pregnancies when mother is of blood group 'O' containing anti A and anti B, fetus is of A, B, or AB group, the maternal antibodies cross placenta to cause hemolysis of fetal RBC

abort to bring to premature end, especially a pregnancy

aborticide 1. the killing of an unborn fetus. 2. an agent that destroys the fetus and produces abortion.

abortifacient any agent causing abortion, e.g. drugs like quinine, ergot and prostaglandins

abortion expulsion of product of conception from uterus before 20 weeks of gestation (viability). ***a. complete***. The product of conception is expelled in full, ***a. habitual*** Spontaneous abortions occurring in three or more successive pregnancies, ***a inevitable*** A condition where cervix is fully dilated and abortion is invariable, ***a. missed*** Retention of dead product of conception with regression of features of pregnancy

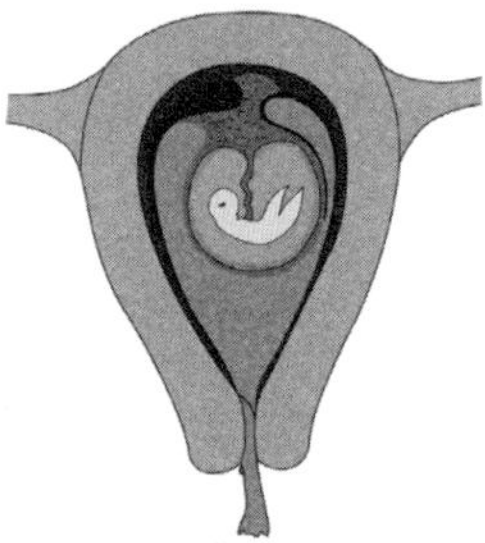

Inevitable abortion

a. therapeutic Interruption of pregnancy for medical and psychological reasons, e.g. carriage of pregnancy harmful to mother's health, genetically diseased fetus unlikely to survive or likely to be grossly malformed, conception arising out of rape or contraceptive failure ***a. threatened*** a condition where bleeding is minimal and cervix is not dilated and abortion may or may not occur

abortion incomplete in which, part of the product of conception has been

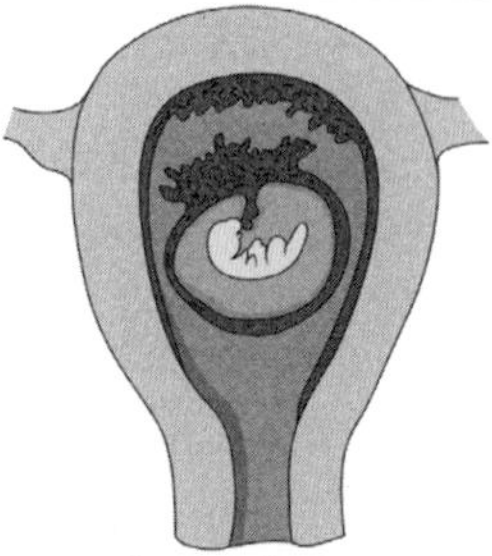

Complete abortion

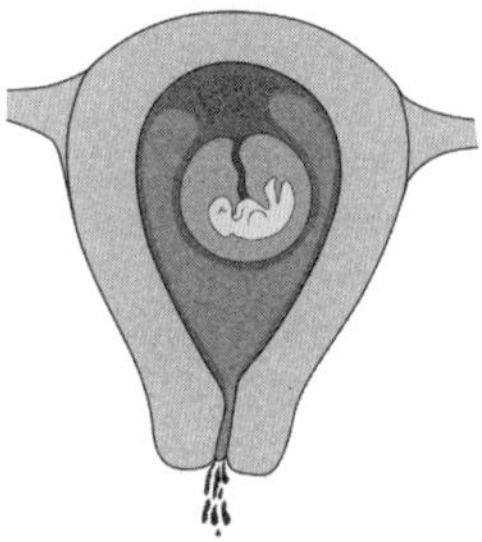

Threatened abortion

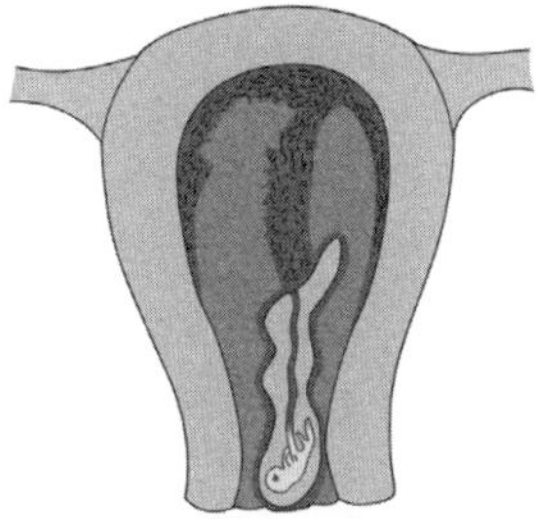

Abortion incomplete

passed but part (usually the placenta) remains in uterus

abortive poliomyelitis an early form of poliomyelitis, characterized clinically by relatively mild symptoms of upper respiratory infection, headache, gastrointestinal disturbances, nausea, and vomiting but which does not progress to involve the central nervous system. Definite diagnosis rests upon isolation of the virus and serologic reactions

abortus the aborted fetus

abrachia absence of arms

abrachius an armless individual

abrasion rubbed or scrapped skin or mucous membrane

abruptio separation. ***a. placentae*** Premature separation of placenta

abscess localized collection of pus; ***a. Bartholin's*** pus in Bartholin's gland near orifice of vagina ***a. pelvic*** In pouch of Douglas

absorbent able to take in or suck up and incorporate; a substance that absorbs or promotes absorption

abstinence voluntary self-denial or forbearance from indulgence of appetites, especially from food, alcoholic drink or sex relations

abulia lack of will power, initiative and drive

abuse misuse or excessive use

acarbia pronounced reduction in bicarbonate of the blood

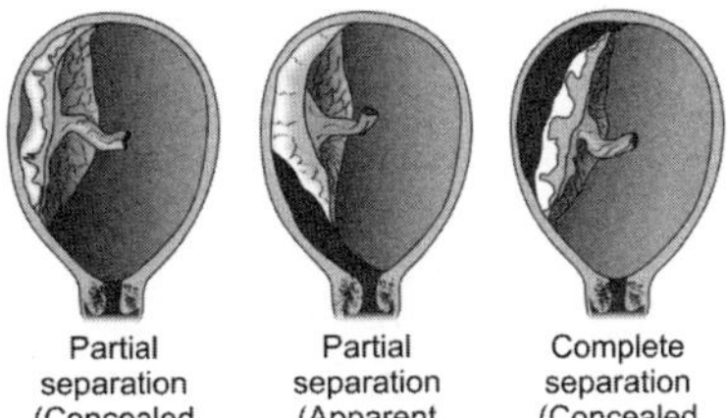

Abruptio placentae

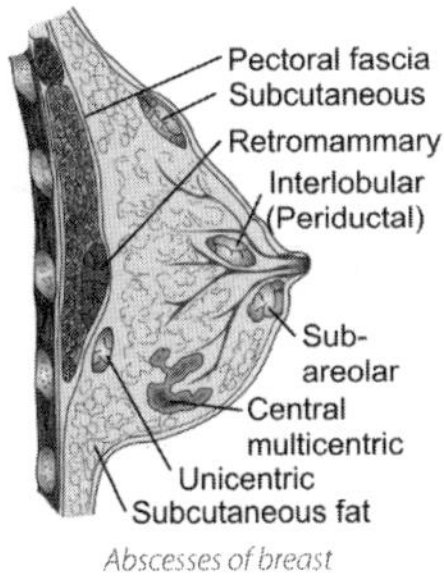

Abscesses of breast

acardia congenital absence of the heart, a condition sometimes present in the parasitic members of conjoined twins

acardiacus a conjoined twin parasitic on its mate or utilizing the placental circulation of its mate and having no heart

acceleration refers to a periodic rise in fetal heart rate from the baseline in response to stress of lowered oxygen availability or fetal movement

accessory extra or supplementary

accoucheur one who conducts delivery

accreta morbid attachment. ***a. placenta*** A placenta attached to uterine muscle due to deficiency of decidua basalis

acetabuloplasty An operation performed to improve the depth and shape of the hip socket in correcting congenital dislocation of the hip or in treating osteoarthritis of the hip

acetabulum a cup-shaped socket in the pelvic bone into which fits the head of femur

acetaminophen analgesic, antipyretic but with weak anti-inflammatory property, potentially hepatotoxic in large doses

acetoacetic acid a ketone produced in liver from fat breakdown

acetylcholine it is a neurotransmitter at cholinergic synapses, responsible for nerve transmission and muscle contraction

acetylcysteine a mucolytic and also antidote in acetaminophen overdose

acheilia congenital absence of the lips

achlorhydria absence of hydrochloric acid in gastric juice

achondroplasia a form of dwarfism with large head, normal trunk but short limbs, of autosomal dominant inheritance

acid a substance which when combined with alkali forms salt

acidfast not readily decolorized by acids after staining, e.g. tuberculosis bacilli and lepra bacilli

acidosis a condition arising from accumulation of acids or depletion of alkalies with decline in blood pH, can be metabolic acidosis (diabetic ketoacidosis, renal failure, lactic acidosis) or respiratory acidosis due to retention of carbon dioxide

acinus a small sac-like dilatation, particularly in a gland

acitretin a metabolite of etretinate, used in treatment of psoriasis

acme the critical stage or crisis of a disease

acne an inflammatory disease of the skin with formation of papules or pustules, involves face, back

acognosia a knowledge of remedies

acoustic relating to hearing or the perception of sound

acquired immunodeficiency syndrome caused by HIV leading to T4 cell destruction, immunodeficiency and opportunistic infections

acrania lack of cranium

acrocephaly malformation of the head consisting in a high or pointed cranial vault due to premature closure of the sagittal, coronal and lambdoid sutures

acrocyanosis the slightly bluish, grayish discoloration of newborn's hands and feet within the first 24 hours of birth

acromegaly a disease due to excess of GH secretion from pituitary in adult

acromion a process of the scapula

acrosome the cap on head of spermatozoon, it contains enzymes for penetration into ovum

actinomyces a fungus, anaerobe causing actinomycosis of jaw, intestine and lungs

actinomycin an antineoplastic agent

active transport movement of ions or molecules across cell membranes against concentration gradient utilizing ATP

acupressure a system of complementary medicine in which points in body are stimulated to cure diseases

acupuncture a system of complementary medicine based on energy lines or meridians running from head to toe through which flow the positive and negative energy. Disequilibrium in energy flow causes disease. Application of fine needles to specific acupuncture points along meridians can rebalance the energy flow

acute developing rapidly and running a short course

acute renal failure sudden and severe renal compromise due to shock, drugs or infection

acute yellow atrophy a rare complication of pregnancy with rapid progressive atrophy of liver with 80% mortality

acyclovir antiviral used in herpes simplex

adactyly congenital absence of finger or toes

adaptation the ability to adjust to changing circumstances

addiction physiologic or psychological dependence on some agents or drug, usually psychotropic

adduct to draw towards center or median line

adenitis inflammation of gland

adenocarcinoma carcinoma from any glandular tissue

adenofibroma a tumor containing connective as well as glandular tissue

adenohypophysis anterior pituitary

adenoid pharyngeal tonsils

adenoma benign tumor arising from gland

adenosine a purine nucleotide consisting of adenine and ribose, component of RNA and used IV in treatment of PSVT, forms adenosine diphosphate, monophosphate and triphosphate

adhesion a fibrous band or structure joining parts to each other

adipocere a waxy substance formed during decomposition of body

A

adiposis obesity, fatty change in organ

adipsia absence of thirst

adjuvant assisting or aiding in any remedy

adnexa appendages or accessory structures, uterine adnexa, the ovaries and fallopian tubes

adolescence the period of development from puberty to cessation of physical growth, i.e. 11 to 19 years

adrenaline a secretion from adrenal medulla, acts as vasopressor

adrenal pertains to adrenal or suprarenal glands

adrenocorticotropic hormone (ACTH) from anterior pituitary that stimulates adrenal cortex

aerobe organism requiring oxygen for survival

aerophagia excessive swallowing of air

aerosol suspension of liquid or solid particles (drugs) in a gas for inhalation

afebrile without fever

affect pertaining to emotional tone or feeling

afferent towards the center, e.g. afferent nerve fibers carrying information from periphery to center

affinity attraction

afibrino genemia absence of fibrinogen in blood causing bleeding as in DIC

aflatoxin toxin produced by *Aspergillus flavus* infecting groundnut seeds causing hepatic malignancy

after birth term used for delivery of placenta and membranes

after pains painful uterine contractions occurring after fetal delivery

AGA Abbreviation for "Appropriate for Gestational Age", when a newborn's birth weight is within the 10th to 90th percentile expected for that length gestation

agar used in culture media, extracted from red algae

agenesis absence of an organ due to nondevelopment

ageusia absence of taste sensation

agglutination aggregation of different particles or cells

agglutinin antibody which aggregates a particulate antigen (agglutinogen) present in sample or on cells

agnathia absence of jaw

agnosia inability to recognize the sensory inputs

agonist a drug that acts on receptor in a manner similar to naturally occurring substance

agoraphobia fear of open spaces

agranulocytosis reduction in number of granulocytes (neutrophils, monocytes, eosinophils), usually drug-induced

agraphia impaired ability to write

air hunger deep sighing respiration due to oxygen lack

airway 1. mechanical device used to secure air passage 2. the passage through which air enters the lungs

alantois membranous sac projecting from ventral surface of embryo that helps to form placenta

ala wing, e.g. sacral ala

albinism congenital absence of body pigmentation—partial or complete (hair, skin, eyes)

albumin the major plasma protein responsible for plasma colloidal osmotic pressure

albuminuria passage of albumin in urine, normally <30 mg/24 hours

albuterol a beta agonist used in bronchial asthma

alcohol organic compounds containing OH group. ***a. ethyl*** The commonly consumed alcohol, excess consumption causing liver damage, neuropathy and cardiomyopathy. Ingestion during first trimester can cause fetal damage. ***a. methyl*** Industrial spirit, accidental ingestion causes fatal acidosis and blindness

aldeslukin recombinant interleukin 2, used in treatment of metastatic renal cancer

aldosterone mineral corticoid from adrenal cortex, essential for sodium and water retention in body and potassium excretion

alendronate a bisphosphonate used for treatment of osteoporosis

alesthesia experiencing a sensation away from site of its occurrence

alexia inability to understand written language due to cerebral lesion

alfentanil opioid analgesic derived from fentanyl

alginate derivative of alginic acid used as absorbent in dressing and for dental impression

algorithm step-by-step method of solving a problem

alkali any compound with pH more than 7, turning red litmus blue, form soap in combination with fatty acids

alkaline phosphatase an enzyme secreted by liver, formed in bone and by neutrophils

alkaloid nitrogenous organic compounds of plants like morphine, atropine

alkalosis base excess in body with loss of hydrogen ions, can be respiratory (excess CO_2 wash out) or metabolic (excess H^+ loss)

alkaptonuria a condition in which urine darkens on standing and there is arthritis

allele one of the two or more forms of a gene at corresponding sites (loci) on homologous chromosomes defining a characteristic

allergy hypersensitive state to some drugs, pollens, food items causing asthma, urticaria, angioedema

alopecia baldness, can be patchy, male pattern, total or universal (entire body)

alopurinol xanthine oxidase inhibitor used in gout

alpha-fetoprotein a plasma protein produced by fetal liver; level increased in hepatocellular carcinoma and germ cell tumors; amniotic fluid AFP is raised in neural tube defect

A

alteplase a tissue plasminogen activator used in thrombolysis of acute MI and thrombotic stroke

alternative medicine a holistic system of healthcare that recognizes interplay of body, mind and spirit in causation of disease

alum a local astringent and styptic, also used as adjuvant in vaccines and toxoids

alveolus a sac-like dilatation

amanita a genus of poisonous mushrooms

amantadin antiviral agent against influenza A; also dyskinetic agent used in Parkinsonism

amastigote the intracellular non-flagellated stage of hemoparasite *Leishmania*

amaurosis blindness without an apparent cause

ambenonium a cholinergic agent used to treat muscular weakness of myasthenia gravis

ambient surrounding or prevailing

amblyopia dimness of vision without detectable organic lesion of eye

amblyoscope an instrument for training amblyopic eye to take part in vision and for increasing fusion of the eyes

ambroxol a mucolytic.

Ambu bag a hand operated, self-reinflating bag used during resuscitation. It is connected by tubing and non-rebreathing valve to a face mask or endotracheal tube and is used for artificial ventilation

amebiasis infection with ameba especially histolytica producing dysentery and liver abscess

ameboma a tumor-like growth in intestine in amebiasis

amelia congenital absence of limb

ameloblast a cell that forms enamel of tooth

amenorrhea absence of menstruation

ametropia condition of eye in which image fails to be focused on retina

amifostine a chemoprotectant used to prevent renal toxicity of cisplatin

amikacin aminoglycoside antibiotic active against aerobic gram-negative bacilli causing UTI and other infections

amino acid protein constituents essential for nutrition

amino caproic acid a plasmin inhibitor, used in bleeding

aminophylline bronchodilator, used in asthma

amlodipine calcium channel blocker used in hypertension

ammonia a colorless gas of pungent odor produced from protein breakdown in intestine, converted to urea in liver

amnesia loss of memory

amniocentesis transabdominal or transcervical puncture of amniotic sac to obtain amniotic fluid for analysis of

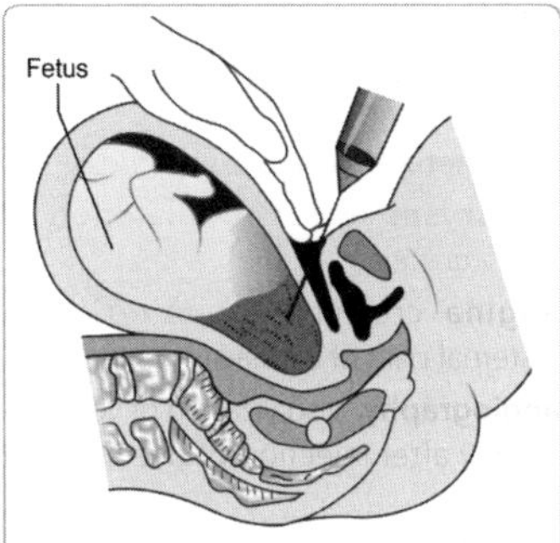

Amniocentesis

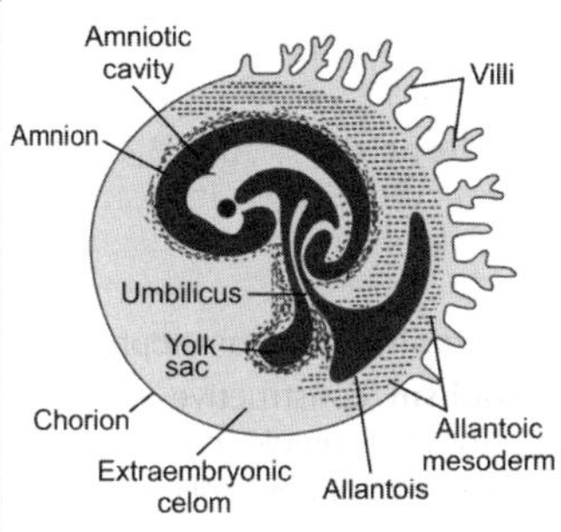

Amnion

alpha-fetoprotein (neural tube defect) and genetic analysis, bilirubin level, L:S ratio, etc. (fetal maturity)

amnion the innermost membrane covering fetus

amnioscope an endoscope introduced through cervix to visualize fetus

amniotic fluid also called liquor amni, surrounds fetus, formed from fetal urine, GI secretions and placental secretion. The amount varies from 500 ot 1500 mL at term

amniotic fluid embolism entry of amniotic fluid to maternal circulation via placental sinuses causing collapse and shock

amniotomy the artificial rupture of amniotic membranes when an amnihook or other rupturing device is introduced into the vagina and a small tear is made in the membranes

amoxapine an antipsychotic agent

amoxicillin semisynthetic derivative of ampicillin, a broad spectrum antibiotic

amphetamine sympathomimetic amine, a CNS stimulant

amphoric sound resembling that made by blowing across neck of a bottle

amphotericin B antifungal antibiotic, effective also against *Leishmania*

ampicillin acid-resistant semisynthetic penicillin

amprenavir a protease inhibitor for HIV

ampulla flask-like dilatation of tubular structure, e.g. Fallopian tube

amrinone a cardiac stimulant used in congestive failure

amsacrine antineoplastic agent

amygdale an almond-shaped structure of brain related to limbic system

amylase an enzyme causing hydrolysis of starch

A

amyloid extracellular amorphous waxy substance stained pink by congo red

amyloidosis a group of diseases characterized by deposition of amyloid in various tissues with organ dysfunction

amyotrophy muscular atrophy

anabolism constructive process of synthesis of complex compounds for cell growth, opposite of catabolism

anaerobe organism growing in absence of oxygen

anagen the first phase of hair cycle in which hair growth takes place

anagrelide an agent used to reduce elevated platelet count

analgesia loss of sensibility to pain

analgia freedom from pain

anaphylaxis immediate hypersensitivity with vascular collapse, bronchospasm, angioedema, pruritus, etc.

anaplasia loss of differentiation of cells leading to tumor formation

anastomosis communication between vessels and hollow tubes

anastrozole antineoplastic agent for breast cancer

anatomy the science of structure of an organism

androgen a hormone that promotes masculinization

anemia reduction in number of red cells or their hemoglobin content

anencephaly congenital absence of cranial vault, i.e. cerebral hemispheres

anesthesia loss of ability to feel pain

anesthesiologist physician specializing in anesthesiology

anesthetize to induce anesthesia

aneurysm localized dilatation of vascular wall

angina crushing agonizing retrosternal pain of cardiac ischemia

angiography visualization of vessel in X-ray after injection of dye into the vessel

angiology science of blood vessels and lymphatics

angioma a tumor whose cells tend to form blood vessels or lymph vessels

angiopathy any disease of blood or lymph vessel

angioplasty dilatation of narrowed vessel segment using inflatable balloon or laser

angiotensin a powerful vasopressor formed from plasma decapeptide angiotensinogen

angular pregnancy implantation of fertilized ovum in the angle where the Fallopian tube enters the uterus

anhidrosis absence of sweat secretion

ankylosis immobility of a joint due to fibrous or bony tissue growth

anode positive electrode to which negative ions are attracted

anomaly deviation from normal

anorexia loss of appetite

anoscope speculum for examining anus and lower rectum

anovulatory cycle menstrual cycle not preceded by ovulation

anovulatory not associated with ovulation

anoxia lack of oxygen

antacid a substance neutralizing gastric acid

antagonist acting opposite, a drug or muscle

ante prefix, meaning before

anteflexion abnormal bending forward, e.g., especially of uterine body at its neck

antemortem before death

antenatal before birth

antenatal period the time of pregnancy from the first day of last menstrual period (LMP) to the start of true labor

antepartum before parturition. ***a. hemorrhage*** Bleeding from genital tract any time after 24 weeks of pregnancy until parturition

anterior fontanel diamond-shaped fontanel located at the juncture of the coronal, frontal and sagittal sutures

anteroinferior infront and below

anterolateral infront and to one side

anteromedian infront and toward midline

anteroposterior passing from front to rear

anterosuperior infront and above

anteversion turning forwards, e.g. body of uterus in relation to vagina

anthelmintic an agent destructive to worms

anthrax infectious disease, contacted from soil or slaughter house

anthropology the study of men; physical, cultural, linguistic and archeologic

antibiosis an association between two organisms that is detrimental to one of them

antibiotic chemical substance produced by microorganisms or synthesized that inhibits growth of other microorganism or tumor cells

antibody an immunoglobulin molecule that reacts with specific antigen that induced its synthesis. Antibody can be complement fixing, blocking and cytotoxic

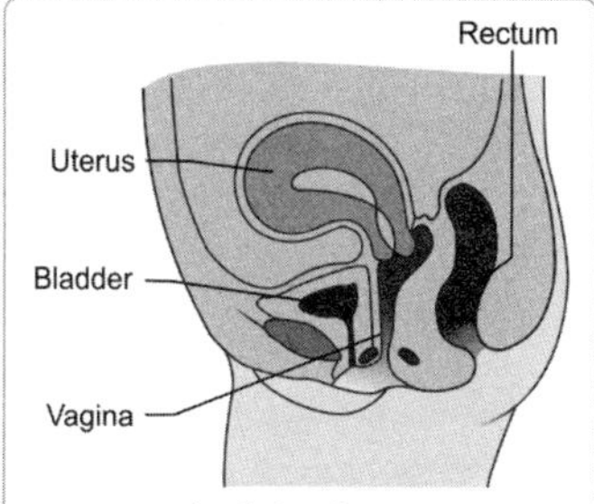

Anteflexion of uterus

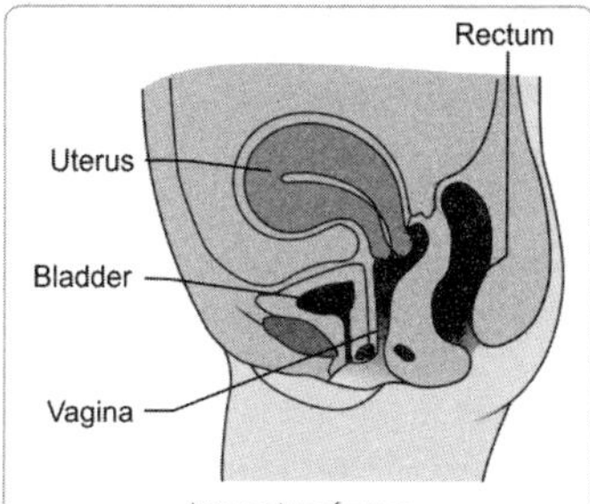

Anteversion of uterus

A

antibody titers a test used to indicate the relative concentration of a particular antibody present in a person's blood. For example, a high rubella titer indicates a person has been exposed to rubella (German measles) and has formed a significant amount of antibody against the rubella virus and therefore, will most likely be able to ward off another attack of the virus without becoming ill

anticholinesterase a drug that inhibits acetylcholine esterase thus potentiating action of acetylcholine, principally used in myasthenia gravis

anticoagulant agent that prevents blood coagulation

anticonvulsant drug that suppresses convulsion

anti D antibody against D antigen, a part of Rh antigen, given to Rh negative mothers conceiving Rh positive baby

antidepressant a drug used to treat depression

antidiuretic a drug that suppresses urine formation

antidote an agent that counteracts the affect of poison

antiemetic drug against nausea and vomiting

antiestrogen substances that block or modify action of estrogen, e.g. clomiphene citrate

antigen any substance which on introduction into body brings about immunity by stimulating antibody production

antihistamine drugs that block tissue receptors for histamine, useful in allergy (H1 receptors) and acid peptic disease (H2 receptors)

antihypertensive an agent that reduces blood pressure by central alfa adrenergic action, peripheral vasodilatation, beta adrenergic blockade, etc.

anti-inflammatory counteracting inflammation

antineoplastic agents that prevent the development, growth and proliferation of malignant cells

antioxidants agents that prevent or inhibit oxidation, e.g. vitamin A, C and E

antipyretic agent effective in treatment of burn

antipyrotic agent that reduces fever

antiseptic agent that prevents sepsis or infection

antiserum serum derived from animal or human body containing antibodies against particular viral or bacterial antigens, e.g. antitetanus serum

antispasmodic agent that relieves spasm

antithrombin any substance that neutralizes thrombin, thus preventing coagulation. Antithrombins are normally present in blood. In their congenital absence, one is prone to thrombosis

antitoxin antibody produced in response to toxin of bacteria

antitussive agent effective against cough

antivenin material (serum product) that neutralizes venom of snake, spider

antroscope an instrument for inspecting maxillary antrum

anuresis absence of urine

anuria failure of the kidneys to secrete urine as in shock due to abruptio placentae, septic abortion

anus opening of rectum to exterior for discharge of feces

aortic regurgitation leakage of blood from aorta into left ventricle during the diastole

aortic stenosis narrowing of aortic valve. Normal valve diameter is 2 cm per square meter

aperient drug that stimulates defecation

aperture an orifice or opening

Apert's syndrome congenital disease with fusion of cranial sutures at birth and webbed fingers

apgar score scoring system designed by Dr Virginia Apgar to assess birth asphyxia

aphakia absence of lens of the eye

aphasia loss of power of speech/ expression

apheresis withdrawal of blood followed by separation of desired component (leukocyte, plasma) and retransfusion of remainder to the donor

apicitis inflammation of apex of tooth

aplasia failure of development

apnea cessation of breathing

apocrine a form of glandular secretion in which the free end of secreting cell is cast off along with secreted product, e.g. mammary and sweat gland

apomorphine a central emetic used to induce vomiting, in poisoning treatment

aponeurosis a sheet-like tendinous expansion connecting muscle to bone

apophysis any bony outgrowth or swelling

apoplexy sudden neurologic compromise due to CVA or collapse due to adrenal hemorrhage (adrenal apoplexy)

apparatus 1. a mechanical device or appliance used in operations or experiments. 2. a group of structures or organs that work together to perform function, e.g. ***a. auditory, a. biliary, a. juxtaglomerular, a. lacrimal***

appendicitis inflammation of vermiform appendix, a very serious condition if occurs during pregnancy as it is drawn up in the abdomen and inflammatory process may progress rapidly

apraxia loss of ability to carry out purposeful movement

aprotinin an inhibitor of proteolytic enzymes, used as antihemorrhagic and to reduce perioperative blood loss during cardiopulmonary by pass

A

APTT activated partial thromboplastin time

aqueduct a canal or passage. ***cerebral a.*** a narrow channel in midbrain connecting third and fourth ventricles

arachidonic acid a polyunsaturated essential fatty acid formed from linoleic acid, a precursor to leukotrienes, prostaglandins and thromboxane

arachnoid resembling spider web, the middle covering of brain and spinal cord between dura and pia matter

arcuate arched or bow-like

ardeparin low molecular weight heparin and anticoagulant and antithrombotic used in deep venous thrombosis

ARDS acute respiratory distress syndrome, adult respiratory distress syndrome

areolar gland (Montgomery's glands). Large modified sweat glands beneath the areola secreting a lipoid material that lubricates the nipple

areola the pigmented area surrounding the nipple

Arnold-Chiari deformity a condition in which the inferior poles of cerebellar hemispheres and medulla protrude through foramen magnum causing hydrocephalus. It is commonly associated with spina bifida and meningomyelocele

aroma pleasant odor

aroma therapy treatment of ailment using highly concentrated essential oils extracted from plants, a form of complementary medicine

arrectores pilorum involuntary muscle in skin connected to hair follicle whose contraction due to cold, fright causes erection of hair and "goose flesh" appearance of skin

arrhythmia abnormal rhythm of heart beat

arteriosclerosis hardening and thickening of arterial walls due to formation of atheromatous plaques

arteritis inflammation of an artery. ***a. giant cell*** occurs in elderly with severe headache, cord like superficial temporal artery with danger of blindness, ***a. takayasu*** pulseless disease, progressive obliteration of brachiocephalic trunk, left subclavian and left common carotid arteries

artery a vessel carrying blood from heart to periphery or lungs

artesunate an antimalarial for resistant Falciparum malaria

arthralgia joint pain

arthritis inflammation of a joint

arthrodesis surgical fusion of a joint

arthrography visualization of interior of a joint after injection of contrast or air

arthropathy any joint disease

artificial insemination introduction of semen to vagina artificially other than coitus to achieve conception

artificial respiration maintenance of respiration by other means, e.g. mouth to mouth or by ventilator

artificial rupture of membranes (ARM) amniotic sac is ruptured via vagina to induce or accelerate labor

ascites accumulation of fluid in the abdominal cavity

ascorbic acid vitamin C

aseptic free from pathogenic bacteria

aseptic technique technique that prevent contamination of operative wounds

aspartame artificial sweetner, 200 times sweeter than sucrose

aspergillus a genus of fungus infecting ear canal and lungs

aspermia lack of or failure to ejaculate semen

asphyxiant an agent, especially gas producing asphyxia

asphyxia suffocation; a neonatorum. Failure of child to breathe after birth

aspiration suction of fluid or air from a cavity; inhalation of foreign substance

assay determination of the amount of a particular constituent in a mixture

asthma airway hyper-reactivity with spasm and narrowing usually due to hypersensitivity

astigmatism ametropia caused by differences in curvature in different meridians of cornea

asymptomatic without any symptoms

asynclitism a parietal presentation of fetal head in which the transversely placed sagittal suture lies close to symphysis pubis or sacrum; the sideways rocking mechanism of fetal descent during labor. It can be anterior or posterior

ataxia failure of muscular coordination leading to disturbance of equilibrium, can be motor or sensory

atelectasis incomplete expansion of lungs at birth or collapse of adult lung

atherosclerosis a sclerodegenerative disease of arterial wall marked by intimal lipid deposit, fibrous tissue accumulation and smooth muscle cell proliferation

athetosis repetitive involuntary, slow, sinuous and writhing movements of hands

atopy genetic predisposition towards immediate hyper-sensitivity

atorvastatin a cholesterol synthesis inhibitor, hypolipidemic agent

atovaquone an antibiotic for pneumocystis pneumonia and malaria

atracurium a nondepolarizing neuromuscular blocking agent used as adjunct to general anesthesia

atresia congenital absence or closure of a normal body opening or passage or tubular structure

atrichosis congenital absence of hair

atrium a chamber

atrophy diminution in size of an organ

atropine anticholinergic belladonna alkaloid used as smooth muscle relaxant, and in Parkinsonism and organophosphorus poisoning

attachment the establishment of a reciprocal relationship between the parents and the newborn after a period of bonding; development of a deeper intimacy, which grows over time

attention-deficit disorder a disease of infancy or childhood, mainly boys characterized by inappropriate attention, hyperactivity and impulsivity

A

attitude the relationship of the fetal head and limbs to its trunk

audiometry measurement of acuity of hearing for various frequencies of sound

augmentin amoxycillin-clavulanic acid

aura a subjective sensation or motor phenomena, usually preceding epileptic seizure

auscultation listening to the sounds produced in the body, i.e. cardiac contraction, air entry-exit from lungs, turbulent flow within vessels and intestinal peristalsis

autism a behavioral disorder in children with poor interpersonal relationship and expression, related to advanced paternal age

autoclave a self-locking apparatus for sterilization of materials by steam under pressure

autocrine a mode of hormone action in which the hormone secreted affects the function of the cell that produced it

autoimmune disease diseases in which antibodies are produced against body's own tissues to cause organ damage, e.g. rheumatoid arthritis, SLE, rheumatic carditis, myasthenia gravis

autoimmunity a state where body produces antibodies against its own cells/tissues

autologous related to self

automaticity capacity of a cell to initiate an impulse without external stimulation

autonomic self-governing

autosomes the chromosomes in the body other than the sex (X and Y) chromosomes

autotrophic self-nourishing

avascular blood less

avitaminosis a state of vitamin deficiency

avulsion tearing away of a structure or part

axilla armpit

axis a line through center of body or about which structure revolves; the second cervical vertebra with its odontoid process around which atlas rotates

axis of birth canal the course taken by fetus during parturition; first downwards and backwards and then downwards and forwards

azathioprine 6 mercaptopurine, anti-neoplastic and immunosuppressive

azatidine an antihistaminic

azelaic acid a dicarboxylic acid used topically in acne vulgaris

azelastine an antihistaminic used as nasal spray in nasal allergy

azithromycin a macrolide, useful against bacteria and anaerobes and tuberculosis

azoospermia absence of spermatozoa in semen

aztreonam a monobactam antibiotic used in gram-negative sepsis

azygos unpaired structure/organ, e.g. ***a. vein***

B. scan a two-dimensional cross sectional display in ultrasound

Babinski's reflex dorsiflexion of great toe and fanning out of other toes on stimulation of lateral part of sole of foot is called positive Babinski's reflex; commonly results from pyramidal tract interruption; also positive in infants below 6 months (before myelination)

baby-blues a common transient mild depression or emotional disturbance affecting the mother after delivery due to hormonal changes, sleep deprivation and emotional let-down

baby-friendly initiative (BFI) part of a global campaign by WHO and UNO childrens fund to encourage breastfeeding. The ten steps of the program are:

- breastfeeding policy is communicated to all staff
- healthcare staff trained to implement the policy
- all pregnant mothers informed of benefits of breastfeeding
- mothers assisted to start breastfeeding half an hour after delivery
- educate mothers to breastfeeding and maintenance of lactation
- neonates be given only breast milk
- 24 hour rooming in
- on demand breastfeeding
- no pacifiers or teats to be given to breastfeed babies
- establishment of breastfeeding support groups. A global award is given for a hospital implementing all 10 steps and has approximately 75% breastfeeding rate and a certificate of commitment when a hospital is working towards the 10 steps

bach flower remedies a system of complementary medicines, based on homeopathic principles, 38 flower remedies are available to treat emotional and psychological disorders

bacillus any rod-shaped micro-organism

bacillus Calmette-Guérin the attenuated vaccine given to infants within first week of birth left deltoid against tuberculosis

bacitracin topically used antibacterial agent

backache any pain in back, due to muscle spasm, disk, ligaments, vertebral body, nerve roots and meninges

backache in pregnancy is usually due to exaggerated lordosis requiring postural correction and lumbar support

baclofen GABA inhibitor used to reduce muscle spasticity

bacteria any microorganism of the class Schizomycetes; can be spherical or ovoid (cocci) rod-shaped (bacilli) or spiral

bacteriophage a virus that infects bacteria

bacteriuria presence of bacteria in urine, significant if concentration exceeds 105 mL

B

bag of membrane the amnion and chorion which contain the liquor amni

Baker's cyst synovial cyst in popliteal fossa

balanoposthitis inflammation of glans and prepuce

ballottment palpatory technique for examining flating, objects, e.g. fetus in uterus, hydronephrotic kidney

bandage a piece of gauze to be wrapped around a body part as dressing

Bandl's ring ring like thickening at the junction of upper and lower uterine segments

barber's itch folliculitis of face mostly by *Staphylococcus aureus*

barbiturates a large group of hypnotic drugs, also used as anticonvulsants, can cause tolerance and dependency

Barlow's test a test to diagnose congenital dislocation of hip (CDA) in the newborn. The baby lies on back both feet pointing towards examiner who grasps each leg with knee and hip flexed, placing middle fingers of each hand over greater trochanter and thumb of each hand on inner aspect of thigh. The thighs are then abducted and the middle finger of each hand pushes the greater trochanter forward. If there is CDH, the femoral head will be felt to 'clunk' as it inters acetabulum. In CDH femoral head can be displaced backwards on slight pressure when the hips are flexed and adducted (Barlow's sign)

barr body sex chromatin mass seen within the nuclei of normal female somatic cells, representing inactivated X-chromosome

barrel chest rounded chest due to air trapping as in emphysema. In normal chest, AP diameter is more than transverse, hence elliptical shape

barrier contraception mechanical barrier to prevent sperm from entering cervical canal, e.g. diaphragm

barrier nursing precaution taken to prevent infection spreading from the patient to other patients and attending nursing staff. Staff wears gown, gloves, masks goggles, overshoes and baby is nursed in separate cubicle

Bartholin's duct duct of sublingual salivary gland that runs parallel with Wharton's duct and opens with it

Bartholin's gland a compound mucus gland lying in lateral wall of vestibule of vagina, at the junction upper and middle one-third

Bart's test antenatal screening test that helps to identify mothers having risk of having a baby with Down's syndrome or open neural tube defect. Serum alpha-fetoprotein, alpha and beta chorionic gonadotro-phin and unconjugated estriol are estimated and if risk is high, amniocentesis is advised

basal body temperature chart daily temperature charting to predict ovulation

basal ganglia four masses of gray matter (caudate, lentiform, amygdaloid and claustrum) lying deep in cerebral hemispheres

basal metabolic rate (BMR) normal value is 40 kcal/m^2/hour, a test of thyroid function

base any substance that accepts hydrogen ion, strong bases feel slippery and are corrosives

basophil a leukocyte having affinity for basic dyes, the cytoplasm containing coarse bluish-black granules and nucleus is pale and bilobed

battered child syndrome physical injuries inflicted upon children

battery unlawful touching of a patient without consent, justification; battery occurs if a surgical or medical procedure is done without prior consent

battledore placenta placenta with the umbilical cord attached to margin rather than center

beclomethasone synthetic corticosteroid

bedsore pressure sore, i.e. ischemic necrosis of tissue especially over bony prominences

belching expulsion of stomach gas through mouth and nose

Bell's palsy sudden unilateral lower motor facial palsy due to swelling/ischemia of the nerve in bony canal

Benedict's test 8 drops of urine is added to 5 mL of Benedict's solution and boiled to see for green, yellow, red precipitate

benign prostatic hypertrophy (BPH) prostatic enlargement in elderly due to hyperplasia causing obstruction of prostatic urethra

benzidine used for test of occult blood in stool (to a solution of benzidine in glacial acetic acid is added 3% H_2O_2 and the stool sample. Appearance of blue color indicates presence of blood

benzodiazepine psychotropic agents with potent hypnotic and antianxiety effects

bereavement loss of loved one or loss of good health, wealth or position leading to depression, anguish

beriberi a vitamin B1 deficiency disease, can be dry or wet types

betadine povidone-iodine

betahistine drug used for vertigo

betalactamase an enzyme produced by certain bacteria that inactivates antibiotics

betamethasone synthetic bezoar accumulation of vegetable or organic fibers (hair) in stomach glucocorticoid

betatron electron accelerator that produces high energy electrons or X-rays

bicarbonate salt of carbonic acid ($NaHCO_3$), used to treat acidosis

biceps a muscle with two heads

bicornis users with two horns due to incomplete union of Müllerian ducts

bifocal eye glasses with lenses for distant and near vision

bigemini group of two beats separated by a long pause, commonly due to regular extra-systoles (e.g. digitalis toxicity)

B

bilateral both sides

bile acid cholic, taurocholic and glycocholic acids that exist as salts in bile and are helpful for intestinal fat absorption (micelle formation)

bile a thick viscid fluid with bitter taste secreted by liver. The bile when secreted in liver is straw-colored but down below is yellow, brown or green in color

bile pigment bilirubin and biliverdin, imparting brown color to urine and feces

bilirubin bile pigment; yellow to orange-colored, can be direct acting when conjugated to glucuronic acid or indirect acting when unconjugated

biliverdin greenish pigment, formed by oxidation of bilirubin

Billing's method a method of family planning where one avoids intercourse during vulnerable period, i.e. 3 days before to 3 days after ovulation when cervical mucous becomes thin to facilitate sperm movement

bimanual examination by both hands

bimanual uterine compression a method of arresting postpartum hemorrhage where left hand on abdomin pulls uterus forward and right hand within forward and right hand within vagina closed to form a fist presses the anterior vaginal wall so that anterior and posterior uterine wall as pressed firmly

bioassay determination of strength of a drug in live animal/humans

bioavailability the rate and extent to which an active drug or metabolite enters the general circulation to be available at the acting site

biochemistry chemistry of living things

biofeedback a training program aimed at controlling in function of autonomic nervous system

biological pregnancy test pregnancy test based on hCG in urine, e.g. gravindex test

biophysical profile a non-invastive test of fetal well-being using ultrasound to monitor fetal heart rate, fetal tone, body movements, breathing movements and amniotic fluid volume

biopsy microscopic examination of tissue taken from body to look for pathological changes

biparietal diameter distance between two parietal eminences of fetal skull, usually 9.5 cm at term measured in ultrasound as an indicator of fetal growth and maturity when biparietal diameter passes through pelvic brim the head is said to be engaged

bipolar in bipolar disease, patient has alternating mania and depression

birth canal the bony and soft tissue structures through which fetus must pass during parturition

birth control prevention or control of conception

birthing chair a chair for delivery which should be titled to 40′ to the vertical immediately before delivery and throughout third stage of labor

birthing room delivery or labor room

birth mark nevus, pigmentation or vascular tumor

birth rate the number of births during one year per 1000 population (crude birth rate) or 1000 female population in childbearing age of 15 to 45 years (true birth rate)

birth weight weight of a baby immediately following delivery normally 3.2 kg in full-term

bisacadyl alaxative

bisacromial diameter distance between two acromion processes on fetal shoulders; usually 12 cm

Bishop's score

criteria	*score*			
	0	*1*	*2*	*3*
cervix				
dilatation(cm)	closed	1-2	3-4	5+
length(cm)	3	2	1	0
consistency	firm	medium	soft	
position	posterior	central	anterior	
head				
cm above ischial spine	–3	–2	–1	0

score below 5 in prime is unfavorable

Bishop's score a method of assessing the favorability of cervix prior to induction of labor

Bitot's spot Triangular, shiny, gray spots on conjunctiva seen in vitamin A deficiency

black measles also called hemorrhagic measles implying a severe hemorrhagic measle eruption

bladder receptacle to hold secretions (urinary bladder, gallbladder)

blanch to lose color. In blanching test, the nail is pressed quickly and then released. When circulation is good, color returns within 5 seconds

Bland diet Diet without irritant foods, e.g. milk, cream, prepared cereals, eggs, lean meat, fish, cheese, custard, cookie, etc.

blastocyst a stage of mammalian embryo next to morula and consists of outer trophoblast to which is attached an inner cell mass. The enclosed cavity is blastocele

blastomere one of the cells resulting from cleavage of a fertilized ovum

bleeding time time required for blood to stop flowing from a pin prick. Normal range 1–3 minutes (Dukes) or 1–9 minutes (Ivy)

blind spot physiological scotoma situated 15'to outside of visual fixation point, corresponding to optic disk

blister collection of fluid within epidermis

block regional anesthesia

1. ***b. epidural*** injection of local anesthetic to extradural space beneath ligamentum flavum for pain relief
2. ***b. paracervical*** injection of local anesthetic into lateral fornices of vagina to block inferior hypogastric plexus for relief of labor pain
3. ***b. pudendal*** local anesthetic injection around ischial tuberosity to block pudendal nerve

blood the fluid with suspended cells and other constituents that circulates within heart and blood vessels providing oxygen to tissues, carrying carbon dioxide for exhalation

blood-brain barrier a barrier membrane, i.e. endothelium and basement membrane, which prevents entry of damaging substances into CNS

blood gas analysis study of pH, ($PaCO_2$) partial (pressure of oxygen, (PaO_2) partial pressure of (CO_2) and (SO_2) oxygen saturation of blood

blood group A genetically determined system of antigens located on surface of RBC. AB and O system is the commonly accepted one. There are 30 Rh antigens too

blood pressure pressure exerted by moving blood on the vessel wall. A value beyond 140/90 mm Hg in those below 50 years and 160/95 mm Hg in those above 60 years is abnormal

blood product products derived from blood, i.e plasma, platelet concentrates, factor VIII concentrate

blood sugar concentration of sugar commonly glucose in blood, normal value 60 to 100 mg/dL

blood urea urea concentration in blood, normal value 15 to 40 mg/dL

blood volume quantity of blood in body, usually 70 mL/kg; decrease in blood volume decreases cardiac output and can cause shock

bloody show rupture of the small cervical capillaries when the cervix begins to dilate and efface; when the mucus plug is lost, the resultant cervical drainage is pink-tinged

body mass index (BMI) weight in kg divided by height in m^2 normal BMI is 20 to 25, below 20 being under weight and above 25 over weight, above 30 obese, above 35 morbidly obese

boil a furuncle, acute inflammation of subcutaneous tissue including glands and hair follicles

bonding the initial attraction and period of exploration between the parents and newborn; becoming acquainted

bone age estimation of biological age based on development of ossification centers of wrist and long bones

bone densitometry method of determining bone density by radiographic or ultrasonic means for diagnosis of osteoporosis

bone marrow bone marrow is highly vascular, pulpy, network of reticular tissue found in the hollow interior of bones. The major function of the bone marrow in adult bones is hematopoiesis or production of new blood cells

borborygmus a gurgling splashing sound heard in abdomen caused by passage of gas

botulin the neurotoxin responsible for botulism

botulism a severe form of food poisoning due to botulinous toxins A, B, C, D, E, F and G

bougie a slender flexible instrument for dilating tubular organs, e.g. urethra

bowleg outward bending of lower limbs (genu varum, due to rickets)

Bowman's capsule a bilayered membrane closely applied to glomerulus functioning as a filter for formation of urine

Boyle's apparatus machine for general anesthesia delivering anesthetic agents as gases, i.e. nitrous oxide, halothane, cyclopropane, etc.

brachial relating to arm, ***b. artery*** continuation of axillary artery along inner side of upper arm ***b. plexus*** a nerve plexus at root of neck formed by C5-C8 and T1 giving rise to median radial and ulnar nerves

bradycardia sinus rhythm <60/minute in adult, <100/minute in a child and <120/minute in fetus

bradykinin a peptide smooth muscle dilator

brain composed of neurons and neuroglia, average weight 1350 to 1400 g of which 2% in spinal cord and 85% in cerebrum, divided into:

1. diencephalons (thalamus, hypothalamus, epithalamus)
2. mesencephalon (tegmentum, crura cerebri, medulla)
3. metencephalon (cerebellum, pons) and
4. telencephalon (cerebral, cortex).

brain death isoelectric EEG for at least 30 minutes with no change in response to sound and pain stimuli; absent respiration and all reflexes (barbiturate, diazepam, methaqualone can produce short periods of isoelectric EEG)

branchial arches five pairs of arched structure that form lateral and ventral walls of pharynx of the embryo from which structures of face and neck are formed

branchial clefts openings between branchial arches

Brandt-Andrews maneuver a method of delivery of placenta and membranes after their descent into vagina. One hand lifts up the contracted uterus, the other hand gently pulls cord down

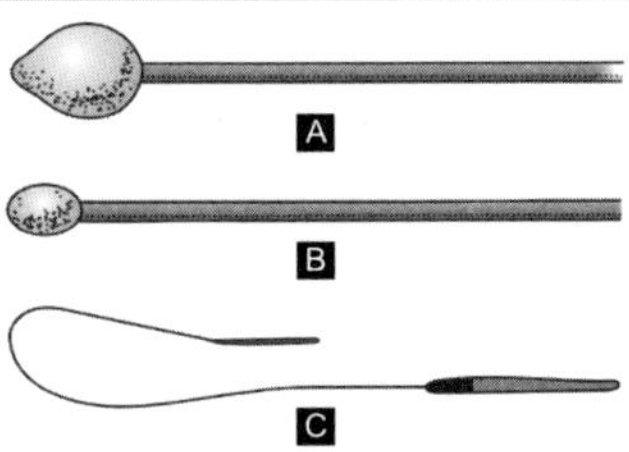

Bougies: (A) Otis bougie a boule; (B) Olive-tipped bougie; (C) Filiform bougies

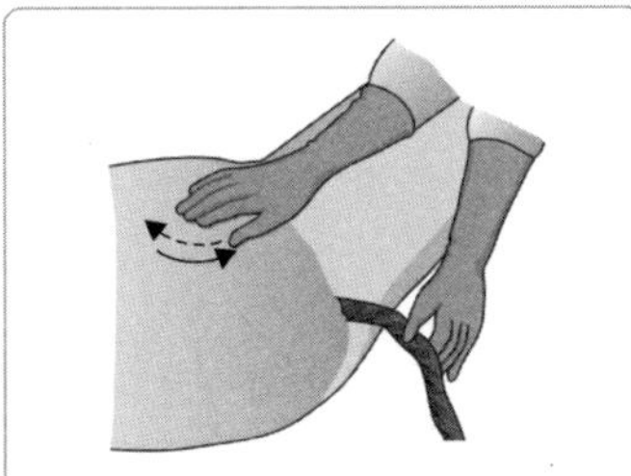

Controlled cord traction (Brandt-Andrews method)

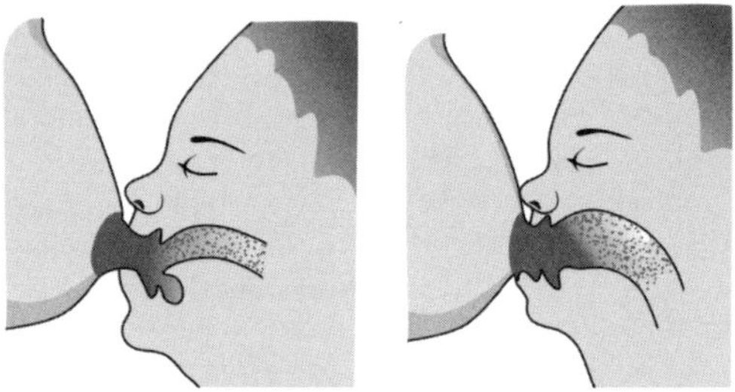

Technique of breastfeeding

brassiere pregnant women should wear well-fitting wide strap brassiere

Braxton Hicks' sign painless intermittent uterine contractions occurring after 3rd month of pregnancy

breast the mammary glands placed anteriorly over 2nd to 6th ribs

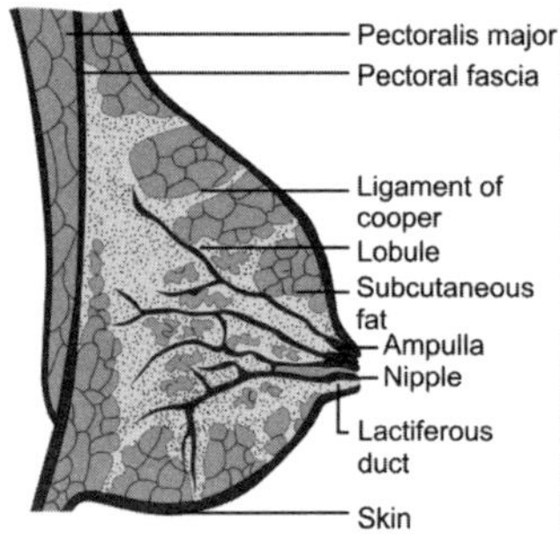

Breast

breastfeeding Feeding of an infant or young child with breast milk directly from female human breasts

breast pump a suction pump for manual expression of milk by vacuum

breech presentation fetal buttocks present at pelvic inlet

bregma that point on skull where coronal and sagittal sutures join

brittle diabetes changing and unpredictable response to insulin leading to ketosis, particularly in childhood diabetes

broad ligaments two folds of peritoneum continuous with that of uterus and extending to pelvic side wall containing Fallopian tubes parovarium ovarian blood vessels and lymphatics

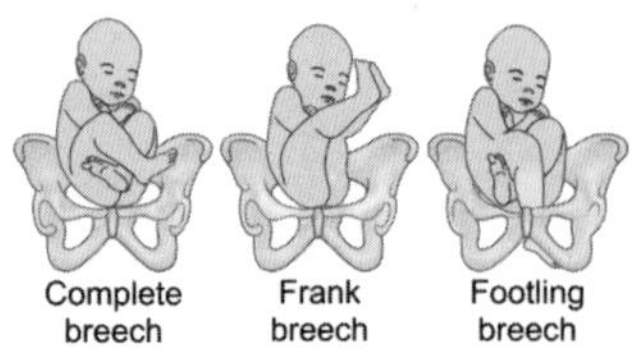

Breech presentation

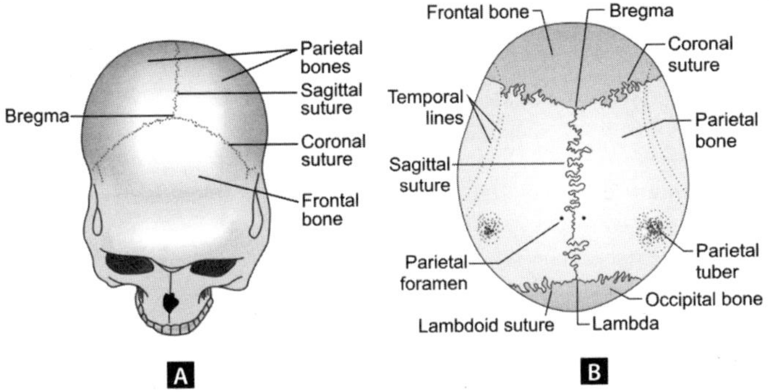

Bregma

bromhexine a sputum liquefier

bromocriptine a dopaminergic ergot derivative that is used in hyper prolactinemia and Parkinson's disease

bronchiectasis chronic irreversible and permanent dilatation of bronchi, may be congenital or acquired

bronchiole respiratory bronchiole is the last division of bronchial tree and continues as alveolar duct into alveolus. Terminal bronchiole is next to last subdivision of a bronchiole

bronchiolitis inflammation of bronchioles, commonly in small children

bronchitis inflammation of bronchioles, commonly in small children

bronchogram radiopaque material opacification of bronchi

bronchopneumonia inflammation of terminal bronchioles and alveoli

bronchopulmonary dysplasia pulmonary fibrosis and impaired oxygen transfer in babies who are ventilated for long that disrupts growth of lungs

bronchoscope an endoscope for visualization of tracheobronchial tree, biopsy and foreign body removal

brown fat a thermogenic layer of adipose tissue of embryonic life present between shoulder blades, behind sternum, in neck, around kidneys. It is utilized by newborn for production of heat

brow presentation a form of cephalic presentation where attitude of head is midway between flexion and extension, the presenting fetal diameter being mentovertical 13 to 13.75 cm which cannot negotiate with pelvis causing obstructed labor contributing factors are anencephaly, hydrocephaly, android pelvis

brucellosis Infection caused by Brucella organism (*B. abortus, B. suis* and *B. melitensis*)

B

bruise injury with effusion of blood into subcutaneous tissue and skin discoloration with intact skin

Brushfield's spots gray or pale yellow spots present at the periphery of iris in Down's syndrome

buccal smear scrapting from oral mucosa examined for Barr bodies

buffer A substance that maintains hydrogen ion concentration in blood. Principal blood buffers are bicarbonates, carbonates, carbonic acid, dibasic phosphates, Hb and plasma proteins

buffy coat a light colored layer containing white cells that forms when blood is centrifused or is allowed to stand in a test tube

bulbocavernous reflex contraction of bulbocavernosus muscle on percussing of dorsum of penis

bulimia excessive and insatiable appetite, bouts of overeating followed by vomiting in young girls

bulla a large blister or skin vesicle filled with fluid

bullaquine an antimalarial

bupivacaine a local analgesic used for epidural intrathecal and paracervical block-duration of action being 2 to 4 hours

Burkitt's lymphoma undifferentiated lymphoblastic lymphoma involving sites other than lymph nodes and RE system, with strong association with EB virus infection

burn an injury to tissues caused by: (a) physical agents, the sun, excess heat or cold, friction, nuclear radiation; (b) chemical agents, acids or caustic alkalis; (c) electrical current. Burn are described as being partial thickness (involving only the epidermis) or full thickness (involving the dermis and underlying structure). Clinically, emphasis is placed on the percentage of shock and prevention of infection and malnutrition needs specials attention

burning foot syndrome burning in the sole of feet due to vitamin deficiency and chronic renal failure

Burns-Marshall technique a method for delivery of head in breech delivery. Once trunk is delivered the baby is allowed to hang by its own weight to aid flexion and descent of head till hairline appears. Then the baby is elevated holding at the ankles that aids in delivery of head, often aided by low forceps

bursa a pad like cavity in the vicinity of joint lined with synovial membrane, acting to reduce friction between tendon and bone

bursitis inflammation of a bursa

busulphan an antineoplastic drug often used in chronic myeloid leukemia

butyrophenone a class of chemicals of which haloperidol is a member antipsychotic agents

Byler's disease inherited disease with cirrhosis and mental retardation in children

byssinosis pneumoconiosis of cotton and textile workers

cachet used for administering medicines with a bitter taste

cachexia a state of ill health, malnutrition and wasting

café-au-lait spot spots of patchy pigmentation of skin, usually light brown in color-characteristic of neurofibromatosis

caffeine an alkaloid of tea and coffee. CNS stimulant, analgesic

calamine a pink powder containing zinc oxide and little ferricoxide, used as protective, astringent

calcaneus the heel bone articulating with talus and cuboid

calciferol vitamin D2, ergocalciferol

calcitonin calcium lowering hormone, used in hypercalcemia, Paget's disease; secreted by D cells of thyroid

calcitriol a sterol of vit D activity, very potent

calcium channel-blockers a group of drugs that act by slowing the influx of calcium ions into muscle cells resulting in decreased arterial resistance and decreased myocardial O_2 demand

calcium most abundant mineral in body, essential for blood, clotting, cardiac contraction and bone formation

calculus any abnormal concretion in the body

Caldwell-Moloy classification the classification of female pelvis as gynecoid, android anthropoid and platypelloid calipers

calf fleshy muscular back part of leg formed by gastrocnemius and soleus

callus localized hypertrophy/thickening of skin at friction or pressure points calorie

cancer malignant tumor which is invasive and metastasizes to new sites by lymph/blood

Candida a genus of yeast-like fungi that develop a pseudomycelium and reproduce by budding

candidiasis infection of skin and mucous membrane by candida early warning signs of cancer

canker ulceration of mouth and lips

cannula a tube for insertion to cavity or into blood vessel, its lumen is fitted by trocar

capsule Gelatin enclosure for drug delivery

caput succedaneum swelling on presenting part of fetal head during labor

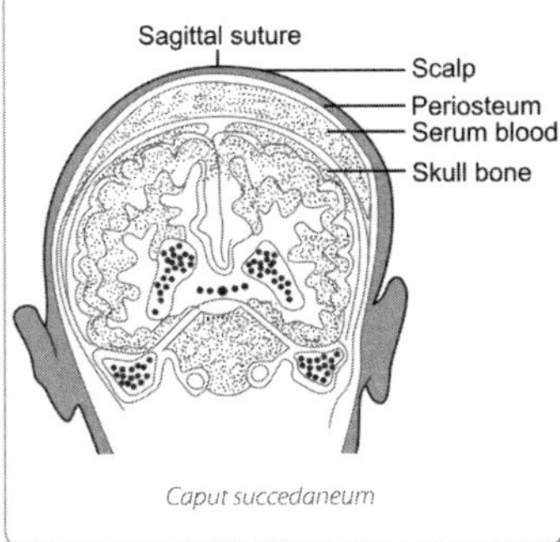

Caput succedaneum

C

carbachol cholinergic drug for producing miosis, also used for emptying bladder

carbamazepine antiepilepsy drug used for temporal lobe epilepsy and trigeminal neuralgia

carbidopa dopa decarboxylase inhibitor, used in combination with levodopa for Parkinsonism

carbimazole antithyroid drug

carbohydrate chemical substances containing carbon, oxygen and hydrogen, e.g. sugar, glycogen, starches, dextrin and celluloses. Sucrose is glucose + fructose; maltose is 2 D glucose; lactose is glucose + galactose

carbon dioxide final metabolic product of carbon compounds present in food. CO_2 combining power is a test of buffer capacity of blood. Solid CO_2(–80°C) used for removal of naevi, telangiectasis, warts, hemorrhoids, etc.

carbon monoxide present in automobile exhaust fumes, displaces O_2 from hemoglobin, hence diminishing O_2 transport

carbon tetrachloride A colorless toxic anesthetic liquid previously used for ankylostomiasis but toxic to liver and kidney

carbuncle Spreading inflammation of deeper skin

carcinoembryonic antigen a class of antigen in fetus and expressed by colonic tumors. CEA level returns to normal after complete removal of colonic tumor

carcinogen carcinoma inducing chemicals, e.g. benzpyrines

carcinoid tumor of Argentaffin cells in the GI tract, bronchi, ovary, secreting serotonin

carcinoma malignant growth of epithelial tissue; basal cell carcinoma is from basal layer of skin, rarely metastasizes (rodent ulcer); epidermoid carcinoma. For tumor on the surface either wart-like or infiltrating. medullary carcinoma. Carcinoma that is soft because of predominance of cells and paucity of fibrosis. Squamous cell cancer. Cancer from squamous epithelium with rolled out everted edges. Scirrhous carcinoma. A form of cylindrical carcinoma with a firm, hard structure

cardiac cycle the period from beginning of one heart beat to beginning of next beat. It comprises atrial systole 0.1 second and ventricular contraction of 3 second relaxation of 0.5 seconds

cardiac failure condition resulting from inability of heart to pump sufficient blood to meet the body needs

cardiac output blood ejected from left/right ventricle per minute, usually 3L/min

cardiac plexus branches of vagus and sympathetic trunk encircling base of heart

cardiac reserve the capacity of heart to increase cardiac output and raise in arterial blood pressure (Marey's law)

cardinal ligament also known as transverse cervical or Mackenrodt's ligaments. Two thickened bands of parametrium fixing cervix to lateral pelvic wall

cardinal movements the predictable sequence of movements through the birth canal that the fetus will go through during labor and birth: descent, flexion, internal rotation, extension, external rotation and expulsion

cardiocentesis puncture of heart

cardiogenesis formation and growth of embryonic heart

cardiogram recording of electrical activity of heart

cardiomegaly enlargement of heart

cardiopulmonary resuscitation emergency medical care to a person whose heart and lung function is going to stop or has recently stopped. Artificial respiration and cardiac massage are the two principal components of CPR

caries attrition of enamel and dentin

caries the decay or death of bone which becomes soft, discolored and porous

carneous mole a mass of blood clot surrounding a dead embryo and retained in uterus

carotene Yellow crystalline pigments of plant and animal tissue, converted to Vitamin A in liver

carotid body a pressure and hypoxia sensitive flat structure present at carotid bifurcation

carpal tunnel the canal beneath flexor retinaculum of wrist in which flexor tendons and median nerve pass

carpal tunnel syndrome pain, tenderness and weakness of muscles of thumb caused by pressure on median nerve in carpal tunnel

carpopedal spasm spasms of hand and feet seen in tetany and hyperventilation

carrier a person who harbors a pathogenic organism without any sign or symptom of disease but is capable of spreading the organism to others

cartilage a type of dense connective tissue capable of withstanding high pressure and tension. Cartilage is avascular and is without nerve supply

caruncle small fleshy growth

casein the principal protein in milk derived from casinogen

cast 1. a solid mold of a part, usually applied for immobilization of fracture, dislocation and severe injuries. 2. in dentistry a positive copy of tissues of jaw over which denture base is to be made. 3. pliable or fibrous matter which mold to the shape of the part in which they accumulate. According to source they can be classified as bronchial, intestinal, nasal, esophageal, renal, vaginal, etc. According to constituents casts can be bloody, fatty, hyaline, granular, waxy, etc.

castle factor also known as Castle's intrinsic factor, it is a small mucoprotein secreted by the gastric parietal cells.

This factor is required to facilitate adequate absorption of vitamin B12 by the stomach. Deficiency of this factor can result in pernicious anemia

castrate to remove or inactivate ovaries or testis

casualty accident/injury/death

catabolism breakdown of complex substances into simpler substances with consumption of energy; opposite of anabolism

cataphasia involuntary repetition of same word

cataplexy the brief sudden loss of muscle control brought on by strong emotion, i.e. excitement, anger

cataract opacity of lens nucleus, capsule or both. Immature stage: lens swollen, anterior chamber shallow; mature stage: lens shrinks, no iris shadow on transillumination cataract can be polar, lamellar, nuclear, cortical, congenital, traumatic, diabetic but senility is the single most common cause

catarrh inflammation of mucous membranes especially of nose and throat

catecholamine biologically active amines like epinephrine and nor epinephrine derived from amino acid tyrosine

catgut suture made up of ship's intestine. Chromium trioxide treatment enhances strength of the suture

catheter a hollow tube for evacuation and injection of fluids. Arterial and venous catheters for recording of pressure, pacing catheter for atrial/ventricular pacing, self-retaining bladder catheter; Tenckoff peritoneal catheter for peritoneal dialysis

cation an ion with positive charge that travels onto cathode

CAT scan computerized axial tomography; computerized X-ray picture of any body part

cat scratch fever febrile disease with lymphadenopathy transmitted by cats

cauda tail or tail-like structure. Terminal portion of spinal cord is cauda equina. Inferior portion of epididymis cauda epididymis

caudal block regional analgesia through sacral hiatus, less reliable than epidural analgesia

causalgia intense burning pain accompanied by trophic skin changes due to injury to sympathetic innervation

caustic an agent particularly an alkali that destroys living tissue

cauterization destruction of tissue by caustic, electric current, freezing, etc

cavity a hollow space in viscus or tooth

cecum the dirated pouch distal to ileum giving off the vermiform appendix

cefadroxil long acting oral cephalosporin

cefotaxime a third generation cephalosporin antibiotic having a broad spectrum of activity, used to treat intra-abdominal infections, bone and joint infections, gonorrhea, and other infections due to susceptible organisms including penicillinase-producing strains

celiac disease intestinal malabsorption syndrome mostly gluten induced

cell kinetics the study of growth and division of cell

cell membrane the envelop surrounding cell, composed of carbohydrate, lipid and protein

cell organelle structures in the cytoplasm like mitochondria, Golgi complex, endoplasmic reticulum, ribosomes, etc.

cell the basis structural unit of all plants and animals containing protoplasm and nucleus

cellular immunity T-cell mediated immune reaction, basis of organ transplant rejection, lepromin test and BCG vaccination

cellulitis inflammation of cellular or connective tissue

central venous pressure the pressure in right atrium indicating adequacy of venous return and blood volume

centrifuge a machine that spins test tubes at high speed, causing heavy particles to settle down to the bottom. RBCs settle down at bottom, and WBCs form a thin layer between RBC and plasma

cephalexin analog of antibiotic cephalosporin

cephalhematoma subcutaneous swelling containing blood found on the head of a newborn baby disappearing within 2 to 3 months

cephalic index maximal length of head divided by maximal breadth × 100

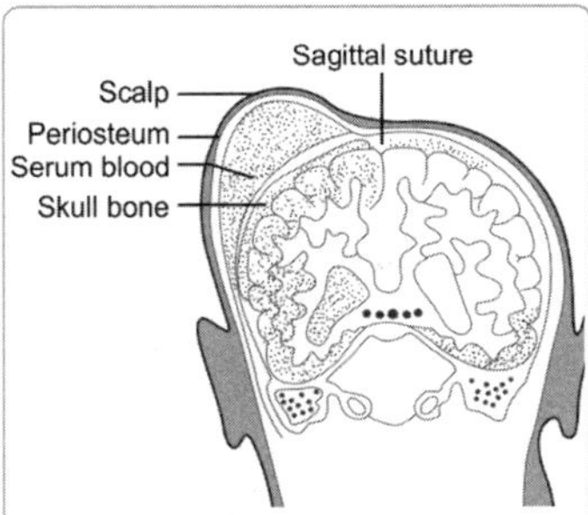

Cephalhematoma

cephalic presentation when the head of the fetus is the presenting part, may be vertex, face, sinciput or brow presentation

cephalometry measurement of the head using various bony points, used to assess growth and in determining orthodontic or prosthetic treatment

cephalopelvic disproportion a mismatch between fetal head and maternal pelvis diagnosed when fetal head does not engage by 36 weeks of pregnancy

cephaloridine an analogue of the antibiotic cephalosporin

cerclage encircling of a part with a ring or loop as in incompetent cervix

cerebellum largest portion of rhombencephalon lying dorsal to pons and medulla oblongata: involved in coordination of fine movements, maintenance of posture, equilibrium, muscle tone, etc.

C

cerebrospinal fever inflammation of brain and meninges

cerebrospinal fluid the cushioning fluid formed in the choroid plexuses of the lateral and third ventricle. Normal amount 100 to 140 mL, specific gravity 1003 to 1008

cerebrovascular accident (CVA) ischemic or hemorrhagic cerebral events due to embolism, thrombosis, vasculitis, aneurysm, A V malformation, etc.

cerebrum consists of two hemispheres united by two commissures; corpus callosum, anterior and posterior hippocampal commissures

cerumen the wax like, soft brown secretion in external auditory canal

cervical dilatation the opening or enlargement of the external cervical os from a few millimeters to 10 centimeters when completely dilated

cervical incompetence a patulous cervix that causes repeated abortion after 12th week of pregnancy

cervical intraepithelial neoplasia (CIN) CIN-I mild reversible CIN-II moderate but reversible CIN-III severe but irreversible or carcinoma in situ demanding surgery

cervical plexus the plexus formed by joining of anterior rami of first four cervical nerves, communicating with sympathetic ganglia

cervical spondylosis degenerative disease of cervical vertebral, disks and articulations often causing cord compression

cervical vertebra first seven bones of spinal column

cervicitis inflammation of uterine cervix

cervix the neck or part of an organ resembling neck

cesarean section an operation for delivery of fetus by putting incision on anterior abdominal wall and uterus after 24th week of pregnancy

cesarean section, lower segment (LSCS) involves horizontal incision on lower uterine segment. Classical caesarean section involves vertical incision on body of uterus with danger of scar rupture in subsequent pregnancies

Chadwick's sign The bluish or purple coloration of the vagina and cervix when pregnancy is presumed.

chalazion distention of a Meibomian gland of eyelid with hard secretions, resembling tumor

chancre hard painless syphilitic primary ulcer on exposed part with slough leather base

chancroid nonsyphilitic venereal ulcer due to *Haemophilus ducrey*

cheilitis inflammation of lips

cheilosis red lips, with fissured angles of mouth commonly due to riboflavin deficiency

chest the body part accommodating heart and lungs

chickenpox varicella infection with vesicles on skin that dry up in 5 to 7 days

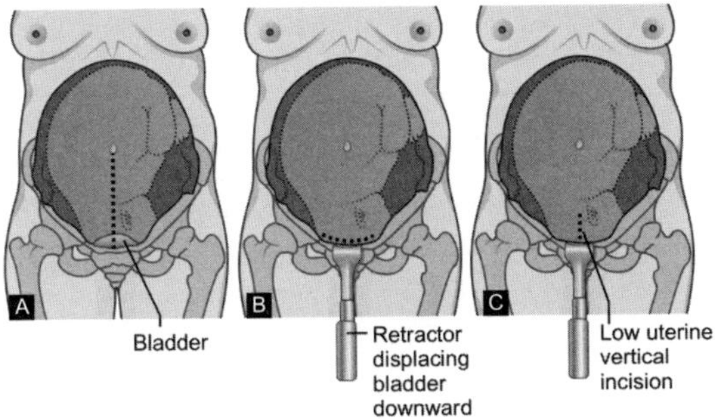

Cesarean sections: (A) Vertical uterine incision (classical incision); (B) Low uterine transverse incision; (C) Low uterine vertical incision

chikungunya an arboviral infection with fever, joint pain and rash

chilblain a form of cold injury characterized by local erythema, itching and often blistering

child abuse direct or indirect harm to children damaging prospect of their development— physical, social, intellectual and emotional

chill shivering with sensation of coldness and pallor of skin

Chlamydia a genus of microorganisms causing ornithosis, lymphogranuloma venereum, trachoma and genital infection

chloasma skin pigmentation (localized) following trauma, idiopathic or pregnancy

chlorambucil cytotoxic agent used to treat CLL, Hodgkin's disease, etc.

chlordiazepoxide a benzodiazepine, used to treat anxiety, alcohol withdrawal syndrome, etc.

chlorhexidine an antiseptic, often used for mouthwash

chloroxazone muscle relaxant

chlorpheniramine an antihistamine agent

chlorphenoxamine drug for Parkinsonism

chlorpromazine tranquillizer used in psychosis

chlorpropamide oral hypoglycemic agent of sulfonyl urea group

chlorthiazide a diuretic

choanal atresia congenital obstruction of the posterior nares (between the nose and throat). Since babies breath mainly through their noses, a baby with choanal atresia will have severe respiratory distress at birth. The immediate treatment is insertion of an oral airway

cholangiography radiography of biliary system

cholangioma tumor of bile ducts

C

cholecystitis inflammation of gallbladder manifesting with fever, chills, upper abdominal pain and mild jaundice, nearly always caused by gallstones

cholecystokinin hormone secreted by duodenum that stimulates gallbladder contraction and pancreatic secretion

cholelithiasis stone formation within gallbladder

cholera profuse watery diarrhea and vomiting with dehydration caused by *Vibrio cholerae*

cholesterol a monohydric alcohol, principal constituent of gallstones and constituent of cell membrane, precursor of cortisol hormones

chondritis Inflammation of cartilage

chorditis inflammation of vocal/spermatic cord

chordoma a tumor along vertebral column composed of embryonic nerve tissue

chorea a movement disorder due to extrapyramidal damage characterized by quasipurposive, involuntary, nonrepetitive limb movements, e.g. Sydenham (rheumatic) chorea, chorea gravidarum, Huntington's chorea

choreoangioma a collection of fetal blood vessels in Wharton's jelly forming a tumor on the placenta, of little clinical significance

choreoathetosis bizarre limb movements of extrapyramidal disease

chorioamnionitis inflammation of membranes covering fetus, i.e. amnion and chorion

choriocarcinoma malignant neoplasm of chorion usually following hydatid mole, abortion or often normal pregnancy

chorion an extraembryonic membrane that covers outerwall of blastocyst from which develop chorionic villi

chorionic gonadotropin a hormone produced by blastocyst stimulating the corpus luteum to produce progesterone to maintain the pregnancy

chorionic villi minute finger-like projections arising from trophoblasts. They have outer syncytotrophoblast and inner cytotrophoblast encasing fetal capillaries, oxygen, transfer from maternal blood to fetal blood and carbon dioxide transfer from fetal to maternal blood occurs across the villi

chorionic villus sampling A procedure to obtain a sample of the chorionic villi from the placenta via aspiration; tests for chromosomal and biochemical disorders during early pregnancy

choroid plexus vascular finger-like folds in pia mater in third, fourth and lateral ventricles of brain forming CSF

christmas factor a thromboplastin activator present in plasma

chromatin it is a DNA structure present in the cell nucleus. Males are chromatin negative and females are chromatin positive (inactivated X-chromosome)

chromatography a method of separating two or more chemical compounds in solution by passing across the surface of an absorbent paper

chromosome the structures containing DNA that store genetic information. There are 22 pairs of autosomes and one pair of sex chromosome in every cell

chyle the protein and fat rich fluid of lymphatic channels drained to left subclavian vein via thoracic duct

cilia hair-like processes projecting from epithelial cells of bronchi propelling up mucus and foreign particles

ciliary process about 70 folds arranged meridionally so as to form a circle, secrete nourishing fluid for cornea, lens and vitreous

ciprofloxacin a quinolone antibiotic against *Chlamydia* and gram-negative organism, be used with caution in pregnancy

circle of Willis the anastomosis at base of brain where posterior cerebral and middle cerebral vessels meet

circulatory failure inadequate cardiac pump action to meet oxygen demand of body tissues. Peripheral circulatory failure means pooling of blood in expanded vascular space consequent to vasodilatation resulting in decreased venous return to heart

circumcision removal of extra prepucal skin covering glans penis

circumduction circular movement performed by the limb, the joint performing the movement is at the apex of the cone

circumvalate papillae v-shaped row of papillae at base of tongue

cirrhosis chronic liver disease characterized by bridging fibrosis, hepatic cell degeneration and regeneration and evidence of portal hypertension

cisapride a dopaminergic drug used for GI motility disorders and in GE reflux

cisplatin antineoplastic agent for treatment of ovarian and testicular tumors

clamp a surgical instrument meant to compress to prevent hemorrhage, e.g. holister clamp for occluding vessels in umbilical cord

Clark's rule a formula for calculating pediatric dose, i.e. weight of the child in lb × adult dose/150

claudication pain in calf muscle during walking due to inadequate blood supply

claustrophobia fear of closed space

clavicle collar bone, articulating with acromion and sternum, can be fractured during birth

clavulanic acid beta lactamase inhibitor, usually combined with synthetic penicillins

claw foot excessively high longitudinal arch of foot with dorsal contracture of toes

claw hand a hand characterized by hyperextension of proximal phalanges and extreme flexion of middle and distal phallanges

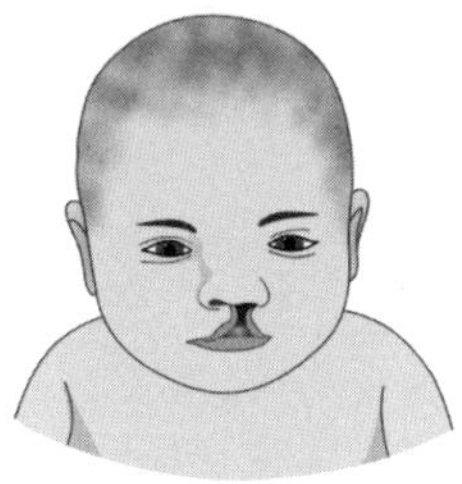

Cleft lip

clean catch method contamination-free urine specimen collection

cleft lip a congenital defect arising from failure of fusion of median nasal and maxillary processes, can be unilateral or bilateral

cleft palate a defect in palate, central or to one side often associated with cleft lip, hampers with ability to suck and with speech

cleidotomy division of fetal clavicles to facilitate delivery

cleptomania impulsive stealing in which motive is not related to value of stolen object

climacteric menopause or end of woman's reproductive ability. Male climacteric points to lessening male sexual activity

clindamycin an antibiotic against gram-positive cocci, implicated to produce pseudomembranous colitis due to resistant Clostridium difficile

clitoridectomy This refers to partial or total removal of the clitoris. This has been defined by the WHO as type I female genital mutilation (type I FGM)

clitoris small erectile body beneath anterior labial commissure of female, homologous to penis of male

clitoris crises involuntary orgasm in female in tabes dorsalis

clobetasol a locally applied steroid

clofazimine antileprotic agent that stains skin

clofibrate lipid lowering agent, may be carcinogenic and causes gallstones

clomiphene clomiphene citrate, a nonsteroidal agent to stimulate ovulation in females and spermatogenesis in males

clonazepam anticonvulsant for myoclonic seizure

clonidine antihypertensive agent, also used for migraine prophylaxis

clonus alternate contraction and relaxation of muscles, sign of upper motor lesion

Clostridium anaerobic spore forming rods common in soil and GI tract of animal and man

clotrimazole antifungal agent for treatment of vulvovaginal candidiasis

clotting formation of jelly-like mass at bleeding site or within vessel due to activation of coagulation factor embedding platelets and RBCs in fibrin mesh

cloxacillin beta lactamase resistant penicillin

clozapine diabenzodiazepine group of antipsychotic agent

clubbing bulbous enlargement of finger and toes tips with exaggerated lateral and longitudinal curvatures. Most commonly found in infective endocarditis, suppurative lung disease, cyanotic heart disease and often congenital

cluster headache nocturnal headache, 2–3 hours after falling asleep, continuing for months associated with watering from eyes

coach A person who assumes the role of advocate and support person for the laboring woman, assists with conditioned techniques for relaxation and breathing

coarctation a stricture, compression of walls

cocaine CNS stimulant, in toxic doses causes CNS depression, cardiac arrhythmia and respiratory depression

coccydynia persistent pain around coccyx

coccygeus one of two muscles arising from ischial spines and inserted into lateral borders of sacrum and coccyx forming part of pelvic floor

cochlea a winding cone-shaped tube resembling a snail shell, winding two and three quarter turns about a central bony axis, organ responsible for hearing

cochlear implant an electronic device that receives sounds and transmits the resulting electric signals to implanted electrodes in cochlea so that the sound is perceived

codeine derivative of opium used as analgesic-hypnotic, cough suppressant

cod liver oil oil extracted from liver of fish rich in Vitamin A and D

cognition awareness with perception, reasoning, judgment, memory, etc.

cohort a group of people who possess a common characteristic

coitus sexual intercourse between male and female

cold common SYN nasal catarrh, acute catarrhal inflammation of mucous membrane of nasal cavity, sinuses and pharynx caused by rhinovirus

cold pack wrapping patient in cold water soaked clothing to reduce fever, for relief of pain and diminution of swelling in bruise

colic spasmodic pain originating from any hollow viscus

colitis inflammation of colon

collagen vascular diseases A group of diseases of blood vessels of unknown etiology manifesting with joint pain, skin rash, muscle ache and bleeding manifestations. Included in this group are SLE, rheumatoid arthritis, systemic sclerosis, etc.

Colles' fracture transverse fracture of distal end of radius with displacement of lower fragment backward, upward and laterally

colon irritable motility disorder of colon manifesting with abdominal pain, frequent small ribbon like stools, usually triggered by anxiety

C

colonoscope a flexible fiberoptic instrument to visualize interior of colon

color blindness defective perception of color; color blindness in which all colors are perceived as gray is called monochromasia

colostrum breast fluid secreted during first 2 to 3 days after delivery, rich in protein, calories and antibodies

colpectomy surgical removal of vagina

colpocele a hernia into the vagina

colpocystitis Inflammation of the bladder and vagina

colpoperineoplasty plastic repair of the vagina and perineum

colpoperineorrhaphy surgical repair of the ruptured vagina and perineum

colpopexy fixation of vagina

colpoplasty also called vaginoplasty. It is the plastic surgery of the vagina

colporrhaphy repair of vagina

colporrhexis a tearing or laceration of the vaginal vault

colposcope a speculum for examining vagina and cervix for early detection of malignancy

colposcopy examination of vagina and vaginal portion of cervix by colposcope, usually to select sites of abnormal epithelium for biopsy in patient with abnormal Pap smear

colpostenosis narrowing of the vagina

colpotomy incision on vaginal wall, e.g. to drain pelvic abscess

colpoxerosis a condition characterized by unusual dryness of the vaginal mucous membrane

coma a state from which patient cannot be aroused by painful stimuli and he does not respond to inner needs

comedo Blackhead, discolored dried sebum plugging an excretory duct of the skin, e.g. acne involving face, back and neck in adolescents

commensal organisms that live in an intimate nonparasitic relationship

commissure a transverse band of nerve fibers passing over the midline in the CNS

communicable disease a disease that may be transmitted directly or indirectly from one person to another

complement a series of enzymatic proteins in normal serum that once activated augment immune mechanisms by leukocyte chemotaxis, and bacterial opsonization

complement fixation some antigen-antibody reactions fix complement for completion of reaction. The process is the basis of Wasserman reaction for syphilis

compliance the property of altering size and shape in response to application of force, weight or release from such force, e.g. pulmonary compliance a measure of the force required to expand the lungs. Children have higher pulmonary compliance in comparison to adults

compound fracture fracture with communication to exterior by breach in the skin

computed tomography a radiological imaging technique that images 1 to 10 mm thick slices of body part

conceptional age age of the fetus calculated from the day of fertilization

conception fertilization of ovum by spermatozoon

condom a contraceptive sheath to be worn by male for contraception

condyloma a wart-like growth in the skin around anus/external genitalia. **c. acuminata** Usually venereal, caused by virus. **c. latum** A mucous patch on the vulva or anus characteristic of syphilis

cone biopsy removal of cone shaped portion of cervix to exclude malignancy confabulation

congenital born with, i.e. malformation present from birth

congenital dislocation of hip (CDH) common to breech delivery and girls, often familial, best confirmed by US

congestion the presence of excessive amount of blood or tissue fluid in an organ or tissue

conjugate paired or joined

conjugation a coupling together. In biology, the union of two unicellular organisms accompanied by an interchange of nuclear material

conjunctivitis inflammation of conjunctiva

connective tissue tissue that binds together or supports the structures of body. Blood, bone cartilage and fibrous tissue are connective tissues

consanguinity blood relationship

consciousness a state of awareness, i.e. orientation in time, place and person

consent granting permission by patient for a procedure

constipation infrequent defecation with passage of unduly hard and dry fecal material, sluggish action of bowels

constriction ring localized annular spasm of uterus usually at junction of upper and lower uterine segments, can form around neck of fetus or causes retention of placenta, rexalation of it may occur with amylnitrite

contact dermatitis Dermatitis due to an irritating or sensitizing chemical

contact mutual touching or apposition of two persons/objects or one who has recently been exposed to contagious disease

contagion communication of disease from one person to another by direct contact

contamination 1. introduction of disease germs or infectious materials into normally sterile objects. 2. radiation in or on a place where it is not wanted

continent capable of controlling urination and defecation or sexual indulgence

continuing professional education periodic updating and refreshing of professional knowledge and skill

continuous positive airway pressure (CPAP) a method of ventilation where pressure of 2 to 5 cm H_2O is generated in respiratory tract by nasal face mask or endotracheal route

contraception prevention of conception

contraceptive any process, device or method that prevents contraception. They include spermicides, estrogen-progesterone pills, and physical barriers like IUD

contracted pelvis pelvis in which brim, cavity or outlet is less than normal causing obstructed labor

contraction stress test a procedure to help measure fetal well-being by stimulating the uterus to contract with oxytocin administration or nipple stimulation and measuring the response of the fetus to the contractions; it can be interpreted as positive, negative or equivocal.

contracture permanent contraction of a muscle due to paralysis/spasm/ ischemia

contrast in radiology radiopaque material to provide a contrast in density between tissue of organ being X-rayed

contrecoup injury injury to one part of brain with lesion on opposite side, e.g. blow to the back of head causing injury to frontal lobes as they are forced against anterior portion of cranial valt

contusion a bruise, injury with subcutaneous hemorrhage but intact skin

convalescence the period of recovery after an illness/operation

convulsion paroxysms of involuntary muscle contraction and relaxation

Cooley's anemia thalassemia major, an inherited disorder of hemoglobin synthesis

Coombs' test a test for detection of antiglobulins in blood, helpful in diagnosis of autoimmune hemolytic anemia

coordination working together of various muscles for performing certain movements

cordocentesis percutaneous umbilical blood sampling under US guidance form study of karyotyping, genetic analysis, IUGR, etc.

corneal transplant either partial thickness or full thickness transfer of cornea from a healthy cadaver, donor to treat corneal opacity obstructing vision

cornea the clear transparent anterior portion of eye covering 1/6 the surface of globe functioning as an important refractive medium. It is composed of 5 layers: Epithelium, Browman's membrane, substantia propria, Descemet's membrane and layer of endothelium

coronal plane plane dividing into front and back portions

coronary angiography opacification of coronary arteries by injection of iohexol or urograffin or any such contrast agent

coronary bypass surgically established shunt between root of aorta and involved coronary distal to block or diverting internal mammary to augment myocardial blood flow

cor pulmonale right heart failure secondary to pulmonary pathology

corpuscle any small rounded body, an encapsulated sensory nerve ending, blood cell

corpus the principal part of any organ or body

corrosive poisoning poisoning by strong alkalies, acid, antiseptics e.g. hydroxides of sodium, ammonium potassium

cortex outer layer of an organ like kidney, adrenal, ovary, lymph node, thymus, cerebrum and cerebellum

cortical necrosis damage to renal cortex due to hypoperfusion as in shock

corticoid steroid hormone secreted by adrenal cortex

corticosterone hormone of adrenal cortex influencing carbohydrate metabolism, Na^+ and K^+ homeostasis

corticotropin (ACTH) the anterior pituitary hormone that stimulates adrenals to secrete glucocorticoids

corticotropin releasing factor the hypothalamic factor regulating secretion of corticotropin

cortisone adrenal hormone, largely inactive till converted to active cortisol; influences metabolism of fat, carbohydrate, protein N^+ and K^+

coryza acute nasal catarrh with profuse watery secretion

cosmetic surgery commonly known as plastic surgery, done to improve appearance, i.e. correction of ugly burns and scars, elephantiasis, localized obesity, pendulous breast, facial wrinkles

cough forceful expiratory effort with closed glottis, to expectorate mucous and foreign body

counseling providing of advice and guideline to a patient by health professional

counterincision a second incision made to facilitate drainage or to reduce tension on the stitches

counterirritant an agent applied locally to produce mild inflammatory reaction to relieve pain of adjacent or deeper structures

couplet care a system in which one nurse cares for the postpartum mother and her newborn as a single unit; it is also known as mother-baby dyad.

couvelaire uterus the appearance of uterus in severe accidental hemorrhage the uterus appearing purplish blue bruised due to entry of blood into myometrium

Cowling's rule age of child on next birthday divided by 24 to give pediatric dose

coxa hip joint. ***c. vulga*** hip deformity with increase in the angle between neck and shaft of femur. ***c. vara*** opposite to coxa vulga

cracked nipple soreness of nipple during breastfeeding if baby is not fixed to nipple correctly

cramp spasmodic painful contraction of a muscle

craniostenosis contracted skull due to premature closure of cranial sutures

craniotomy perforation and crushing of fetal skull to aid in delivery of dead fetus

C

creatine methylglycocyamine, a colorless substance excreted in urine, combines with phosphate to form creatine phosphate

Crede's method expulsion of placenta by putting downward pressure on the uterus through anterior abdominal wall and squeezing uterus but inversion is a danger

crepitation crackling sound heard 1. in lungs in pneumonia, 2. movement of fractured bones, 3. in soft tissues in anaerobic gas forming infections and in 4. subcutaneous emphysema

cretin hypothyroidism in babies manifesting as rough skin, mental subnormality, potbelly, coarse features, hypoactivity and delayed dentition

Creutzfeldt-Jakob disease a neurodegenerative disease caused by prion

cri-du-chat syndrome a chromosomal deletion disorder characterized by cry like a cat, microcephaly, mental retardation, dwarfism and laryngeal defect

crib a small bed with high legs and sides for infant and babies

Crohn's disease regional enteritis, a granulomatous inflammation involving all the three coats of small intestine and often colon

cromolyn sodium disodium chromoglycate, useful in bronchial asthma, mast cell stabilizer

cross-fertilization Fusion of male and female gametes from different persons

cross matching a test for compatibility in blood transfusion where donor red cells are matched with recipient plasma and vice versa

croup laryngitis marked by barking cough, stridor, and respiratory difficulty usually due to formation of diphtheritic membrane

crowning showing of fetal head in vulva during parturition

crown-rump length a measurement in US to assess fetal age in uterus

cryoprecipitate precipitation of immune complexes in patients with autoimmune diseases when their serum is stored in cold

cryopreservation preservation of biological material, e.g. sperm, organs, tissue, plasma in subzero temperature

cryosurgery tissue destruction by application of cold probe (–20°C or below) as to control pain, bleeding, e.g. hemorrhoidectomy, tonsillectomy, conization of cervix, thalamotomy

cryptomenorrhea monthly subjective symptoms of menstruation without vaginal bleed usually due to unperforated hymen

culture propagation of microorganisms or living tissue in special media

currett a spoon-shaped scrapping instrument used in dentistry, gynecology and orthopedics

Cushing's syndrome symptoms arising out of hypercortisolism with buffalow hump, stria hypertension and weight gain

cyanocobalamin vitamin B12 deficiency causes anemia, neuropathy and CNS degeneration

cyanosis bluish discoloration of skin due to raised (>5 gm%) of reduced hemoglobin in blood

cyst a closed sac or pouch with a definite wall containing fluid, semisolid material

cystic fibrosis inherited disease of exocrine gland affecting respiratory tract, pancreas and intestine characterized by dry viscid mucus respiratory infection, pancreatic insufficiency, increased sodium content of sweat, SYN: mucoviscidosis

cystitis inflammation of urinary bladder

cystocele protrusion of urinary bladder into vaginal volt

cytokines a chemical substance secreted by activated macrophages and lymphocytes influencing inflammation and repair

cytology study of cell structure and function. Vaginal and cervical cytology can indicate hormonal status and malignancy potential

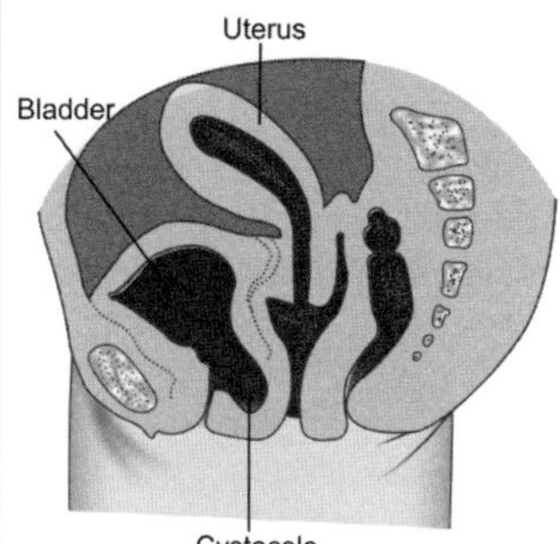

Cystocele

cytomegalic inclusion disease a viral disease causing encephalitis, retinitis and fetal death

cytoplasm protoplasm of a cell excluding nucleus, contains mitochondria

cytotrophoblast the inner cell layer of blastocyst becoming less obvious after 20th week

D

danazol a progesterone used in endometriosis and fibroadenosis of breast

dandruff seborrhea, exfoliation of epidermis of scalp with white greasy, dry scales

Dandy-Walker syndrome congenital hydrocephalus due to blockage of foramen of Luschka and Magendie

dapsone a sulfa drug used for leprosy

Darier's disease (keratosis follicularis) a congenital disorder characterized by verrucous popular growths that coalesce into plaques of various sizes on scalp, face, neck and trunk

DDT dichlorodiphenyl trichloroethane (chlorophenothane) an insecticide used in mosquito control

deafness complete or partial loss of ability to hear

death permanent cessation of all vital functions including that of brain, heart, lung

death rate number of deaths per 1,000 population in a given time

decadron dexamethasone, a long acting corticosteroid

decidua endometrium of uterus during pregnancy with outer compact layer and inner spongy layer

decidual cast the expulsion of the decidua intact in the shape of uterine cavity, following the death of the ovum in an ectopic pregnancy

deciduoma uterine tumor containing decidual tissue, when malignant termed choriocarcinoma

deciduous teeth primary dentition of 20 teeth that erupt between 6 months and 3 years

Chart: Eruption of deciduous (milk) teeth

Upper	*Eruption*	*Lower*	*Eruption*
Central incisor	5–7 Mths	Second molar	20–30 Mths
Lateral incisor	7–10 Mths	First molar	10–16 Mths
(Cuspid) canine	16–20 Mths	(Cuspid) canine	16–20 Mths
First molar	10–16 Mths	Lateral incisor	8–11 Mths
Second molar	20–30 Mths	Central incisor	6–8 Mths

Chart: Eruption of permanent teeth

Upper	*Completed by*	*Lower*	*Completed by*
Central incisor	9–10 yr	Third molar	18–25 yr
Lateral incisor	10–11 yr	Second molar	13–16 yr
(Cuspid) canine	12–15 yr	Second premolar (Bicuspid)	13–14 yr
First premolar (Bicuspid)	12–13 yr	First premolar (Bicuspid)	12–15 yr
Second premolar (Bicuspid)	12–14 yr	First molar	6–7 yr
First molar	6–7 yr	(Cuspid) Canine	10–13 yr
Second molar	14–16 yr	Lateral incisor	9–10 yr
Third molar	18–25 yr	Central incisor	8–9 yr

decision analysis a logically consistent approach to the common clinical problem of needing to make a decision when its consequences cannot be foretold with certainty. The biological variation, inconsistent drug response and poor clinical outcome data on many drug/therapeutic procedures make decision analysis a charter so that patient can be foretold in advance all about the possible outcome of treatment and he can choose the one he thinks the best

decision making the process of using all the informations available about a patient and arriving at a decision concerning therapeutic plan

decompensation failure of heart to maintain adequate circulation to meet oxygen demand of tissues

decongestant reducing congestion or swelling

decubitus ulcer skin ulceration due to prolonged pressure, commonly over bony prominences

deep transverse arrest obstruction to passing down of fetal head during second stage of labor resulting from occipitoposterior position in first stage

deep vein thrombosis thrombosis of deep veins in the leg threatening pulmonary embolism. It is of particular danger during puerperium

defecation bowel evacuation

defecation syncope syncope occurring during or immediately after defecation

defeminization loss of female sexual characteristics

defibrillation stoppage of fibrillation of heart by drugs or electrical current

deflexion partial or nonflexion of fetal head as in persistent occipitoposterior position

deformity an alteration in the natural form or alignment of an organ

degeneration deterioration in organ structure or function

dehydration excessive fluid loss or inadequate fluid intake resulting in hemoconcentration and renal failure

deletion the loss of genetic material from one chromosome

delirium a state of mental confusion in which patient is disoriented for time and place with illusions and hallucinations. This may occur during fever, after head injury, drug intoxication, etc.

delivery childbirth

deltoid muscle the prominent muscle covering shoulder—attached to deltoid ridge of humerus

delusion a false belief inconsistent to ones knowledge and experience, and with evidence to contrary

demand feeding feeding when baby appears hungry and not according to fixed time table

dementia global impairment of intellectual function (cognition) interfering with social and occupational activities

demineralization loss of minerals, such as calcium and phosphorus, from bone

D

demography statistical and quantitative study of characteristics of human population like size, growth, density, sex, age, etc.

dengue a group of B arbovirus disease caused by bite of *Aedis egypti* mosquitoes, characterized by fever, myalgia, lymphadenopathy and often purpuric spots

denominator in obstetrics, a particular point on the presenting part of the fetus used to indicate its position in relation to maternal pelvis

dental plaque a gummy mass of microorganisms and minerals that grows on the crown and causes dissolution of enamel and tooth substance

dentition the type, number and arrangement of teeth in the dental arch

dentrifice a powder or other substance used for cleaning the teeth

deodorant an agent that masks or absorbs foul odor

deoxyribonucleic acid a protein consisting of deoxyribose, phosphoric acid, two purine bases (adenine and guanine) and two pyrimidines (thymine and cytosine), principally present in cell nucleus, principal protein of genes and chromosomes

dependence psychic raving for a drug that may or may not be accompanied by physiological dependence

depletion removal of substances, like water, electrolyte, blood, from the body

depression 1. altered mood with loss of interest in pleasurable activities, feeling of worthless, excessive guilt, self-reproach, suicidal ideation 2. lowering of a part, 3. decrease in the activity of a vital organ

dermatitis inflammation of skin, may be allergic, actinic, infective, exfoliative, etc. characterized by redness, itching, etc.

dermoid cyst a nonmalignant cystic tumor containing ectodermal elements like skin, hair and teeth

descent downward movement of fetal head during labor; often measured in fifths

desensitization prevention of anaphylaxis usually by administering repeated small doses of the agent causing anaphylaxis/allergy

detoxify to remove toxic quality of a substance. To treat toxic overdose of a drug/alcohol

detrusor external muscular coat of urinary bladder

developmental milestones development of skills like crawling, sitting, laughing, walking in infants and children

dexamethasone synthetic glucocorticoid

dextran a plasma volume expander, a polysaccharide fermented from sucrose

dextroamphetamine an isomer of amphetamine, a CNS stimulant

dextropropoxyphene analgesic with high addiction potency

Table: Developmental milestones

Age	*Ideal body wt.*	*Height*	*Body surface*	*% Adult dose*
Newborn	3.4 kg	50 cm	0.23 m	12.5%
1 month	4.2 kg	55 cm	0.26 m	14.5%
3 months	5.6 kg	59 cm	0.32 m	18%
6 months	7.7 kg	67 cm	0.4 m	22%
1 year	10 kg	76 cm	0.47 m	25%
3 years	14 kg	94 cm	0.62 m	33%
5 years	18 kg	108 cm	0.73 m	40%
7 years	23 kg	120 cm	0.88 m	50%
12 years	37 kg	148 cm	1.25 m	75%

dextrose $C_6H_{12}O_6$ (SYN: glucose), a simple monosaccharide sugar

diabetes a general term for diseases causing excessive urination

diadanosine an antiviral used in HIV infection

diagnosis the term used to denote the name of disease or diseased process using scientific and skillful methods

diagonal conjugate an internal measurement of pelvis taken from promontory of sacrum to the lower border of symphysis pubis normally measuring 12.5 cm subtracting 1.3 cm from this gives true conjugate

dialysis the process of diffusing blood across a semipermeable membrane to remove toxic materials

diameter distance from one point to another diagonally opposite point on the perimeter of a sphere

diamox acetazolamide, a carbonic anhydrase inhibitor

diaphoretic agents that increase sweating/perspiration

diaphragmatic hernia a condition when the diaphragm does not close completely and the abdominal contents slip into the thoracic cavity; causes respiratory distress in the newborn

diaphragm the musculomembranous wall separating abdomen from thoracic cavity. It contracts with each inspiration permitting descent of base of lung. The attachment is to 6th rib anteriorly and 11–12th ribs posteriorly. Diaphragmatic contraction aids in defecation, parturition and urination by increasing intra-abdominal pressure. It becomes spasmodic in hiccough and sneezing. Contribution of both diaphragms to respiratory inflow is 40% and nerve supply is by phrenic nerves

diaphysis the middle part of long bone

diarrhea frequent passage of unformed watery stool due to inflammation, irritation, retention, emotion, etc.

D

diastole that period of cardiac cycle (usually of 0.5 sec) during which the heart dilates, ventricles fill with blood

diastolic pressure the period of least pressure in the arterial vascular system

diathermy the therapeutic use of a high frequency current to generate heat within some part of body

diatom one group of unicellular microscopic algae seen in lungs of patients with antemortem drowning

diazepam antianxiety benzodiazepine useful in treatment of cocaine poisoning, status epilepticus, convulsion and a variety of anxiety disorders

Dick test a skin test for susceptibility to scarlet fever similar to Schick test for diphtheria

diclofenac analgesic anti-inflammatory agent

dicumarol an anticoagulant that increases prothrombin time

dicyclomine an anticholinergic agent

didelphic pertains to double uterus

dienestrol synthetic estrogen

dietetics the science of applying the principles of nutrition to the feeding of individuals or groups

diet food substances normally consumed in the course of living

diethylstilbestrol a synthetic estrogen

dietician one who provides dietary guidelines in treatment of disease and to maintain good health

differential blood count determination of number of each variety of leukocytes in one microliter of blood

diffusion a process by which various gases intermingle as a result of incessant motion of their molecule i.e. there is always a tendency of molecule or substances (gas, liquid, solid) to move from a region of high concentration to a low concentration

digestion the process by which food is broken down by enzymatic action into absorbable forms

digitalis cardiotonic glycoside that increases myocardial contraction and refractory period of A-V node

digital radiography radiography using computerized imaging instead of conventional film or screen imaging

dihydroergotemine vasoconstrictor used in migraine

dilantin a derivative of glyceryl urea (diphenyl hydantoin sodium) used as antiepileptic best for clonic/tonic clonic seizure

dilatation and curettage cervical canal dilatation and scraping of uterine cavity

dilatation and evacuation cervical canal dilatation and evacuation of product of conception by suction/forcep

dilatation expansion of a vessel or an orifice

dilators insturments used to dilate canals, cavities or openings

diltiazem calcium channel blocker, useful for ischemic heart disease

dimenhydrinate a drug for control of dizziness, vomiting and nausea

dimorphism the quality of existing in two different forms. ***d. sexual*** having some properties of both sexes, e.g. hermaphrodites

diphtheria acute infectious disease, characterized by fever, sore throat, cervical lymphadenopathy and formation of gray pseudomembrane at the site of infection, i.e. tonsil, pharynx, larynx, nose, etc. Causative agent is club shaped *Bacillus*, *Coryne bacterium diphtheriae*

diplegia paralysis of legs and hands of one side

diplococci cocci always found in pairs; can be encapsulated (pneumococci) intracellular gonococci)

dipstick A chemical impregnated paper strip used for analysis of chemical constituents in urine

disaccharide a carbohydrate formed of two simple sugars, e.g. lactose sucrose and maltose

disc a rounded flat plate. ***d. intervertebral*** a layer of fibrocartilage in between vertebral bodies

discharge the flow of substances from body. ***d. vaginal*** white mucoid non-irritating vaginal discharge during pregnancy, if profuse irritating or offensive, investigation be advised

disease lack of ease, illness or suffering; can be hereditary, autoimmune infective, degenerative or malignancy

disengagement the emergence of fetal head from within the maternal pelvis

disinfectant a substance that prevents infection by killing pathogenic organisms

disinfection the process of making rooms/linens/organs germ free. The common methods of disinfection are by autoclaving, boiling in water, ethylene oxide/formaldehyde gas, alcohol, iodine, phenols, etc.

dislocation displacement of any part

disodium edetate a chelating agent used to treat hypercalcemia

disorientation inability to be aware of time, place and person

displacement removal from normal position. Normal uterus is antiflexed and anteverted. Retroversion and prolapse are displacements

disproportion lack of proper harmony in size between two parts. ***d. cephalopelvic*** disparity between fetal head and maternal pelvis through which it has to pass

dissect to split, to go into detail, to separate various parts of cadaver

disseminated intravascular coagulation (DIC) a coagulation disorder with bleeding tendency due to consumption of clotting factors and platelets due to thrombin generation in blood stream

dissociation separation of complex compounds into simpler ones

distal farthest from the center, from a medial line

D

distance space between two objects

distillation condensation of vapor that has been obtained from a liquid heated to volatilization point

diuresis passage of large amounts of urine

diuretic an agent that increases formation of urine

diurnal daily

diverticulum a pouch or sac in the wall of a hollow organ

dizygotic pertaining to or derived from two separate zygotes, e.g. ***d. twins***

dizziness a sensation of unsteadiness or whirling

doctor to teach, a person qualified to practice medicine

doderleins bacillus a nonpathogenic *Lactobacillus* of vagina producing lactic acid from glycogen metabolism to maintain vaginal pH of 4.5

dolicocephalic having a skull with long anteroposterior diameter

domiciliary within or at home

dominance 1. genetic quality through which one gene of pair of allele expresses, while the other is suppressed. 2. preferred hand or side of body. 3. in psychiatry, the tendency to control others

domperidone antiemetic, increases gastric motility, useful in dyspepsia

donor one who donates blood, tissue or an organ for use in another person

dopamine a vasopressor catecholamine and neurotransmitter, also implicated in some forms of psychosis and abnormal movement disorder

Doppler a method to measure blood flow in arteries and veins

dorsal pertains to back, opposite of ventral

dose amount of medicine/radiation to be given at one time

double blind trial a test for the real effect of new drug or treatment in clinical practice. Neither the patient nor the administering staff knows about the placebo and new drug

double contrast examination radiographic examination in which both a radiopaque and a radioluscent contrast medium are used simultaneously to visualize internal anatomy

douche a current of vapor or stream of hot/cold water directed against a part

Douglas pouch peritoneal space lying between uterus and front of rectum

doula a woman who serves other women

Down syndrome congenital anomaly due to trisomy 21 manifesting with mental retardation, skeletal anomalies and light yellow spots at periphery of iris

doxycycline broad spectrum tetracycline used in bid dose

drainage the free flow of fluid from a wound/cavity

dramamine diphenhydramine, an agent for vertigo

drepanocyte sickle cell

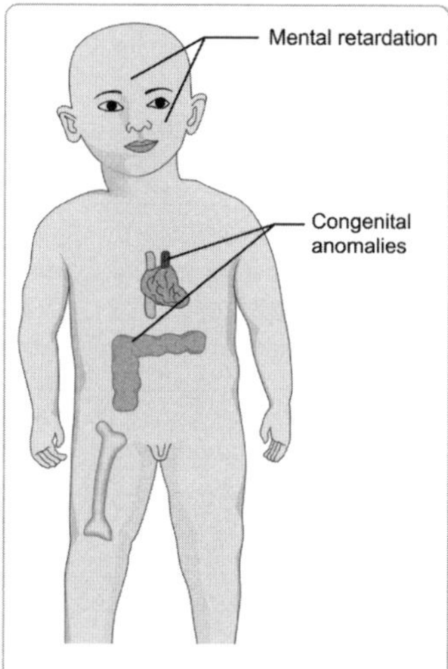

Down syndrome

dressing protective or supportive covering for injured part

droplet infection infected particles coming as spray from patient's mouth and nose

drowsiness the state of almost falling asleep

drug abuse self-administered drug overuse

drug addiction a condition caused by excessive or continued use of habit forming drugs

drug interaction interaction between drugs taken concurrently

drug rash rash produced in some individuals by intake or application of drugs

drug reaction adverse and undesired reactions to a substance

Dubowitz score a method for assessment of gestational age

Duchenne's muscular dystrophy a form of childhood muscular dystrophy

Ducrey's bacillus small rod-shaped organism found in pairs, causative agent of soft sore

duct a narrow tubular vessel or channel to convey secretions from gland

ductus arteriosus the channel communicating ascending aorta to left pulmonary artery in the fetus

ductus venosus a fetal blood vessel that connects the umbilical vein and the inferior vena cava

duffy system a blood grouping system

duodenum the first part of small intestine from pylorus to jejunum, about 10" long

dura mater the outer membrane covering the brain and spinal cord

duration of pregnancy averages 266 days from conception to delivery and 280 days (40 weeks or 9 months plus 7 days) from last menstrual period to delivery

dwarf an abnormally short or undersized person

dydrogesterone orally effective synthetic progestin used mainly in diagnosis and treatment of primary amenorrhea and dysmenorrhea

dysentery inflammation of mucosal lining of GI tract with passage of blood, pus and mucus in stool

dysfunctional labor occurs when there is a problem with the frequency, duration and intensity of uterine contractions, and/or the resting tone of the uterus between contractions

dysgenesis defective development

dyslexia inability to interpret written language even though vision is normal

dysmenorrhea painful menstruation

dyspareunia painful sexual intercourse experienced by females

dyspepsia imperfect digestion with abdominal bloating, heart burn, flatulence, anorexia, nausea, etc. can be gastric, hepatic, biliary, alcoholic in origin

dysphagia difficulty in deglutition, can be due to spasm of pharyngoesophageal musculature, stricture, neoplasm, paralysis

dysphasia impairment of speech both articulation and comprehension

dysphoria excessive depression feeling without apparent cause

dysplasia abnormal tissue growth/differentiation

dyspnea labored or difficulty in breathing either due to vigorous physical activity, anemia, cardiac or pulmonary disease

dyspraxia a disturbance in the programming, control and execution of volitional movements

dystocia Abnormal or difficult labor or delivery. Used to refer to weak or ineffective uterine contractions; may also be used to describe the situation in which the shoulders of a baby in vertex presentation become trapped after delivery of the head (shoulder dystocia)

dystonia increased muscle tone

dystopia displacement of any organ

dystrophy defective muscle power, nutrition and metabolism

dysuria painful micturition either due to concentrated acid urine, urinary crystals/concretions, urinary infections, pelvic pathology and prolapse uterus

Eales' disease retinal vein thrombophlebitis with recurrent hemorrhages into retina and vitreous

early deceleration a transitory decrease in the fetal heart rate caused by head compression, which stimulates the vagus nerve to slow down the heart rate

Ebstein's anomaly downward displacement of septal leaflet of tricuspid valve with gross tricuspid regurgitation

ecchymosis collection of blood beneath the skin causing discoloration

eccrine sweat glands sweat glands of skin with density of over 400 per sq. cm on the palms and about 80 per sq. cm on thigh

echocardiography the technique of imaging the cardiac structures non-invasively through passage of ultrasound

echoencephalogram recording of midline shift of brain structures by ultrasound waves

eclampsia coma and convulsion occurring after 28th week of pregnancy and in immediate postpartum

econazole a topical antifungal agent

ecstasy methylenedioxymeth-amphetamine (MDMA) a hallucinogen widely abused, can cause cardiac arrhythmia, hepatotoxicity, hyperthermia, DIC

ecthyma a shallow skin lesion with crusting, often followed by pigmentation and scarring

ectoderm the outer layer of cells in developing embryo giving rise to skin, teeth, nervous system, organs of special sense, pituitary, pineal and suprarenal glands

ectomorph linear slender body build with poor musculature

ectopia malposition or displacement

ectopic pregnancy implantation of fertilized ovum outside the uterine cavity, can be abdominal, tubal or ovarian with liability for rupture and hemorrhage

ectopic rhythm any abnormal or irregular cardiac rhythm

ectropion eversion of eyelid margin

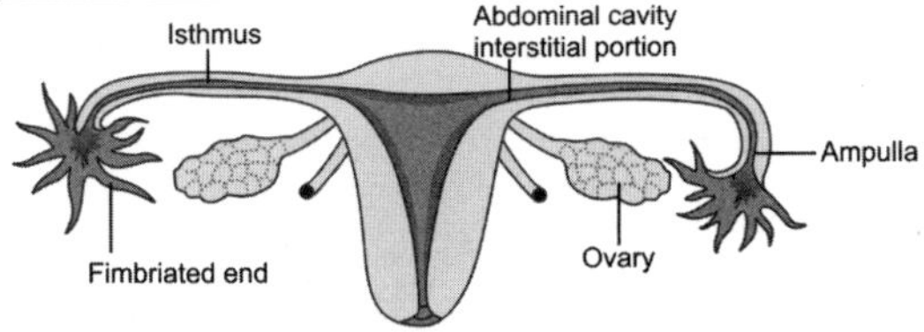

Sites of implantation in ectopic pregnancy

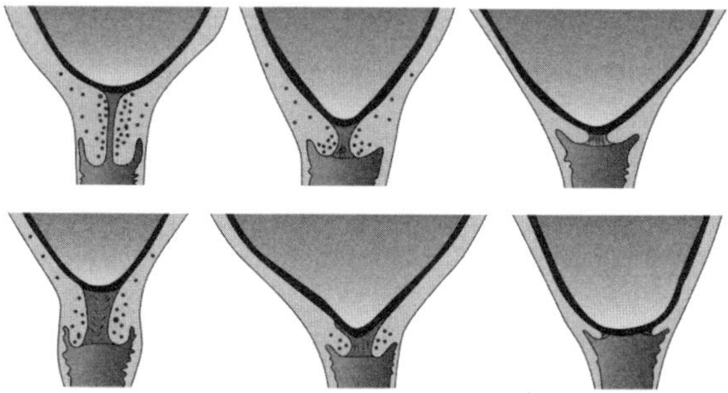

Effacement

eczema acute or chronic cutaneous lesion with erythema, papule, vesicles and crusts leading to itching, lichenification and pigmentation: mostly atopic or allergic

edema excessive tissue accumulation water, either localized or generalized, can be due to poor venous drainage, lymphatic obstruction, increased venous pressure (CHF), hypoalbuminemia or increased water retention

Edward's syndrome trisomy 18 with peculiar facies, congenital heart disease and mental retardation

effacement dilatation of cervix and stretching of birth passage

effect result of an action or force. ***e. cumulative*** drug effect on repeated administration of a drug

efferent carrying away from a central organ

effleurage a form of abdominal massage which can reduce pain perception during labor

effluent fluid discharged from sewage treatment or industrial plant

effusion escape of fluid/air into a cavity, e.g. hydropneumothorax, chylothorax, pleural effusion

Ehler-Danlos syndrome an inherited disorder of elastic connective tissue characterized by fragile hyperelastic skin and hypermobile joints

Eisenmenger's complex in a case of congenital heart disease with left to right shunt (ASD, VSD, PDA, etc.) when the pulmonary vascular resistance equals or exceeds systemic resistance it is called Eisenmenger's complex

ejaculation ejection of seminal fluid from male urethra

elastic bandage bandage that can be stretched to exert continuous pressure

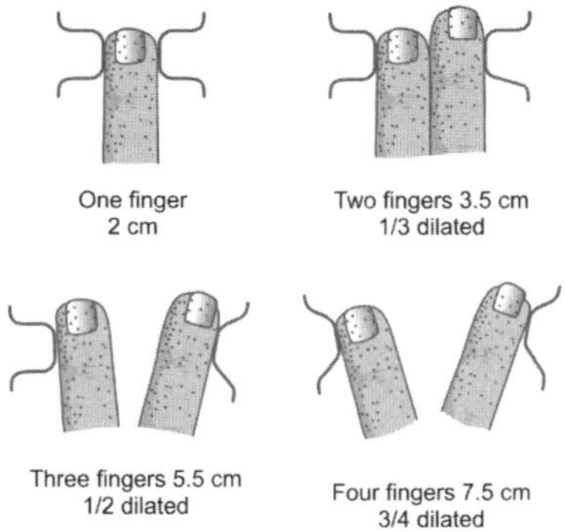

Clinical estimation of dilatation of cervix

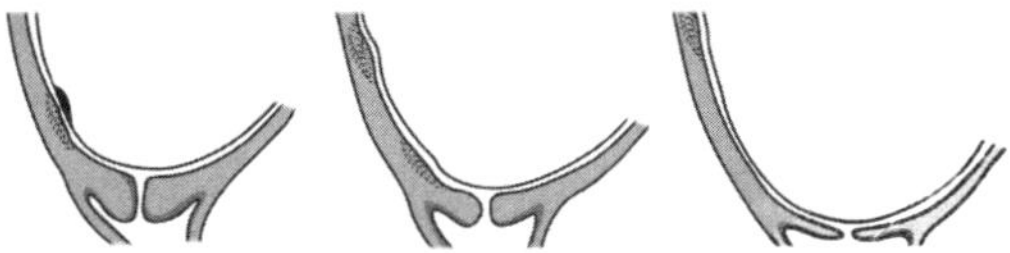

Dilatation and effacement of cervix

elastic cartilage yellow cartilage of epiglottis, pharynx, external **ear**, auditory tubes

elective therapy a planned convenient therapy/operation

electrocardiogram (ECG) record of electric activity of heart

electrocardiograph the machine used to record electrocardiogram

electrocoagulation electrode coagulation of tissue by means of a high-frequency current in a medium intervening between an electric conductor and the object to which the current is to be applied

electroencephalogram (EEG) recording of electrical activity of brain through surface electrodes

electrolysis dissolution of tissue by electric current e.g. destruction of hair follicle

electrolyte 1. a solution which conducts electricity. 2. ionized salts in blood, tissue fluids and cells

electronic fetal monitoring a type of monitoring in which information about the fetal heart rate and the laboring woman's uterine contraction pattern is continually assessed; can be either direct (invasive or internal) or indirect (noninvasive or external)

E

electrophoresis the movement of charged colloidal particles as a result of changes in electric potential

elephantiasis hypertrophy of skin and subcutaneous tissue due to lymphatic stasis, e.g. in filariasis that involves scrotum, penis, legs, breasts and hands

elimination diet a diet regime used to determine which foods cause allergic response. Offending food then is discovered when one by one food is gradually introduced into diet

emaciation to become excessively lean

embolism obstruction to blood flow by mass of red blood cells and fibrin mesh. Atrial fibrillation and pelvic-leg vein thrombosis predispose to embolism

embolus a mass of undissolved matter in blood vessel, may be clot, fat, air bubble, clumps of bacteria, amniotic fluid

embryo 2nd through 8 weeks of fetal development

embryogeny the growth and development of an embryo

embryology the science that deals with origin and development of an organism

embryonic plate that portion of inner cell mass of the blastocyst from which the embryo itself is formed

emergency cardiac care (ECC) care necessary to deal with an acute cardiopulmonary event like infarction, arrhythmia, pulmonary embolism

emetic agent producing vomiting, e.g. apomorphine

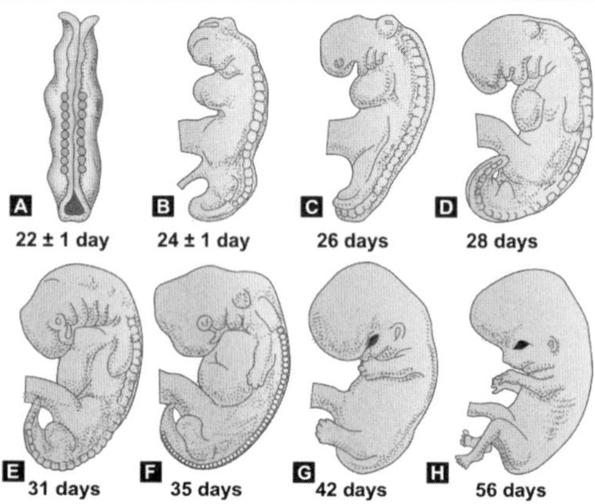

Human embryo at various stages of development

emetine ipecac derivative, used for extraintestinal amebiasis

emmenagogue any substance that can induce menstrual bleeding

emphysema 1. pathological distension of tissues by air/gas. 2. chronic pulmonary disease with dilatation of airspaces beyond terminal bronchioles

emulsion a mixture of two liquids not mutually soluble

enalapril an ACE inhibitor used in hypertension and congestive heart failure

enamel hard glistening white substance forming a covering on crown of teeth

encephalitis inflammation of brain parenchyma, manifesting with changes in level of consciousness, increased intracranial pressure, sensory motor dysfunction

encephalopathy any dysfunction of brain

encephalocele protrusion of brain substance through a cranial defect

encephalogram X-ray of brain with air injected into ventricular system

encopresis condition associated with constipation and passage of watery colonic content across the hard fecal mass, mimicking diarrhea

endarteritis inflammation of intima of an artery resulting from syphilis, trauma, infective thrombi

endemic a disease occurring repeatedly in a particular population conferring some immunity and hence low mortality

endocarditis inflammation of endothelial lining of heart chambers and heart valves; may be due to invasion of microorganisms or abnormal immunologic response

endocervicitis inflammation of mucus lining of endocervix

endocervix the mucous membrane lining the cervical canal

endocrine gland glands secreting directly into blood stream

endogenous produced or arising from within a cell or organism

endometriosis proliferation of endometrium at ectopic sites, i.e. sites other than uterine cavity

endometritis inflammation of endometrium

endometrium the mucous membrane lining the body of uterine cavity

endorphins polypeptides produced in the brain tissue that bind to opioid receptors and block them there by producing analgesia. The most important is beta endorphin

endosalpingitis inflammation of lining of Fallopian tubes

endoscope a device containing optical system for observing or conducting surgery in hollow structures like abdomen, pelvis

endotoxic shock cardiovascular collapse due to endotoxin (lipid A) produced by gram-negative sepsis particularly *E. coli*, *C. aelchii* and often betahemolytic streptococci

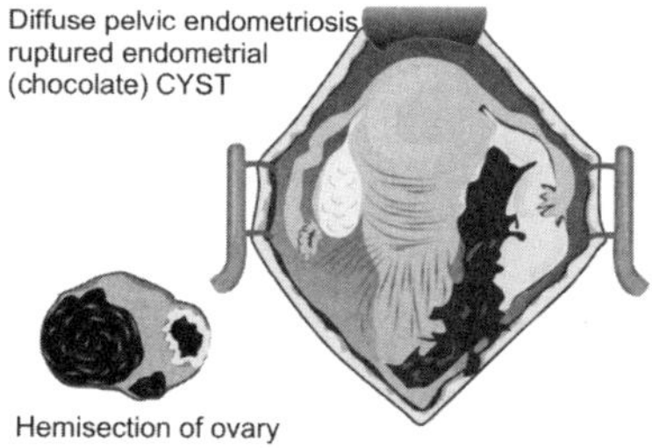

Endometriosis

endotracheal tube an airway catheter inserted into trachea for ventilation, resuscitation and during general anesthesia

enema stimulation of bowel activity by introduction of soothing, cleansing and chemical agents into rectum. Drugs can be given as enema, e.g. steroids in ulcerative colitis, paraldehyde

energy the capacity of a system in doing work

engagement in obstetric descent of presenting part into true pelvic cavity, i.e. the part is immobile

engorgement of breasts painful accumulation of milk in breast after delivery with lymphatic and venous stasis and edema, best relieved by breastfeeding or application of dry dark green cooled cabbage leaves

enkephalins polypeptides produced in brain that bind to opioid receptors to produce analgesia

enteral tube feeding feeding patient with a tube passed into stomach

enteric coated tablet or capsule coated with special coating that only dissolves in intestine

enterocele herniation of upper posterior vaginal wall where a portion of small bowel bulges into the vagina

enterocolitis inflammation of intestine and colon

entonox nitrous oxide and oxygen 50% each premixed in one cylinder used as an analgesic in labor

enuresis involuntary passage of urine in bed after the age of 5 years, often a familial tendency

enzyme complex proteins catabolizing reactions but without being changed themselves, can be synthesizing, coagulating, branching, debranching, digestive, fermenting, glycolytic, lipolytic, mucolytic

enzyme induction increase in enzyme level due to its increased production or decrease degradation. Drugs commonly causing hepatic enzyme induction are barbiturates

enzyme-linked immunosorbent assay (ELISA) a test to detect antigen or antibody, hormones

eosinophil granular leukocyte staining with acid stain eosin

eosinophilia increased blood eosinophil count beyond 6 to 8% or 300/cmm

ephedrine sympathomimetic agent used locally as decongestant and systemically for bronchodilation and raising blood pressure

epicanthus a vertical fold of skin extending from root of nose to the median end of eyebrow covering inner canthus and caruncle

epidemic appearance of a disease in a high proportion not expected for a community in a geographical area

epidemiology science concerned with study and analysis of interrelationship of factors that determine disease frequency

epidermolysis bullosa a severe blistering skin disease often autosomal dominant inheritance

epididymis a small long convoluted organ lying behind testes and containing the ducts of testes. It ends in spermatic duct

epididymitis inflammation of epididymis, usually as a complication of gonorrhea, syphilis, tuberculosis, mumps, filariasis, etc.

epidural analgesia a form of pain relief by injection of bupivacaine into extradural or peridural space best suited for first and second stage of labor; sudden hypotension is a danger leading to fetal hypoxia

epigastrium region over pit of the stomach

epiglottis leaf-shaped flat membrane covering entrance of larynx during swallowing

epilepsy recurrent paroxysmal electrical dysfunction of brain characterized by altered consciousness and motor/sensory phenomena

epinephrine hormone of adrenal medulla, synthesized from phenylalanine having ionotropic, bronchodilator and sympathomimetic effects

epiphora abnormal over flow of tears either due to excess secretion or blockage of lacrimal duct

epiphysis an ossification center separated from parent bone by a cartilage in infants and children; an indicator for assessment of bone age

episiotomy incision of perineum to facilitate delivery and avoid laceration

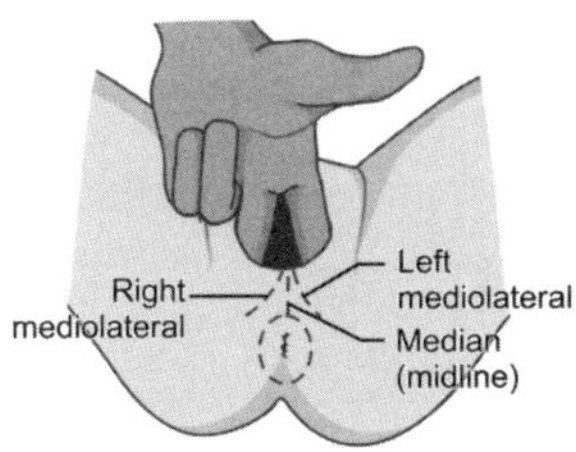

Types of episiotomies

E

epispadius congenital opening of urethra on dorsal aspect of penis or clitoris

epistaxis bleeding from Kiesselbach's area of nose

epithelia tissue those tissues covering outer surface of body and lining the internal passages or cavities. The cells lie in close proximity of each other with little intercellular substance

epithelioma malignant tumor arising from epithelium, e.g. skin or mucous membrane

Epsilon-aminocaproic acid synthetic substance, antifibrinolytic, used to check bleeding

epstein's pearls small white epithelial spot at junction of hard and soft palate in neonates

eradication complete elimination of disease

Erb's palsy paralysis of muscles supplied by C5 and C6

erection swelling, hardness and stiffness of penis on sexual arousal/ physical handling

erethism excessive excitation or irritation

ergometrine the alkaloid from ergot commonly used oxytocic to augment uterine contraction to prevent post partum hemorrhage

ergonomics the science concerned with how to fit a job to man's anatomical, physiological and psychological characteristics in a way that will enhance human efficiency and well-being

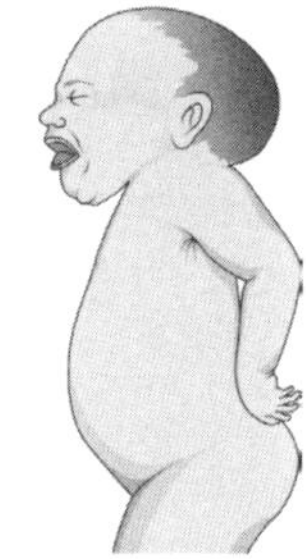

Erb's palsy (affected arm rotated inwardly)

ergonovine meleate an ergot derivative used in treatment of migraine. It also stimulates contraction of uterus

erosion destruction of surface layer

erotism sexual desire

erysipelas spreading inflammation of skin and subcutaneous tissue accompanied by systemic disturbance

erythema toxicum neonatorum an urticarial condition affecting newborns in the first few days of life, the lesions consist of dead white papules, grainy to the touch, with or without surrounding areas of redness

erythroblastosis fetalis hemolytic disease of newborn usually due to Rh incompatibility or ABO mismatching

erythrocyte the nonnucleated biconcave disc of 7.7 micron, matured red blood cell containing hemoglobin, involved in oxygen transport

erythropoiesis formation of red blood cells

erythropoietin an alfaglobulin secreted by kidney that stimulates erythropoiesis

Escherichia coli gram-negative bacillus of intestine causing diarrhea, urinary infection and endotoxic shock

esophageal atresia a condition in which the esophagus ends in a blind pouch or narrows into a thin cord; usually occurs between the upper and the mid-third of the esophagus

esophagus the musculomembranous tube extending from pharynx to stomach

essential hypertension hypertension without an identifiable cause

essential oils highly concentrated oils extracted from plants used in aroma therapy

estradiol $C_{18}H_{24}O_2$ steroid hormone of ovary with estrogenic properties

estrogen substance having estrogenic activity, i.e. development of female sex characteristics, cyclic changes in endometrium and vaginal epithelium, breast changes

estrone $C_{18}H_{22}O_2$ natural estrogenic hormone less active than estradiol but more active than estriol

estrus the cyclic period of sexual activity in mammals; during estrus animal is said to be in heat

ethambutol antitubercular bacteriostatic agent

ethamsylate a hemostyptic used to control bleeding

ethics moral principles or standards governing conduct

ethinylestradiol an estrogenic hormone, very potent

ethionamide bacteriostatic second line antitubercular drug

ethionine progestational agent used in contraception

ethylchloride C_2H_5Cl volatile liquid used for topical anesthesia

ethylene diaminetetraacetic acid (EDTA) a chelating agent

ethylene oxide C_2H_4O a fumigant. Also used for sterilizing articles that cannot withstand heat

etodolac a pain killer

eucapnia Normal CO_2 concentration in blood

eugenics the science dealing with genetic and prenatal influences that affect the expression of certain characteristic in offsprings

euphoria exaggerated feeling of wellbeing

Eustachian tube 4 cm long mucus lined tube extending from middle ear to pharynx

euthanasia mercy killing; dying easily, quietly and painlessly; ending one's life with an incurable disease

euthyroid normal thyroid function

evacuate to discharge especially bladder and bowel

eventration removal of contents of abdominal cavity, partial protrusion of abdominal contents through an opening in the abdominal wall

eversion turning outwards

E

evidence-based medicine evaluation, risk benefit and analysis of prescribing or adopting particular form of therapy

Ewing's tumor diffuse endothelioma causing a fusiform swelling of long bone

exacerbation aggravation of symptoms

exchange transfusion transfusion and withdrawal of small amounts of blood until blood volume is entirely replaced; used in autoimmune hemolytic anemia, hyperbilirubinemia

exercise in pregnancy gentle exercises including yoga, aquatic exercises taken during pregnancy

exercise performed activity of muscles

exfoliation the shedding of cells

exhalation the process of breathing out

exomphalos a herniation of umbilicus along with abdominal contents covered with peritoneum

exotoxin toxins produced by microorganism to surrounding medium

expected date of delivery (EDD) 9 months and 7 days from LMP; for long cycles add days in excess of 28 days and for short cycles subtract days less than 28

expulsion forcible driving out, e.g. of fetus from uterus

exsanguinations excessive blood loss to the point of death

extension movement by which both ends of a part are pulled apart

external os the opening of cervix into vagina

external version a procedure to change malpresentation to normal position, e.g. turning breech to cephalic or transverse or oblique to longitudinal lie

extrauterine pregnancy embedding of the fertilized ovum outside uterine cavity, i.e. ovary, Fallapion tube, abdominal cavity

extravasation exit of fluid from its normal channel to surrounding

extremity the terminal part of anything, an arm or leg

extrinsic of external origin. ***e. factor*** a factor secreted from stomach for absorption of vit B12

extroversion eversion, turning inside out

extubation removal of tube, e.g. laryngeal

exudates a protein rich fluid, high in cell count; can be pus, catarrhal, hemorrhagic, fibrinous

Fabry's disease an inherited disorder of metabolism with accumulations of glycolipid in tissues

face anterior part of head from forehead to chin, composed of 14 bones

face presentation a cephalic presentation in which head and spine of fetus are extended with mentoanterior or mentoposterior position. Persistent mentoposterior can cause obstructed labor

facet a small, smooth area on a bone or hard surface

face to pubis persistent occipitoposterior

facial nerve seventh cranial nerve supplying facial muscles, platysma, submandibular and sublingual glands, and carrying taste sensations from anterior two thirds of tongue

facial palsy paralysis of facial muscles leading to drawing of angle of mouth to healthy side, improper closure of eye; can follow forcep delivery but spontaneous recovery is usual factor

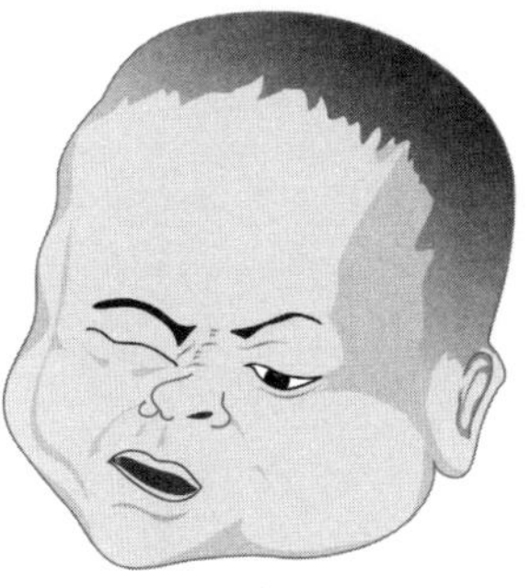

Facial palsy

facies the expression or appearance of the face; certain congenital syndromes present with a specific facial appearance

factitious disorder feigning illness

factor coagulation factors essential for blood coagulation; a group of serine proteases

Fahrenheit a temperature scale with freezing point of water at 32º and boiling point at 212º point

failure loss of function of an organ

faint temporary loss of consciousness due to cerebral ischemia

Fallopian tube the oviducts 10 cm long extending from ovaries to uterus

Fallot tetralogy congenital cyanotic heart disease characterized by over riding of aorta, infundibular stenosis, right ventricular hypertrophy and a ventricular septal defect

false labor uterine contractions causing pain but no dilatation of cervix

false negative a test indicating that the disease is not present when actually it is present

false pelvis the region between brim of true pelvis and iliac crests

false positive a test indicating that the disease is present when in fact it is not

false ribs the lower five pair of ribs that do not unite directly with the sternum

famciclovir antiviral agent for herpes

familial disease occurring more frequently in a family than would be expected by chance

family 1. a group of individuals descending from a common ancestor 2. a group of people living in a household who share common attachments, such as mutual caring, emotional bonds, common goal, etc. 3. in biology, the division between an order and genus

family planning planning and spacing of child birth according to wishes of the couple rather than to chance

famotidine H_2 receptor blocker, used for peptic ulcer disease

farsightedness an error of refraction in which parallel rays are focused at a point behind retina, so that near objects are not seen clearly

fascia fibrous membrane covering, supporting or separating muscles, uniting skin with underlying tissue

fat adipose tissue of body serving as energy reserver, providing fat-soluble vitamins

fatigue feeling of tiredness resulting from continuing activity

fatty acids omega-3 unsaturated fatty acids present in fish and certain vegetables, not synthesized in body. They reduce platelet adhesiveness and lower serum triglyceride; hence used in coronary artery disease prevention

favism hereditary hypersensitivity to a kind of bean, vicia faba characterized by fever, hemolytic anemia, vomiting common to patients of G6 PD deficiency

febrile convulsion convulsion precipitated by fever

feces excreta, stool

feculent resembling stool

fecundity fertility, ability to produce children

female condom a pouch made of polyurethane, which lines the vagina and external genitalia

female woman, sex that produces ova

feminism male developing secondary sexual characteristic of female

feminization testicular an apparent female with genetic characteristic of male due to tissue resistance to androgenic hormones secreted by testes

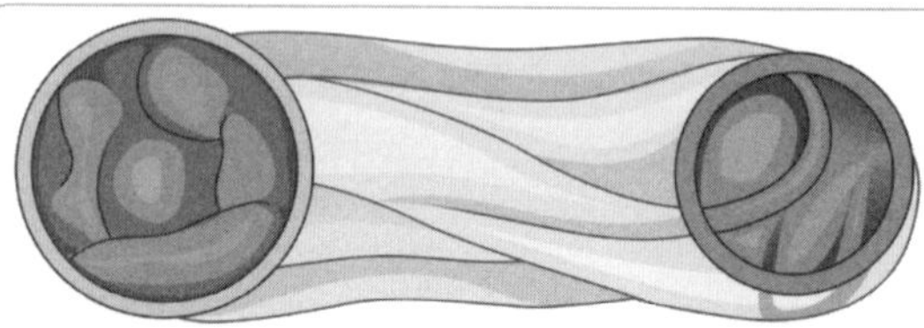

Female condom

femoral pertaining to femur. ***f. artery*** the continuation of external iliac artery to thigh. ***f. vein*** continuation of popliteal vein and continues up as external iliac vein

femur the thigh bone 20" long in adults, articulating with ileum at hip and with tibia at knee

fenestra an aperture frequently closed by membrane

fentayl citrate synthetic potent analgesic

fern pattern palm leaf (arborization) pattern of cervical mucus when allowed to dry on a glass slide; dependent on salt concentration in mucus which is further dependent upon amount of estrogen in the mucus. This test is only positive in mid cycle. If positive in late cycle, indicates lack of progesterone

ferokinetic study of absorption, utilization, storage and excretion of iron

ferritin iron-phosphorus protein complex containing about 23% iron, the principal tissue storage form of iron

ferroprotein important oxygen transferring enzyme

ferrous bivalent iron

fertile capable of producing offspring ***f. period*** 1. 9 days around ovulation, i.e. 5 days before and 3 days following ovulation 2. reproductive life of woman, i.e. 15 to 45 years

fertility ability to reproduce

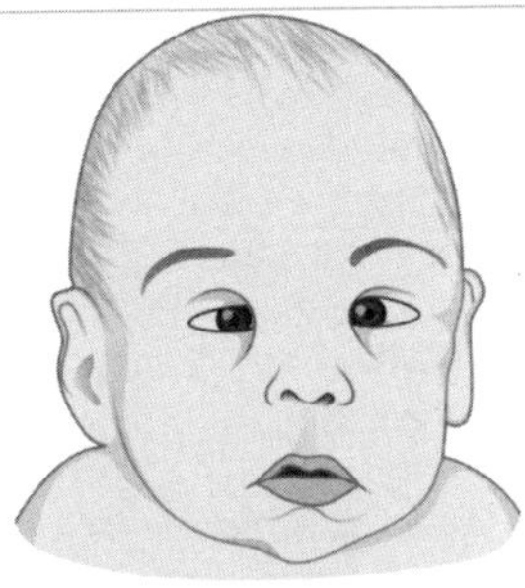

Fetal alcohol syndrome

fertilization union of ovum with spermatozoa or union of male and female gametes in plants

fetal alcohol syndrome birth defects and mental retardation in babies born to alcoholic mothers who continued alcohol ingestion during first trimester

fetal bradycardia the fetal heart rate is less than 120 beats/minutes during at least a 10-minute period of continuous monitoring

fetal circulation oxygenated blood from placenta passes via umbilical vein and ductus venosus to inferior vena cava by passing liver and then to right atrium and then via foramen ovale to left atrium, left ventricle and aorta. Some blood from right atrium also enters right ventricle and pulmonary artery to be shunted to aorta via ductus arteriosus. Blood to placental villi are returned via the two umbilical arteries which are continuation of bypogastric arteries

F

fetal distress fetal hypoxia manifesting with tachycardia or bradycardia, exaggerated or slowness of fetal movement and meconium-stained liqour demanding immediate delivery; can be due to maternal shock, eclampsia, CPD, intrauterine infections, cord round the neck, fetal anemia placenta previa, uterine hypertonicity

fetal heart rate acceleration an increase in the fetal heart rate that occurs during a uterine contraction, with the fetal heart rate decreasing to its previous rate as the contraction subsides

fetal heart rate baseline average fetal heart rate between periodic rate changes (accelerations or decelerations). The baseline fetal heart rate is the average fetal heart rate during any 10-minute period. The normal baseline range is between 120 and 160 beats per minute

fetal heart rate deceleration a decrease in the fetal heart rate that occurs in response to a uterine contraction. There are three types of decelerations (early, late and variable)

fetal heart rate variability the beat-to-beat changes that occur in the baseline fetal heart rate

fetal lie relationship of the fetus to the long axis of the mother. There are three possible lies: longitudinal, transverse and oblique

fetal position the relationship of the landmark on the presenting fetal part to the front, sides or back of the maternal pelvis

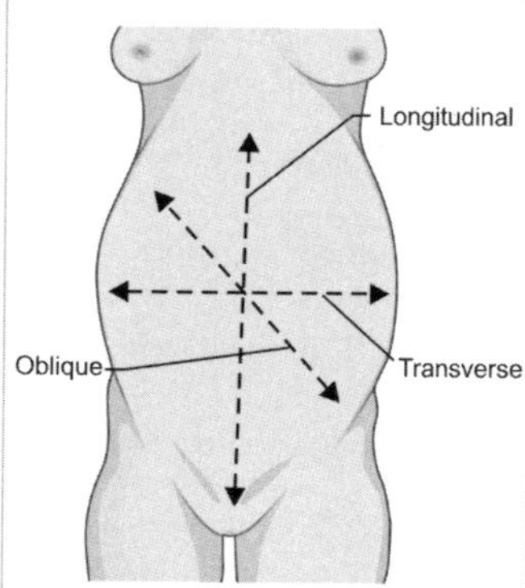

Fetal lie

fetal presentation part of the fetus, which lies at the pelvic brim or in the lower pole of the uterus

fetal skull composed of two frontal bones separated by frontal suture, two parietal bones separated by sagittal suture and separated from frontal bones by coronal suture, occipital bone separated from parietal bone by lambdoid suture. Anterior fontanelle lies at junction of frontoparietal bones and 2 posterior fontanella at junction of occipitoparietal bones. Base of skull is formed by 2 temporal bones, ethmoid and sphenoid bones and contains foramen magnum transmitting spinal cord

fetal surveillance methods to assess and monitor the wellbeing of the fetus during pregnancy, labor and birth; includes fetal biophysical profile, biochemical assessments, amniocentesis, genetic studies,

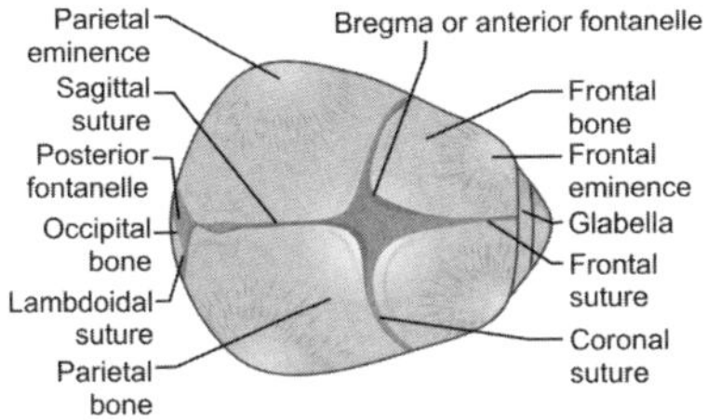

Fetal head at term showing fontanels and sutures

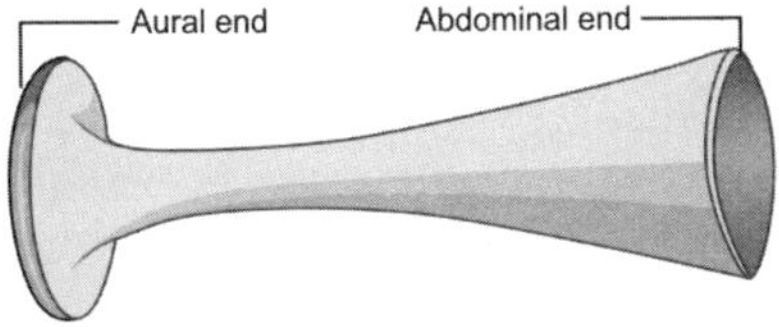

Pinard's fetal stethoscope

antenatal testing, fetal movement counting, non-stress testing, contraction stress testing and clinical assessments

fetoprotein a fetal antigen often present in adults. Amniotic fluid fetoprotein level can indicate about fetal wellbeing and maturity. Level is increased in defects of neuroaxis. Increased levels in adults indicates hepatoma

fetoscope a flexible optical device of fiberoptic material used for direct visualization of fetus in utero

fetotoxic materials toxic to developing fetus, e.g. alcohol sedatives, tetracycline, tobacco

fetus child in utero from third month to birth

fever elevation of body temperature above 37º (98.6ºF). Rectal temperature is 0.5 to 1ºF higher than oral temperature. Body calorie expenditure is increased by 12% for each 0ºC of fever

fiber a thread-like structure. ***f. dietary*** the portion of undigested food stuff giving bulk to stool and preventing constipation. High fiber diet is good for diabetes and prevents colon cancer

fibrillation spontaneous contraction of individual muscle fibers

fibrinogen a coagulation protein of plasma that is precursor of fibrin

fibrinolysis dissolution of fibrin

fibrin whitish filamentous protein formed by action of thrombin on fibrinogen. Fibrin entangles RBC and platelets to produce the clotting

F

fibrocartilage a type of cartilage in which the matrix contains thick bundles of white or cartilaginous fibers, found in the intervertebral discs

fibrocystic disease of pancreas fibroid cystic fibrosis

fibroid fibromyoma of uterus which may grow inwards or outwards to become subperitoneal

fibroma encapsulated, irregular, firm, slow growing connective tissue tumor. Can arise within muscle, breast, uterus (cause menorrhagia)

fibromatosis simultaneous development of multiple fibromas

fibromyositis inflammation of muscle and surrounding connective tissue; a nonspecific illness characterized by pain, tenderness and stiffness of joint capsule

fibromyxoma a fibroma that has undergone partial myxomatous degeneration

fibronectin a group of proteins whose presence in cervical secretion may act as marker for preterm labor

fibroplasias the formation of fibrous tissue as in healing of a wound. ***f. retrolental*** a condition characterized by retinal vascular proliferation and turtuosity and presence of fibrous tissue behind lens leading to detachment of retina

fibrosis abnormal fibrous tissue formation

fibula the outer and smaller bone of leg, often sacrificed in bone grafting

filariasis a chronic disease due to Filaria species

fimbria finger-like projections as that of fallopian tube

fine motor skills skills pertaining to synergy of small muscles of hand

fingerprint an imprint made by the cutaneous ridges of fingers, used for the purpose of identification

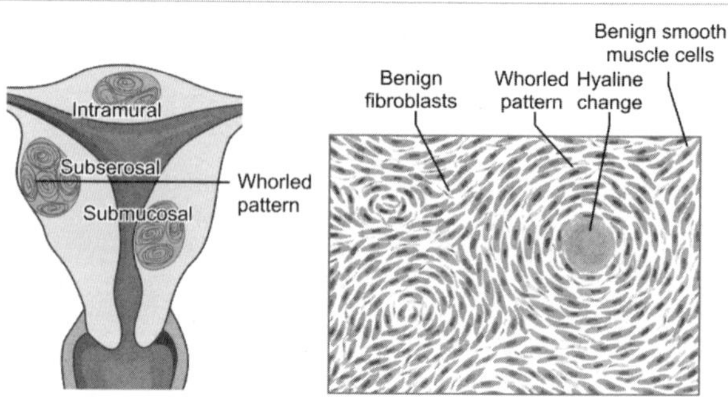

Fibroid

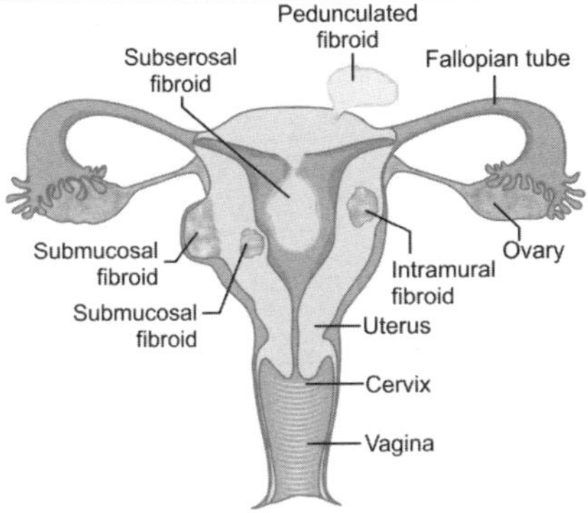

Uterine fibroids

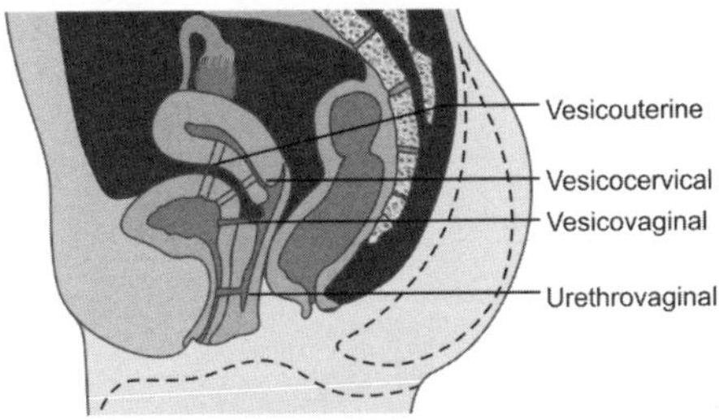

Types of genitourinary fistula

first aid emergency assistance to injured/sick individuals prior to physician's care or transportation to hospital. Common situations necessitating first aid are: foreign body, coma, convulsion, burn poisoning, etc.

fission splitting into two or more parts, a method of a sexual reproduction in bacteria, protozoa and other lower forms of life

fissure a groove or natural division, cleft or slit, break in enamel of tooth, crack like sore, deep furrow in an organ like brain, liver, spinal cord

fistula an abnormal free passage from cavity/or inner organ to exterior/ another organ

flaccid paralysis with loss of muscle tone, reduction or loss of tendon reflexes, atrophy of muscles, usually due to lesion of lower motor neuron

flagellum a hair-like motile process on a protozoon

F

flail chest a condition arising from fracture of a number of ribs, at many points, resulting in the flail rib segment moving in paradoxically with inspiration and out with expiration

flail joint joint with excessive mobility due to paralysis of acting muscles

flat foot an abnormal flatness of sole and loss of arch on inner side of foot

flat pelvis a pelvic in which AP diameter is much shorter than transverse diameter, e.g. platypelloid and rachitic pelvis

flatulence excessive formation or passage of gas from GI tract

flatus expulsion of gas from anus. Average person excretes 400–1200 cc of gas everyday, containing hydrogen, methane, skatoles, indoles, carbon dioxide, small amounts of oxygen and nitrogen. Flatulogenic foods are milk, legumes, fried items

flatus tube a rectal tube which is pushed to facilitate expulsion of gas

flexion the act of bending forward

floss to use dental floss or tape to remove plaque or calculus

fluconazole an antifungal, used in vaginal candidiasis

fluid amniotic yellowish fluid of specific gravity 1.006 composed of albumin, urea, water mixed with lanugo, epidermal cells, vernix casceosa, and meconium

fluid cerebrospinal fluid found in central canal of spinal cord, in the ventricles of brain and in the subarachnoid space

fluid synovial fluid contained within synovial cavities, bursae and tendon sheaths

flumazenil benzodiazepine receptor antagonist; antagonizes actions of benzodiazepines on the central nervous system; used in reversal of sedative effects of benzodiazepines

flunarizine calcium channel-blocker for migraine

fluorescence property of certain substances to emit light when exposed to ultraviolet radiation

fluorescent treponemal antibody test (FTABS) test for syphilis using fluorescent antibody

fluorosis chronic fluorine poisoning causing mottling of tooth enamel, and hyperlucency of bone

folinic acid the active form of folic acid

follicle a small secretory sac or cavity

follicle stimulating hormone hormone of anterior pituitary stimulating spermatogenesis in male and maturation of Graffian follicle in female

follow-up the continued care or monitoring of a patient after the initial visit or examination

fomentation a hot, wet application for relief of pain or inflammation

fomite objects that transmit infectious organisms by contamination

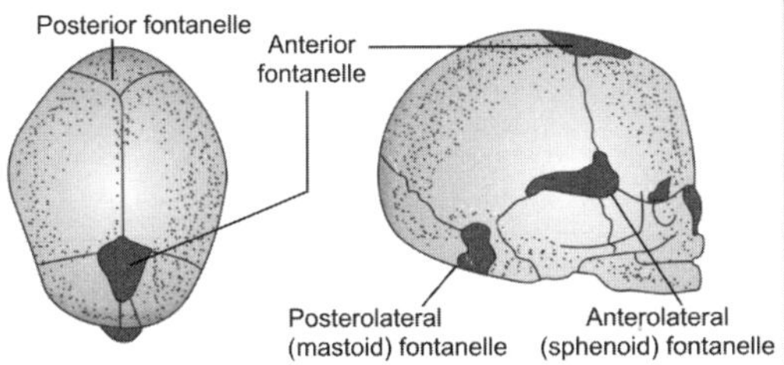

Fontanels

fontanel unossified space lying between cranial bones of the skull

food allergies allergic reactions resulting from ingestion of food to which one has become sensitized. Common offenders are milk, egg, shellfish, chocolate, oranges, etc.

food and drug administration (FDA) in USA, an official regulatory for food, drugs, cosmetics and medical devices; a part of Department of Health and Human Services

food poisoning illness resulting from ingestion of foods containing poisonous substances, e.g. mushroom poisoning, insecticides contaminating food, milk from cows that have eaten some poisonous plants, ingestion of putrefied or decomposed food

food requirement requirement of calorie and protein depending upon age, muscular work and environment. Average active healthy (70 kg) man requires 2700 cal/day and average healthy woman 2000 cal/day. Persons in sedentary work require less calories. Protein requirement of adult is 1 gm/kg, of their ideal weight. Pregnancy and lactation demand 15–25% extra calories. In growing children, protein requirement is 2–3 g/kg/day

foot terminal portion of lower extremity

foot drop plantar flexion of foot due to paralysis of muscles in anterior compartment of leg (lateral popliteal palsy)

footling presentation a type of breech presentation where feet lie in advance of buttocks

foramen a passage, opening, an orifice, a communication between two cavities. ***f. ovale*** the septal opening between the atria of the fetal heart that closes soon after birth

forceps pincers for holding/extracting. ***f. obstetrics*** forceps used to extract the fetal head from pelvis

foreskin the prepuce, i.e. skin covering glans penis

forewater the liqour amni contained in membranes below the presenting part of fetus

fornix anything of arched or vault-like shape

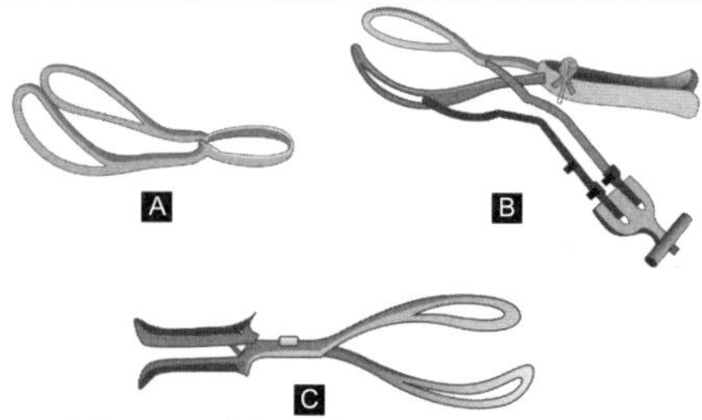

Different types of obstetric forceps: (A) Short-curved forceps; (B) Axis traction forceps; (C) Kielland's forceps

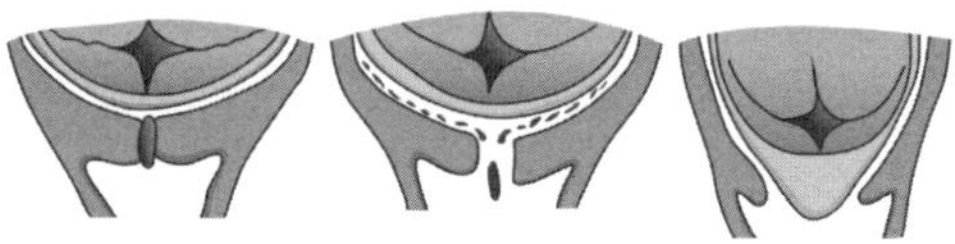

Formation of bag of membranes and forewaters

Fothergill's operation operation for uterine prolapse

fourchette transverse band of mucous membrane at the posterior commissure of vagina

four Ps the four forces of labor including passage, passenger, power and psyche

Fowler' position semisitting position with angulation of upper portion of body at 45–60°, knees may or may not be bent

fracture dissolution in continuity of bone

freckle small brownish or yellowish pigmentation of skin free radical

frenulum linguae a fold of mucous membrane that extends from floor of mouth to the inferior surface of tongue along midline

friable easily breakable

Friedman test one of the biological tests of pregnancy

frigid cold irresponsive to emotions or lack of sexual desire in women

frigidity partial or complete inhibition of sexual excitement

frontal lobe 4 main convolutions infront of central sulcus of cerebrum

frontal plane plain parallel with the long axis of body and at right angles to the median sagittal plane

frontal sinus a pair of hollow assymetrical spaces in the frontal bone above the orbits, filled with air and lined by mucous membrane

frost bite freezing and death of a body part due to cold exposure

fructose $C_6H_{12}O_6$ fruit sugar monosaccharide akin to glucose

fugue a dissociative disorder in which a person acts in normal manner but has complete amnesia for that period of action

fulguration destruction of tissue by high frequency electric sparks

full-term in obstetric child born between 38–41 weeks of gestation

fulminating violently explosive, a disease very severe and sudden

fumigation use of poisonous gases for destroying living organisms like rats, mice, etc. root disinfection

fundal height height of the fundus of the uterus, which is measured in centimeters from the top of the symphysis pubis to the top of the uterus. It is used to assess growth and development of fetus during pregnancy

fundal pertaining to uterine fundus

fundoplication surgical reduction in size of opening into fundus of stomach, used in treating reflux esophagitis

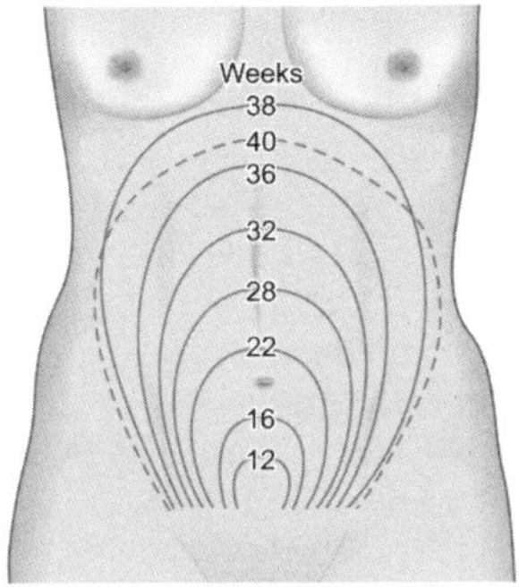

Fundal height

fungus plant-like organism including yeasts and molds but without chlorophil, hence of having parasitic or saprophytic existence

funnel chest sternal depression resembling funnel

funnel pelvis a pelvis that narrows from above downwards, characteristic of android pelvis

furosemide loop diuretic, kaliuretic

furunculosis condition resulting from boil

furunculosis condition resulting from boil

fusion Meeting and joining together

G

GABA gamma aminobutyric acid, a neurotransmitter

gabapentin an antiepileptic agent

gag (1) an instrument to hold open the jaws. (2) to retch or attempt to vomit. g. reflex. Elevation of soft palate and retching on touching the pharynx or back of tongue

Gairdner head box a box placed over baby's head into which additional oxygen is provided to increase oxygen concentration of inspired air

gait manner of walking

galactagogue agent promoting secretion of milk

galactocele a tumor caused by occlusion of a milk duct; hydrocele containing milk-like fluid

galactorrhea excessive flow of milk; continuation of lactation even without childbirth

galactose $C_6H_{12}O_6$ a monosaccharide, isomer of glucose converted to glycogen in liver

galactosemia an autosomal recessive inborn error of metabolism characterized by inability to convert galactose to glucose due to absence of enzyme galactose-1 phosphate uridyl transferase. Symptoms are diarrhea and vomiting with failure to thrive after birth. Infants urine contains high galactose. Intrauterine diagnosis possible from amniocentesis

galea aponeurotica the tendon of occipitofrontalis forming a layer of scalp

Galen's vein these veins run through the tela choroidae formed by the joining of the terminal and choroidal veins. They form venacerebra magna, that empties into straight sinus

gallbladder pear-shaped sac on under surface of right lobe of liver holding bile and discharging. It into common bile duct through cystic duct during digestion

gallstone concretion formed in the gallbladder or common bile duct, commonest being cholesterol stone. Excess of cholesterol or decreased bile acid concentration in bile help to precipitate cholesterol leading to stone formation

gamete intrafallopian transfer (GIFT) a form of in vitro fertilization where sperm and ovum are placed in Fallopian tube

gamete the reproductive units of male and female

gamma globulin immunoglobulin fraction in plasma containing IgG, IgA, IgD and IgE

gamma rays electromagnetic waves of extremely short wave length emitted by radioactive substances having high tissue penetration

ganglion 1. mass of nerve tissue composed principally of nerve cell bodies lying outside brain and spinal cord 2. cystic tumor developing in a tendon or aponeurosis

gangrene dead devitalized tissue due to cut off of blood supply or overwhelming infection

Gardnerella a genus of gram- negative rod shaped bacteria inhabiting vagina *(G. vaginalis)* producing thin grey vaginal discharge with fishy odor

Gardner's syndrome familial polyposis of colon, an autosomal dominant condition with propensity for development of carcinoma

gargoylism congenital condition characterized by dwarfism, kyphosis, and skeletal abnormalities with mental retardation

gas gangrene gangrene caused by *Clostridium welchii* that produces gas in necrosed tissues. It can involve uterus following criminal abortion

gastrectomy surgical removal of a part or total stomach

gastric analysis analysis of gastric contents to determine quality of secretion, amount of free and combined hydrochloric acid, absence or presence of blood, bile duct, etc.

gastric juice digestive juice of gastric glands containing HCl pepsin, mucin, small amount of inorganic salts, intrinsic factor, pH is 0.9 to 1.5 total acidity being equivalent to 30 mL of 1/10 N HCl

gastric lavage emptying out of stomach contents to relieve hiccup; before anesthesia for fear of aspiration and in intestinal obstruction, removal of ingested poisons

gastric ulcer ulcer in the stomach

gastrin a group of hormones secreted by antral mucosa that circulating via blood stimulate gastric HCl secretion. Gastrins also affect secretory activity of pancreas, small intestine

gastritis inflammation of stomach characterized by epigastric pain, vomiting and dyspepsia. Gastric mucosa may be atrophic or hypertrophic. Dietary indiscretion, excessive indulgence in alcohol, *Campylobacter* are responsible

gastrocolic reflex peristaltic wave in colon induced by entrance of food into stomach

gastroenteritis inflammation of stomach and intestinal tract manifesting with epigastric pain, vomiting, fever and dysentery

gastroenterology the branch of medical science dealing with diseases of digestive tract and related structures like esophagus, liver, gallbladder and pancreas

gastroesophageal reflux reflux of acid contents of stomach into lower esophagus due to obesity, hiatus hernia, anticholinergic use, pregnancy, etc.

gastroschisis congenital opening of the abdominal wall allowing the abdominal organs to protrude

gate theory the hypothesis that painful stimuli can be prevented from reaching higher centers for recognition by stimulation of sensory nerves, a key mechanism explaning acupuncture analgesia

gelatin a protein derivative of collagen, used in X-ray films to suspend silver halide crystals, used in capsule making

G

gene basic unit of heredity lying in chromosomes. Their mutation gives rise to new characters

gene splicing in genetic molecular biology, the substitution of a portion of a DNA is spliced into the DNA of another gene

genetic counseling the application of knowledge of genetics in providing advice to parents to have offsprings free of hereditary disease

genetic engineering the synthesis, modification or repair of genetic DNA by synthetic means

genetics the study of heredity and its variation

gene transfer transfer of gene from one person to another for repair of inherited defect in the recipient

Geneva convention 1864 declaration in Geneva that the sick and wounded victims of war including persons involved in their care like doctors, nurses, ambulance drivers, stretcher bearers are neutral and would not therefore be target of military action

genitalia reproductive organs

genotype the hereditary combination of genes, which makes up a person

gentamicin an antibiotic from fungi of genus Micromonospora

gentian violet a dye derived from coal tar, having anti-infective and antifungal property used as stain in cytology and histology.

genu knee

genus in biology taxonomic division between species and family

German measles *see Rubella*

germ an organism that causes disease

germicidal agent destructive to germs

gestational diabetes mellitus (GDM) glucose or carbohydrate intolerance of variable severity which develops or is discovered during the present pregnancy; the condition subsides at the completion of pregnancy.

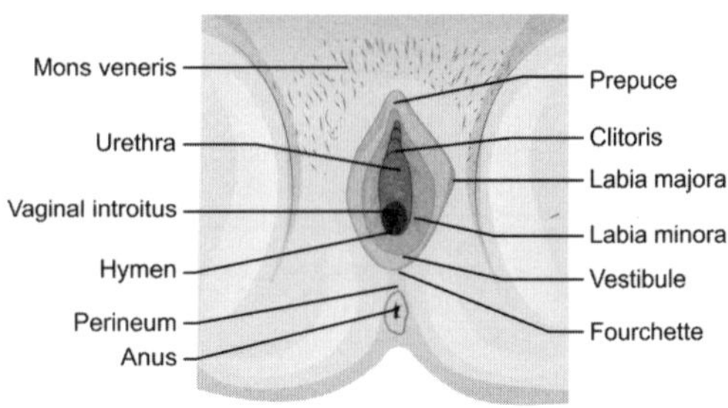

Female external genitalia

gestational period the number of completed weeks of pregnancy calculated from the first day of the last menstrual period

gestation assessment assessment of fetal age and maturity by ultrasound

gestation time span from conception to birth usually 259 to 287 days

gesture a body movement that assists in expression of thoughts (body language)

g. female labia majora/minora, clitoris, fourchette, vestibular gland, Bartholin's gland, vagina, uterus, two Fallopian tubes and two ovaries

Ghon's focus sharply defined peripheral lesion in X-ray chest with hilar lymphadenitis, a feature of primary Kochs

giardia a flagellated protozoa inhabiting intestinal mucosa

gibbus humped back, commonly due to compression fracture, collapse

giddiness light-headed sensation

Giemsa stain a stain for staining blood smears for differential count and detection of parasitic microorganisms

gigantism excessive physical development due to increased growth hormone secretion, late fusion of bones (eunuchoid gigantism)

Gigli's operation pubiotomy or symphysiotomy

Gigli's saw a fine wire instrument for sawing bone

gingivitis inflammation of gums characterized by redness, swelling and tendency to bleed

girdle structure that resembles a circular belt or band

glabella that portion of frontal bone lying between the superciliary arches just above root of nose

gland a secretory organ

glans the head of the clitoris/penis

Glasgow coma scale a scale for evaluating and quantitating the degree of coma by determining the best motor response, verbal and eye opening to standard stimuli. A score of 9 or greater bears better prognosis

glaucoma raised intraocular pressure which can end in blindness. Narrowing of filtration angle, and sclerosis of canal of Schlemm, ocular diseases are responsible

glibenclamide a sulfonylurea for diabetes

globulin simple protein present in blood

glomeruli cluster of capillary vessels enveloped in Bowman's capsule in cortex of kidney

glomus a small round mass made up of tiny blood vessels and found in containing many nerve fibers

glossitis inflammation of tongue; can be acute, painful or chronic, due to infection or avitaminosis (B complex group)

glottis larynx with the two vocal cords and the intervening space, the rime glottides

glucagon polypeptide hormone secreted by alfa cells of pancreas that raises blood sugar and relaxes smooth muscles of GI tract

G

glucocorticoid a class of adrenal hormones that are released in response to stress and effect carbohydrate and protein metabolism

glucose called D-glucose, the primary fuel of human body, in tissue either converted to glycogen, or fat or is oxidized to CO_2 and H_2O

glucose tolerance test a test performed by giving 1.5 g/kg wt of glucose to a patient orally in empty stomach and then examining blood samples every ½ hr for 2 hours. The test helps to assess ability of patient to metabolize glucose and is of primary importance in diagnosis of prediabetic states and hyperinsulinemia

glucosuria abnormal amount of sugar in urine

glucuronyl transferase the liver enzyme that converts toxic fat-soluble bilirubin to water soluble form

glutaraldehyde a sterilizing agent effective against all microorganisms

glutathione a tripeptide of glutamic acid, cystine and glycine, important for cellular respiration

gluten-free diet elimination of gluten from the diet by exclusion of all products prepared from wheat, rye, barley and oats

glycerin $C_3H_8O_3$. a trihydric alcohol present in chemical combination in fats used extensively as a solvent, preservative and emolient

glycerol used as osmotic cathartic in brain edema and as suppository

glyceryl the trivalent radical of glycerol

glycogen polysaccharide; the storage form of carbohydrate in the body (liver and muscle)

glycopyrrolate an anticholinergic drug used in preanesthetic medication to reduce GI and bronchial secretions

glycosuria presence of glucose in the urine resulting from insulin deficiency, reduced renal threshold, excessive glycogenolysis or adrenopituitary disorders

goblet cells a unicellular gland seen in intestinal and respiratory tract, that secretes mucus by rupture of cell wall

goiter an enlargement of thyroid gland

gonad a generic term referring to male and female sex glands (testes and ovary)

gonadal disgenesis congenital disorder with failure of ovaries to respond to pituitary gonadotropin stimulation resulting in amenorrhea, failure of sexual maturation and short stature. Webing of neck, cubitus valgus may be present. Genetic pattern is 45 XO (SYN: Turner's syndrome)

gonadotropin secreted by anterior pituitary as FSH and LH, called interstitial cell stimulating hormone in male (ICSH). ***g. chorionic*** produced by chorionic villi of placenta

gonorrhea contagious inflammation of genital mucous membrane manifesting with burning micturition, painful induration of penis in males, vaginitis and cervicitis in females. Can cause salpingo-oophoritis ending in tubal blockage and sterility in female and chronic prostatitis in male. Can spread to blood to involve principally the joints

Goodel's sign softering of the cervix during pregnancy

gout hereditary metabolic disease of uric acid metabolism with hyperuricemia and arthropathy

Graafian follicle a mature follicle of ovary which on rupture discharges the ovum. Within the ruptured Graafian follicle, the corpus luteum develops

graft transplanted tissue in a part of body for repair of a defect

Gram's stain a staining method for microorganisms dividing them into two broad classes; Gram-positive and Gram-negative

grande multigravida woman in her fourth or subsequent pregnancy

grandiose in psychiatry, urealistic and exaggerated concept of self-worth, importance, ability, power and wealth

grand mal a generalized seizure with loss of consciousness and convulsive limb movements

granular cast coarse or fine granules or casts, sometimes yellowish, soluble in acetic acid, seen in inflammatory and degenerative nephropathies (chronic renal failure)

granulation formation of granules often by outgrowth of capillaries

granuloma a granular tumor or growth of lymphoid and epithelioid cell. It occurs in various infectious disease like leprosy, yaws, syphilis, etc.

granulosa cells the cells lining Graafian follicle, secreting estradiol

granulosa lutein cells granulosa cells after ovulation that secrete estradiol and progesterone

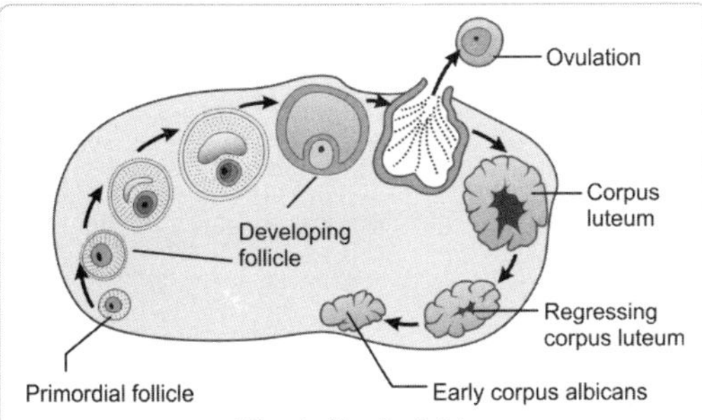

Life cycle of Graafian follicle

G

gravid pregnant

gravidity refers to the total number of a woman's pregnancies regardless of their duration

gravity property of possessing weight, the force of earth's gravitational attraction

gray matter nervous tissue lying peripherally in brain and somewhat centrally in spinal cord where myelinated fibers do not predominate

gray scale display the display of texture of tissue in ultrasound

gray syndrome of newborn ashen gray color, vomiting, cyanosis and flaccidity of newborn when treated with chloramphenicol

griseofulvin an antifungal antibiotic given orally

groin inguinal region, area between thigh and trunk

growth hormone anterior pituitary secretion that regulates human growth; SYN: somatotropin

grunting audible sound made by the newborn on expiration often indicating respiratory distress

gumma encapsulated granulomatous tumor with central necorsis, characteristic of tertiary syphilis seen in skin, liver, testis, brain and bone

gum the fleshy tissue covering the alveolar process of jaw

Guthrie test a blood test for diagnosis of phenylketonuria often done on breast fed babies between 6 to 14 days

gut the bowel or intestine

gynandroid hermaphrodite

gynandromorphism mosaic of male and female sexual characteristics

gynecoid resembling female

gynecology the study of disease of female reproductive organs including breast

gynecomastia abnormally large mammary tissue in male (<2.5 cm in dm) often secreting milk

gyri the raised convolutions of brain surface

habit a motor pattern following frequent repetition or an involuntary act that comes as a reflex action

hair a thin keratinized and cornified structure arising from hair follicle, the shaft of hair has 3 layers, the outer cortex containing the pigment melanin. Hair of eyebrow has life of 3 to 5 months and that of head 2 to 5 years with continuous turnover

hairy tongue tongue covered with hair like papilla with threads of *Aspergillus* or *Candida*

halcinonide a corticosteroid

half life 1. time required for radioactive substance to reduce to one-half its energy due to metabolism or excretion 2. time required for radioactive nuclei undergoing decay to lose half their radioactivity 3. time taken by body to inactivate half of the administered drug/chemical (biological half life)

hallucination a sense of false perception

haloperidol antipsychotic agent used in schizophrenia

halothane fluorinated hydrocarbon used as general anesthetic

Halsted's operation an operation for inguinal hernia; operation for breast cancer

Halsted's suture interrupted suture for intestinal wounds

hamartoma disorganized self-limited, benign growth of normal tissue, when occurring in blood vessels called hemangioma, common to lungs and kidneys

handicap a disadvantage resulting from impairment or disability that prevents fulfillment of the role

hand presentation hand may present in transverse/oblique lie or in compound presentation

hangover headache, depression, fatigue and irritability present sometimes after consumption of alcohol or CNS depressant haploid

hapten that portion of an antigen determining its immunological specificity

haptoglobin mucorprotein accepting hemoglobin in plasma on release in hemolytic conditions. Hence haptoglobin is decreased in hemolytic disorders and increased in certain inflammatory conditions

Hartmann's solution a solution of 0.6 gram NaCl, and 0.31 gram sodium lactate in 100 mL of water used for fluid and electrolyte replacement

hashish an extract from flower, stalk and leaves of *Cannabis sativa*, smoked or chewed for its euphoric effect

hay fever allergic rhinitis usually caused by airborne pollens, fungal spores

headache acute or chronic pain over the skull not confined to any nerve distribution

head circumference the circumference is 33 cm for a well-flexed head and 35 cm for deflexed head

heaf test a form of tuberculin testing

healing restoration to normal mental or physical state

H

health a state of complete mental, physical and social wellbeing, not being mere absence of disease or infirmity

health education educational program aimed for improving and maintaining good health

health hazard any substance, condition or circumstances not conducive to good health

hearing aid an apparatus amplifying sound, worn by persons with impaired hearing

heart a hollow muscular 4-chambered contractile pump in the chest cavity, the principal organ of circulating system

heartburn retrosternal pain due to acid peptic disease

heart lung machine a machine that takes over functions of heart and lung during open cardiac surgery

Hegar's dilators a type of cervical dilator

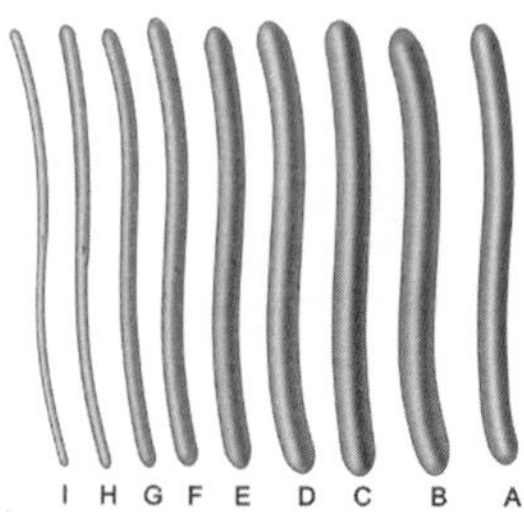

Hegar's dilators

Hegar's sign softening of lower part of uterus in early pregnancy allowing fingers to meet in bimanual examination, a test of early pregnancy

Hellin's law 1 in 89 birth is twins, 1 in 892 birth is triplet and 1 in 893 birth is quadruplets

HELLP syndrome a complication of pregnancy characterized by hemolysis, raised liver enzymes and low platelet

helminthiasis an infestation with worms

hemangioma 1. a benign neoplasm characterized by blood vascular channels. A cavernous hemangioma consists of large vascular spaces. A capillary hemangioma consists of many small blood vessels. 2. a benign tumor composed of newly formed blood vessels

hematemesis vomiting of blood

hematochezia passage of bloody stool

hematocrit (Packed-cell volume) 1. the percentage of the total blood volume composed of red blood cells (erythrocytes). Normal values are 42 to 45%. (2) The percentage of the total volume of a blood sample that is taken up by the red blood cells. Normal values: children, 32 to 65%; adult men, 42 to 53%, adult women 38 to 46%

hematology the scientific study of blood and blood-forming tissues. ***h. tests*** diagnostic tests of the blood and its constituent parts

hematoma a mass of blood in the tissue as a result of trauma or other factors that cause the rupture of blood vessels. ***h. subdural*** a collection of extravasated blood trapped below the dural membranes of the brain causing pressure on the brain, resulting in pain and neural dysfunction. Subdural hematomas may be life- threatening

hematometra accumulation of blood in uterus

hematuria blood in the urine. ***h. gross*** visible evidence of blood in the urine. It may occur from neoplasms of the kidney and bladder, hemorrhagic diathesis, hypertension with renal epistaxis, or acute glomerular nephritis. ***h. microscopic*** the demonstration of hematuria during the microscopic examination of centrifuged urine. It may result from the same causes as gross hematuria or from toxicity of drugs, embolic glomerulitis, vascular diseases, or chronic glomerular nephritis

heme the pigmented, iron containing, nonprotein portion of the hemoglobin molecule

hemiplegia paralysis of one half of body

hemisphere either half of the cerebrum or cerebellum

hemoconcentration an increase in the number of red blood cells resulting from a decrease in the volume of plasma.

hemodialysis a method of removing poisonous substances, urea creatinine, etc. from plasma by passing the patient's blood across semipermeable membr-anes, SYN: hemoperfusion

hemodynamics study of blood circulation

hemoglobin the iron containing protoporphyrin IX, responsible for carriage of oxygen from lungs to tissues

hemolytic anemia anemia resulting from hemolysis of red blood cells

hemolytic disease of newborn ABO or Rh incompatibility resulting in hemolysis, anemia, jaundice, edema and hepatic enlargement

hemolytic uremic syndrome characterized by microangiopathic hemolytic anemia, acute nephropathy and thrombocytopenia in children usually preceded by upper respiratory illness or GI upset

hemophilia a sex-linked hereditary disorder of coagulation with prolonged clotting time, repeated hemarthrosis and bleeding from nose or after trivial trauma. There is deficiency of factor VIII

hemorrhage bleeding either external or internal. ***h. antepatrtum*** bleeding after 28 weeks of gestation and before onset of labor. ***h. accidental*** retroplacental bleeding. ***h. postpartum*** bleeding in excess of 500 mL after child birth

hemorrhagic disease of newborn bleeding from nose, umbilical stump in newborn due to inadequate prothrombin synthesis (premature fetal liver/ poor bacterial flora)

hemorrhoid dilated tortuous veins in the anorectal region

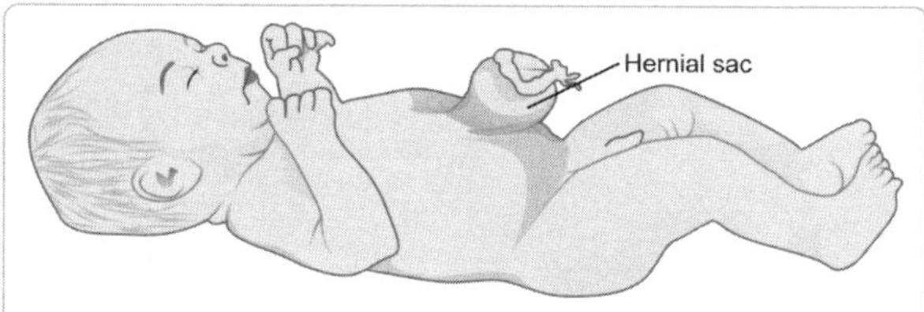

Umbilical hernia

hemosalpinx bleeding into Fallopian tube

heparin a polysaccharide produced by mast cells of liver and basophils, inhibits conversion of prothrombin to thrombin

hepatic coma impaired CNS function due to liver dysfunction. Coma results from increased serum ammonia, false neurotransmitters and middle molecules, the toxic products of protein metabolism. Common precipitating factors are high protein diet, bleeding into GI tract (varices), infections, electrolyte imbalance, diuretics and drugs. Mousy odor, flapping tremor and EEG changes are characteristic

hepatitis B vaccine a recombinant vaccine with hepatitis B surface antigen given as 20 μg dose—3 doses, to persons at high risk

hepatitis inflammation of liver, causative agents include viruses (hepatitis A, B, C delta agent) bacteria, alcohol, drugs and autoimmune disease. Common symptoms and signs are nausea, vomiting jaundice, fever and hepatomegaly

hepatoma a primary malignant tumor of liver

hepatomegaly an enlargement of liver, may be upward or downward, commonly due to alcohol, hepatitis, amebiasis, congestive failure, infectious fevers, etc.

hereditary genetic characteristic transmitted from parent to offspring

hernia protrusion of an organ or part of it through a defect in the wall surrounding it

heroin an extract of morphine with strong analgesic and addictive potential. Acute intoxication produces euphoria, respiratory depression, hypotension and hypothemia

herpes vesiculated eruptions caused by herpes virus

heterogenous composed of different kinds of substances

heterologous 1. composed of tissue not normal to the part. 2. tissue cell or blood obtained from a different individual/ species

heterosexual one whose sexual orientation is to members of opposite sex

heterozygote an individual with different alleles for a given characteristic

hexachlorophene polychlorinated phenol, antiseptic disinfectant

Hick's sign Intermittent painless uterine contraction occurring after third month of pregnancy

high blood pressure blood pressure above the normal range of age. Usually 140/90 mm Hg if below 50 years and above 160/90 if above 60 years

hindwater in labor, the amniotic fluid is divided into fore and hindwaters. Fore-water is ahead of descending part and hind-water surrounds body

hippocrates Greek physician who first established the scientific basis of medical practice, hence known as father of medicine

Hippocratic oath the oath hippocrates exacted from his students which reads like "I will follow that system of regimen which, according to my ability and judgement, I consider for the benefit of my patients, and abstain from whatever is deleterious and mischiveous. I will give no deadly medicine to any one if asked nor suggest any such counsel, and in like manner I will not give to a woman a pessary for abortion. With purity and holiness I will pass my life and practice my art, into whatever houses I enter, I will go into them for the benefit of the sick, and I will abstain from every voluntary act of mischief and corruption, and further from seduction of females or males, of freemen and slaves. Whatever in connection with my professional practice, or not in connection with it, I see or hear in the life of men, which ought not to be spoken of abroad, I will not divulge, as reckoning that all such should be kept secret. "While I continue to keep this Oath unviolated, may it be granted to me to enjoy life and the practice of this art, respected by all men in all times. But should I trespass and violate this Oath may the reverse be my lot"

Hirschsprung's disease a dynamic megacolon due to failure of development of myenteric plexus in the rectosigmoid area of colon

hirsutism excessive hair growth in women

histamine a derivative of histidine that is secreted by mast cells and is responsible for triple response

histocompatibility the ability of cells to survive without any immunological influence or interference; important in blood transfusion and tissue transplantation

histology study of minute structure, composition of tissue and organs

history taking a detailed synopsis of history including life style, habits, medications, past surgical obstetric complications that help to plan of management for current pregnancy

HIV I human immunodeficiency virus I

HIV II human immunodeficiency virus II

H

HIV wasting syndrome wasting of body, a feature of HIV infection

hoarseness a rough quality of voice due to simple chronic laryngitis, vocal cord palsy or infiltration of vocal cords

Hodge pessary a pessary used to maintain position of uterus after correction of retroversion

Hodgkin's disease a lymphoproliferative disease with painless lymphadenopathy, hepatosplenomegaly, and often relapsing fever. Reed-Sternberg's giant cells in lymphnode biopsy are characteristic

Hogben test a pregnancy test based on injection of pregnant lady's urine to dorsal lymph sac of toad; when gonadotropic hormone is present, the toad ovulates 8 to 15 hours after injection

holistic medicine comprehensive and total care of a patient, taking into account his physical, mental, social economic and spiritual needs

holter monitor an ECG recording system capable of recording ECG for 24 hours, particularly useful for recording arrhythmias, and silent ischemia

Homan's sign pain in the calf on passive dorsiflexion of great toe, an evidence of deep vein thrombosis

homeopathy a system of alternative medicine

homeostasis state of equilibrium of internal environment of the body

homogeneous uniform in structure, composition or nature

homologous having the same structure or pattern

homosexual individual attracted to a person of same sex; female homosexuality is known as lesbianism

homozygous having a pair of similar genes

hookworm the intestinal parasite inhabiting duodenum and jejunum and sucks blood for its nourishment

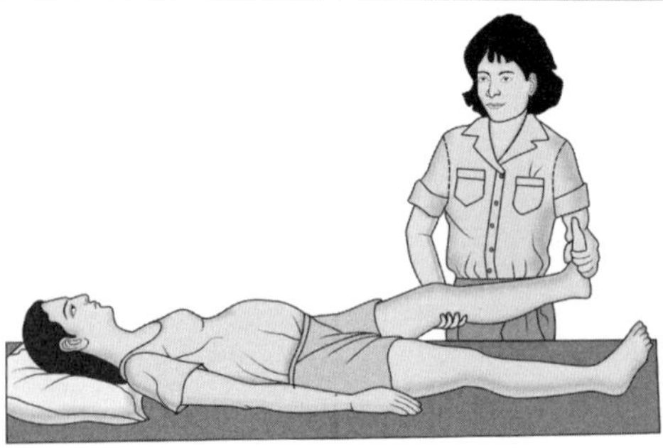

Homan's sign

hormone a chemical substance secreted to bloodstream with specific regulatory action

Horner's syndrome myosis, ptosis, enophthalmos and loss of sweating overaffected side of face due to paralysis of cervical sympathetic trunk

host the organism on which the parasite lives and draws its nourishment

hot water bag a rubber or plastic bag for application of dry heat or keeping moist applications warm

hourglass constriction a constriction ring in uterus occurring during third stage of labor and causes placental retention

human insulin insulin prepared by recombinant DNA technology using *E. coli*

human placental lactogen placental secretion that helps to prepare the breast for milk secretion

humerus bone of upper arm that articulates with scapula above and radius-ulna below

Huntington's disease mucopoly saccharidosis II

Hutchinson's teeth a feature of congenital syphilis in which the lateral incisors are peg-shaped and the central incisors are notched

hyaline it refers to any alteration within cell or in the extracellular space, which gives a homogenous, glassy, pink appearance in histologic sections stained with hematoxylin and eosin

hyaluronic acid an acid mucopolysaccharide forming the ground substance

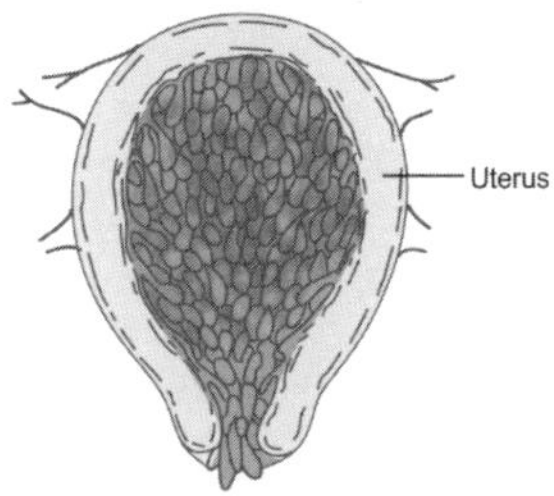

Hydatidiform moles

of connective tissue; functioning as a binding and protective agent

hyaluronidase an enzyme that deploymerizes hyaluronic acid, thereby increases permeability of connective tissues

hydatidiform mole degenerative process of chorionic villi with formation of multiple cysts within uterus

hydralazine antihypertensive acting through vasomotor center in CNS

hydramnios an excess of liquor amnii around the developing fetus

hydrocele fluid accumulation in tunica vaginalis testes or in any sac-like cavity

hydrocephalus increased content of CSF within the ventricles resulting from decreased absorption of CSF, its increased production or blockage to its circulation resulting from developmental anomalies, infection, injury or tumor

hydrochloric acid produced by oxyntic cells of gastric glands, serves to convert pepsinogen into pepsin, dissolves and disintegrates nucleoproteins, precipitates caseinogen, hydrolyzes sucrose, inhibits bacterial multiplication, etc.

hydrocortisone a steroid hormone of adrenal cortex

hydronephrosis collection of fluid in renal pelvic caliceal system usually due to obstruction to urine flow, ultimately causing atrophy of renal parenchyma

hydrophobia morbid fear for water, synonym for rabies in which attempt to drink water causes spasm of pharynx due to CNS irritation

hydrops fetalis severe edema of the fetus due to Rh/ABO incompatibility

hydrosalpinx distended Fallopian tube due to accumulated secretions

hygiene study of methods and means of preserving health

hymen a fold of mucous membrane that partially covers the entrance to vagina

hyoscine scopolamine

hyperacidity excess of acid in stomach

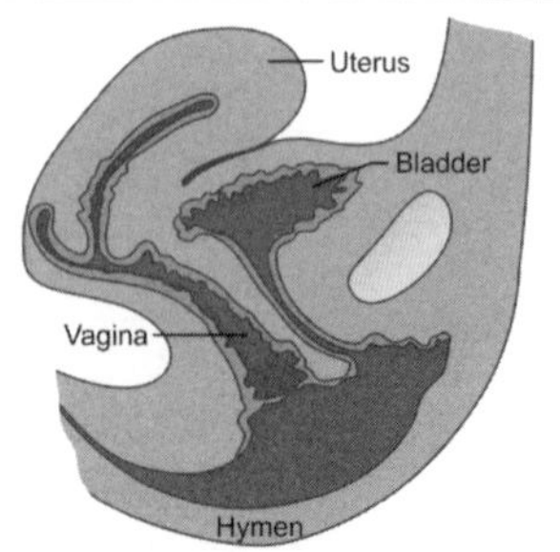

Hymen

hyperbilirubinemia a condition when there is an excessive amount of bilirubin in the blood; excessive levels can lead to brain damage

hypercalcemia excessive amount of calcium in the blood (>12.2 mg%) either idiopathic or secondary to malignancy, prolonged recumbency, vit D intoxication, etc.

hyperemesis gravidarum severe vomiting of early pregnancy due to hydatidiform mole

hyperesthesia increased sensitivity to sensory stimuli especially pain and touch

hyperglycemia accumulation of amino acid glycine in blood manifesting with mental and growth retardation

hyperkalemia serum potassium exceeding 5 mEq/L

hyperlipoproteinemia increased lipoprotein content in blood due to increased synthesis or decreased breakdown

hypermenorrhea abnormal increase in duration or amount of menstrual blood loss

hypernatremia excess sodium content of blood (>150 mEq/L)

hyperplasia excessive growth of normal cells with normal tissue architecture

hyperprolactinemia amenorrhea, galactorrhea produced by increased serum prolactin due to hypothalamic pituitary dysfunction

hyperpyrexia body temperature exceeding 106°F (41.1°C)

hypersplenism enlarged spleen with enhanced removal of blood components from circulation

hypertelorism abnormal width between two paired organs, usually the eyes

hypertension blood pressure considered abnormally high for an age

hyperthermia unusual high fever; a treatment modality by which foreign protein is introduced into body to raise body temperature

hyperthyroidism increased production of thyroid hormones with palpitation weight loss, stare BMR

hypertonic having high osmotic pressure or having greater than normal tension

hypertonic uterus labor contractions lasting longer than 90 seconds, caused by too much stimulation of the uterus

hypertrophy nontumorous enlargement of an organ or structure due to increase in size or number of cells

hyperuricemia increased serum uric acid (8 mg%)

hyperventilation increased rate and depth of inspiration and expiration

hyperviscosity excess adhesiveness or stickiness property of fluid, commonly blood

hypervitaminosis excessive vitamin content of body tissues, commonly involves, fat-soluble vitamins like A, D, E and K; usually secondary to excess ingestion

hypervolemia abnormal increase in volume of circulating blood

hypnotic drugs that cause insensitivity to pain by inducing hypnosis

hypocalcemia decreased plasma calcium manifesting with stridor and tetany

hypocapnea decreased CO_2 tension in blood

hypocarbia decreased CO_2 in blood

hypochlorhydria decreased HCl secretion in stomach often indicative of malignancy of stomach

hypochondriac abnormal and excessive fear of disease

hypochondrium part of the abdomen below the lower ribs

hypochromasia lack of hemoglobin in RBC SYN: hypochromia

hypodermic inserted under the skin

hypogammaglobulinemia decreased gammaglobulin concentration in blood leading to frequent infections; can be congenital or acquired (AIDS)

hypogastrium region below the umbilicus, between the right and left inguinal regions

hypoglycemia decreased blood glucose below 50 mg% manifesting as tremor, sweating, weakness, etc.

hypomagnesemia decreased plasma magnesium with neuromuscular excitability

hypomenorrhea decreased menstrual flow

hyponatremia decreased blood sodium concentration (<130 mEq/L)

H

hypoparathyroidism insufficient parathormone production with hypocalcemia and tetany

hypopituitarism diminished pituitary hormone secretion secondary to pituitary destruction by tumor, infraction, compression resulting in secondary dysfunction of thyroid, adrenal, testis/ovary and growth disturbance in children

hypoplasia underdevelopment of a part or organ

hypospadias abnormal urethral opening, either in the under surface of glans, penile shaft or in perineum

hypostasis diminished blood flow or circulation

hypotension abnormally low blood pressure

hypothalamus the portion of diencephalon comprising the ventral wall of third ventricle and adjacent structures responsible for regulation of body temperature, sugar and releasing and inhibiting hormones. It is the principal center for integration of sympathetic and parasympathetic activities

hypothermia subnormal (below 96ºF) body temperature, induced for open heart surgery and neurological procedures

hypothyroidism deficiency of thyroid hormones causing thick coarse hair, dry, thick inelastic skin, hoarse voice, obesity, depressed muscular activity, slow pulse and hypercholesterolemia. Mental retardation and growth failure may occur in children (cretinism)

hypotonia loss of muscle or arterial tone

hypotonic refers to solutions which are more dilute than physiological saline. ***h. buterus*** weak ineffective uterine contraction causing prolongation of labor

hypotonic labor occurs during the active phase of labor causing ineffectual contractions and a lack of progression of labor

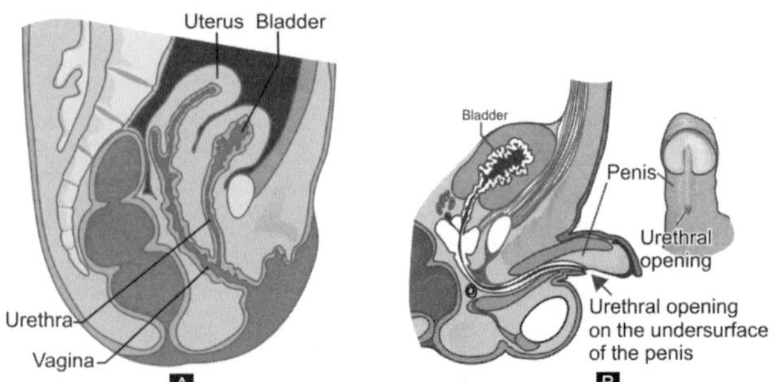

(A) Hypospadias in newborn female; (B) Hypospadias in newborn male

hypovolemia diminished circulating blood volume

hypovolemic pertaining to hypovolemia. ***h. shock*** or hemorrhagic shock can occur following antepartum or postpartum hemorrhage

hypoxemia insufficient oxygen content of blood

hypoxia decreased O_2 concentration in inspired air

hysterectomy *h. supracervical* operation in which only the main body of the uterus is removed, to the level of the internal os, leaving the cervix in place. Also called as subtotal hysterectomy. ***total h*** removal of the entire uterus

hysterectomy surgical removal of uterus either by abdominal or vaginal route. It can be subtotal, total or radical. In radical hysterectomy (Wertheim's operation) uterus, tubes, ovaries, adjacent lymph nodes and part of vagina are removed, usually done in stage I and II cancer cervix

hysteria a conversion disorder in which patient transforms longstanding mental conflict into somatic symptoms. There is no organic disease to account for the symptoms. Patient is amnesic for the period of illness as the primary consciousness reasserts itself

hysterography recording of frequency and intensity of uterine contractions

hysteromyomectomy excision of uterine fibroid

hysterosalpingectomy excision of uterus and tubes

hysterosalpingography X-ray visualization of uterus and the tubes by introduction of contrast media

hysterosalpingostomy anastomosis of uterus with the remaining healthy portion of Fallopian tube after excision of diseased part

hysterotomy incision of uterus as in evacuation of mole, dead fetus or cesarean section

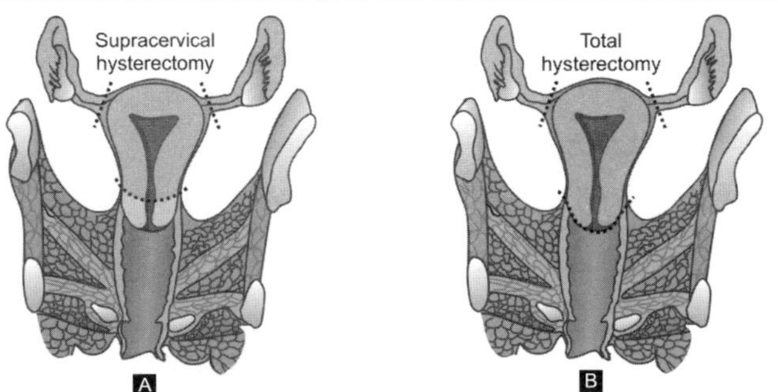

(A) Supracervical hysterectomy; (B) Total hysterectomy

iatrogenic adverse body effect induced by drug, procedure or the doctor

ibuprofen a nonsteroidal anti-inflammatory agent

icebag a watertight bag to hold ice for cold sponging over bruised or sprained area

ichthammol a reddish-brown viscous fluid acting as an antiseptic, often used in ear-dressing and skin applications

ichthyosis condition in which skin is dry, scaly resembling fish skin. Ichthyosis vulgaris is hereditary

icterus pertains to jaundice

identical exactly alike

identity the physical and mental characteristic by which an individual is known and recognized

ideology a philosophy, the science of ideas and thoughts

idiocy severe mental deficiency due to defective mental development, the cause of which may be genetic, vascular or birth asphyxia

idiopathic a disease without recognizable cause

idoxuridine antiviral agent; used for herpes infection of eye in the form of ointment 2%

IgA principally present in exocrine secretions like milk, saliva, intestinal secretions and tear. Hence it protects against mucosal invasion by pathogenic organism. IgE is secreted by mast cells and is responsible for allergy, asthma, eczema, etc. IgG is the principal immunoglobulin and is the major antibody against bacteria, viruses and fungi. IgM is formed during early period of antigenic stimulation or infection

ileocecal valve A muscular ring at the terminal ileum that regulates passage of food from small intestine to large intestine and prevents re-entry of food back into small intestine

ileum lower 3/5 of small intestine from jejunum to ileocecal valve. Average length 15 to 31 feet

ileus a form of intestinal obstruction due to intestinal muscle paralysis, spasm or obstruction in intestinal lumen, e.g. meconium ileus of newborn

iliac crest upper free margin of hip bone or ileum

iliac region inguinal region on either side of hypogastrium

iliac spine one of the four spines of ilium namely the anterior and posterior inferior spines, and the anterior and posterior superior spines

ilium the upper broad part of innominate bone

illusion inaccurate perception, misinterpretation of sensory impressions; when an illusion becomes fixed, it is called delusion

imaging production of image of an object by X-ray, ultrasound, magnetic resonance, etc.

imatinib anticancer agent for chronic myelogenous leukemia (CML)

imbalance loss of balance usually between opposing body forces

imipramine a tricyclic antidepressant, also used in migraine and enuresis

immature not fully developed or mature

immune protected from or resistant to disease due to development of antibodies

immune system a biochemical complex that protects the body against pathogenic organisms and other foreign bodies. The system incorporates the humoral immune response, which produces antibodies to react with specific antigents, and the cell-mediated response, which uses T cells to mobilize tissue macrophages in the presence of a foreign body. The immune system also protects the body from invasion by creating local barriers and inflammation. The principal organs of the immune response system include the bone marrow, the thymus, and the lymphoid tissues

immunity state of being protected against disease either by previous infection or by vaccine. ***i. acquired*** immunity due to active or passive immunization. ***i. cell-mediated*** the T cells interact with antigen with a delayed response as seen in graft rejection or infection with tuberculosis, leprosy. ***i. natural*** immunity conferred by natural inherent factors like race, species. ***i. passive immunity*** due to transplacental transfer of maternal antibodies, antibodies secreted in milk or injection of hyperimmune specific sera

immunization the process of rendering a person immune by active (toxoid, inactivated, killed organisms) or passive process

immunoassay assay of concentration of a substance by using the reaction of an antigen with specific antibody

immunoglobulin proteins capable of acting with antigens; can be IgG, IgA, IgE, IgD and IgM

immunological pregnancy test test based on hCG in urine hCG antibodies are added to urine so also latex particles covered with hCG. In absence of pregnancy, there will be agglutination

immunology study of immunity to disease

immunosuppressant agent suppressing body immune response, usually employed in treatment of autoimmune diseases

impaction condition of being tightly wedged into a part, e.g. tooth impaction, impaction of feces in bowel

impairment any loss or abnormality of psychological, physiological or anatomical structure or function

imperforate without an opening. In imperforate hymen, the menstrual blood accumulates behind to cause hematocolpus. In imperforate anus, the infant has absolute constipation

impetigo inflammatory skin disease marked by formation of pustules which rupture with crust formation, may occur in crops, are contagious. ***i. herpetiformis*** a rare pustular eruption of unknown etiology that occurs especially during pregnancy and in association with hypocalcemia

implant introduction into body tissues, drugs or prosthesis, e.g. knee implant, drug implant

impotency inability of male to achieve erection, can be anatomic (defect in the genitalia), atonic (paralysis of nervi erigentis), functional or vasculogenic

impregnate saturate, to make pregnant

impulsion idea to do something or commit some act suddenly imposed upon the subject that tortures him until the accomplishment of that act

inborn error of metabolism a hereditary disease caused by deficiency of a specific enzyme

incarcerated confined, constricted, constriction as in hernia, incarceration of retroverted gravid uterus—the uterus is imprisoned under sacral promontory

incest coitus between close relatives

incidence the frequency of occurrence of any event or condition over a period of time in a specified population

incidental hemorrhage bleeding from vagina due to extraplacental causes like cervical polyp, erosion, vaginitis, etc.

incise to cut, as with a sharp instrument

incompatible not being in harmony

incompetence inadequacy in function of a part or organ or commonly a valve (ileocecal, mitral, aortic, pulmonary, venous, etc.)

incompetent cervix a condition in which the cervix dilates prematurely, causing a spontaneous abortion or preterm delivery

incomplete abortion abortion in which placenta is retained

incontinence inability to retain urine, feces because of sphincter laxity

incontinence stress (urinary) leaking of urine during coughing, sneezing, laughing, lifting, etc.

incoordination inability to produce harmonious, rhythmic muscular movement

incubation interval between exposure to an infection and appearance of first symptoms; in bacteriology period of culture

incubator 1. enclosed crib in which temperature and humidity are controlled for nursing premature babies 2. apparatus for maintaining bacterial culture

indigenous native to a country or region

indigestion imperfect digestion manifesting as nausea, vomiting, heart burn, belching, etc.

indomethacin antiprostaglandin agent with anti-inflammatory, analgesic and antipyretic properties

induction the process of facilitating labor with oxytoxic drugs

inertia 1. sluggishness, lack of activity 2. in physics, tendency of body to remain in its state uptil acted upon by external force. ***i. uterine*** absence of uterine contractions

inevitable that which cannot be avoided ***i. abortion*** abortion is sure to occur and unavoidable

infant from time of birth to one year of age. ***i. preterm*** born prior to 37 weeks of gestation. ***i. post-term*** born after 42 weeks of gestation. ***i. term*** born between 38 to 41 weeks of gestation

infanticide killing of an infant

infant mortality rate the number of death of infants below 1 year of age for every 1000 live births registered in a given year

infarct area of necrosis consequent to cessation of blood supply

infection tissue invasion with pathogenic agent that produces injurious effect. ***i. acute*** infection appearing suddenly. ***i. chronic*** infection having protracted course. ***i. concurrent*** existence of two or more infections at the same time. ***i. cross*** transfer of one disease from one hospitalized patient to another. ***i. droplet*** infection acquired through microorganisms disbursed to air via breath or nasobronchial secretion. ***i. pyogenic*** infection by pusforming organisms. ***i. lowgrade*** mild inflammation without pus formation

infectious disease disease caused by an infecting agent, not necessarily contagious

infertility inability to conceive. ***i. primary*** not conceived in past. ***i. secondary*** had conceived but aborted

infiltration the process of passing into or through a substance or space

inflammation tissue reaction to injury with vasodilatation, exudation, leukocyte migration followed by healing. ***i. acute*** rapid onset and short course. ***i. catarrhal*** inflammation of mucous membrane with excessive mucous secretion. ***i. exudative*** inflammation with extreme vasodilatation, and large accumulation of blood cells. ***i. granulomatous*** inflammation with excessive granular tissue production as in tuberculosis, syphilis and systemic fungal infections

influenza a viral acute contagious upper respiratory infection

influenza virus vaccine vaccine containing inactivated influenza virus A and B; given every year with different strains of A and B

infrared rays invisible heat rays beyond the red end of spectrum, of 7500 to 150,000 AU used for local application of heat and pain relief

infundibulum 1. funnel-shaped passage or structure. 2. tube connecting the frontal sinus with middle nasal meatus. 3. stalk of pituitary gland. 4. peritoneal end of Fallopian tube. 5. upper end of cochlear canal

infusion liquid substance introduced into body vein

ingestion intake of food or the process by which cells take foreign particles

inguinal canal the canal ½" long, providing passage for spermatic cord in the male and round ligament of uterus in the female. A potential source of weakness; may serve as site of inguinal hernia and undescended testis

inguinal ring interior and exterior openings of inguinal canal, termed as internal and external inguinal rings

inhalation the act of drawing in the breath, vapor or gas into the lungs

inhaler device for administering medicines by inhalation

inheritance something hereditary, acquired through eggs and sperms

inhibition 1. restraint of a function. 2. in physiology slowing or stopping the function of an organ. ***i. competitive*** inhibition by competing with cell receptors. ***i. psychic*** arrest of an impulse, thought, action or speech

iniencephalus congenitally deformed fetus in which brain substance protrudes through a fissure in the occiput

injection forcing a fluid into body via vessel or skin. ***i. epidural*** injection of anesthetic agent into epidural - space. ***i. hypodermic*** injection of substance beneath the skin. ***i. alveolar*** dental infiltration of anesthetic agent. ***i. intramuscular*** injection directly into muscles, e.g. thigh, deltoid, glutei. ***i. intra-articular*** injection into joint space. ***i. z. track*** an injection technique, the needle taking a Z track to make the injected fluid difficult to track back (see Figure)

inlet pelvic the barrier the entrance to the true pelvis

innate something natural, belonging from birth

inner cell mass the group of cells in the cavity of blastocyst from which the amniotic membrane and fetus develop

innervation nerve supply, distribution and function of nervous system. ***i. collateral*** outgrowth of nerves from adjacent nerves, once the original nerve supply is damaged. ***i. reciprocal*** an innervation mechanism by which if flexors are stimulated, the extensors are inhibited

innominate bone the hip bone composed of ilium, ischium and pubis

innominate nameless

inoculate to inject microorganism, serum or toxic materials into body

inoculation the process of being inoculated

inquest investigation into cir-cumstances, manner and cause of health

insanitary not conducive to health

insemination fertilization of ovum, semen discharge into vagina during coitus

insertion 1. placement or implanting of something into another. 2. distal end of muscle attachment through which it moves a part

insidious used to denote the onset of a disease so silently without patient's awareness

insomnia lack of sleep

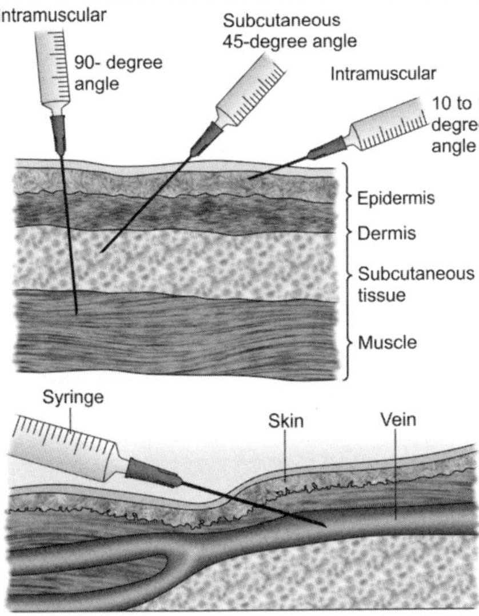

Intramuscular, subcutaneous, intradermal and intravenous injections

inspection visual examination

inspiration sprinkling with powder or a fluid

instillation slowly pouring or dropping a liquid into body cavity

insufficiency inadequacy of function. ***i. adrenal*** decreased adrenal function. ***i. aortic***. imperfect closure of aortic leaflets with back flow. ***i. cardiac*** poor cardiac pump function. ***i. coronary***. diminished blood flow through coronary vessels. ***i. hepatic*** hepatic insufficiency with cholemia. ***i. mitral*** inefficient mitral valve closure with backflow of blood into left atrium during ventricular systole. ***i. respiratory*** hypoxemia and hypercarbia due to poor pulmonary function

insufflate the act of blowing into or pumping air into a cavity/lung as in infants

insulin Hormone secreted by the beta cells of islets of Langer-hans of pancreas. ***i. human*** synthesized by recombinant DNA technology using *E. coli*. ***i. monocomponent*** highly purified insulin containing impurity 10 parts per million. ***i. isophane*** (NPH) intermediate acting insulin with 18 to 28 hours of action

insulin pump a battery driven pump delivering insulin subcutaneously into abdominal wall according to preset program

insulin shock hypoglycemic shock due to overdose of insulin

interaction the process of two or more things acting on each other

intercourse sexual union; social interaction between individuals or groups

intercurrent intervening

intermission interval between two paroxysm of disease

intermittent fever fever in which there is complete absence of symptoms between paroxysms

intermittent positive pressure breathing, assisted breathing in patients of respiratory failure, myasthenia gravis

internal injury any injury not visible from outside

internal os the opening through which cervical canal communicates with body of uterus

internal version usually internal podalic version that aims at converting oblique lie longitudinal

intersex a person having both male and female sex characteristics but genetically either male or female

intertrigo superficial dermatitis of the skin folds

interval space, time or period between two objects or happenings. ***i. AV*** interval between beginning of atrial systole and ventricular systole. ***i. cardioarterial*** time between apex beat and radial pulse. ***i. isometric*** time between onset of ventricular systole and opening of semilunar (aortic-pulmonary) valves. ***i. lucid*** brief remission of symptoms in head injury and psychosis. ***i. PR*** period between onset of P wave and beginning of QRS complex. Normal-less than 0.2 sec. ***i. QR*** period between onset of Q wave and peak of R wave. ***i. QRS*** QRS duration from beginning of Q wave to end of S wave. Normal 0.12 sec. ***i. QT*** interval between beginning of Q wave and end of T wave

intestine the alimentary canal extending from pylorus to anus. The small intestine is 7 meter long and the large intestine 1.5 meter. Cecum is the beginning of large intestine and appendix (3-4" long) is attached to it. The duodenum is 8 to 10" long; jejunum 9 feet and ileum 14 feet. In the wall of the small intestine are Brunners glands, crypts of Lieberkuhn and Peyer's patches

intracellular within a cell, ***i. organism*** those organisms that invade cell, e.g. *Gonococcus*. ***i fluid*** the fluid within cell

intracranial within the cranium. ***i. pressure*** the pressure exerted by CSF with subarachnoid space and ventricles of the brain

intragasrtric balloon placement of inflatable balloon in stomach to treat obesity

intrapartum occuring during childbirth

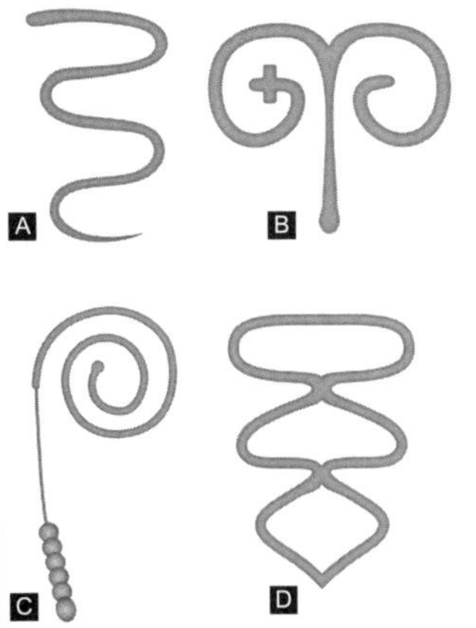

First generation IUDs: (A) Lippes loop; (B) Safe T-coil; (C) Margulies spiral; (D) Dana supers

intraperitoneal within peritoneal cavity. ***i. transfusion*** introduction of Rh negative blood into peritoneal cavity of Rh positive fetus

intrauterine contraceptive device copper or other metalic device placed within uterus to prevent conception

intrauterine within the uterus

intravenous infusion injection of colloid or crystalloid solutions into a vein to treat hypovolemia or maintenance

intraventricular hemorrhage cerebral hemorrhage in a preterm baby

intrinsic factor substance present in the gastric juice that facilitates absorption of vit B12

introitus entrance into a canal or cavity

intubation to insert a tube, e.g. into larynx

intussusception swelling up or enlarging

in utero (Latin) Inside the uterus

inversion reversal of normal relationship; turning inside out. ***i. uterine*** uterus is turned inside out with internal surface protruding at vagina, a serious complication of placental delivery and causes of post-partum bleeding

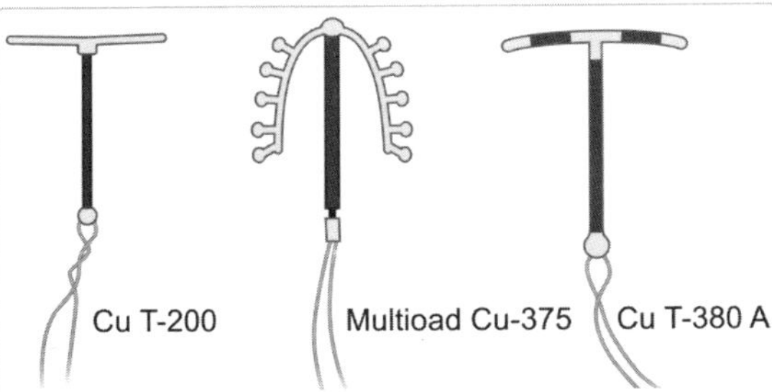

Second generation IUDs

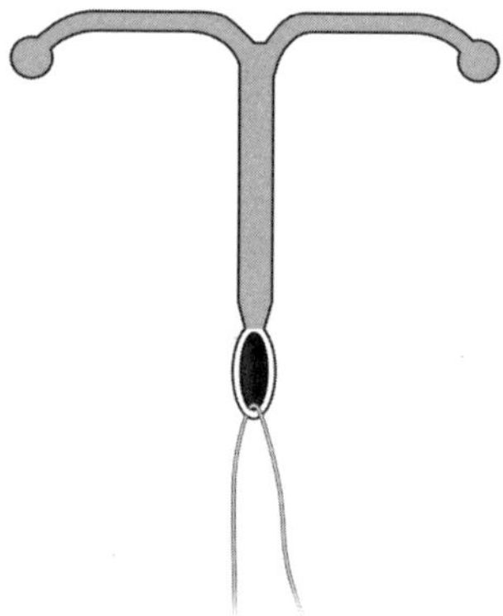

Levonorgestrel intrauterine system

in vitro outside the living body, e.g. tests done in laboratory involving isolated tissue or cell preparation

in vivo within the living body or organism

involution turning inward, reduction in size of uterus following delivery, the retrogressive change in vital processes after their functions have been fulfilled

iodide a compound of iodine, e.g. pot iodide

iodine tincture preparation of iodine in alcohol and water

ion a particle carrying an electric charge. Ions carrying positive charge aggregate near cathode and those with negative charge near anode

iontophoresis introduction of various ions into the skin by means of electricity

ipratropium bromide an anticholinergic given by inhalation in bronchial asthma

iris the organ between lens and cornea. ***i. bombe*** bulging of iris forwards with annular posterior synechia

iritis inflammation of the iris, with photophobia, lacrimation, irregular pupil, dull-muddy looking iris. ***i. plastic*** iritis with fibrinous exudate

iron-dextran injectable form of iron

iron a metallic element existing as Ferrous (Fe^{++}) and Ferric (Fe^{+++}) forms, essential part of hemoglobin and myoglobin. Adult requirement of iron is 0.5 to 1 mg per day; manganese, copper and cobalt are necessary for proper utilization of iron

irradiation therapeutic application of X-ray, radium as in malignancy

ischemia lack of blood supply

ischiocavernosus an erectile muscle extending from ischium to penis or clitoris

ischiococcygeus coccygeus muscle forming posterior portion of levator ani

ischiorectal fossa pararectal fat-filled fossa bounded laterally by obturator internus and ischial tuberosity, posteriorly by gluteus maximus and medially by levator ani

isoantigen a substance present in certain individuals that stimulates production of antibody in other members SYN: alloantigen

isochromosome a chromosome with arms that are morphologically identical and contain the same genetic loci

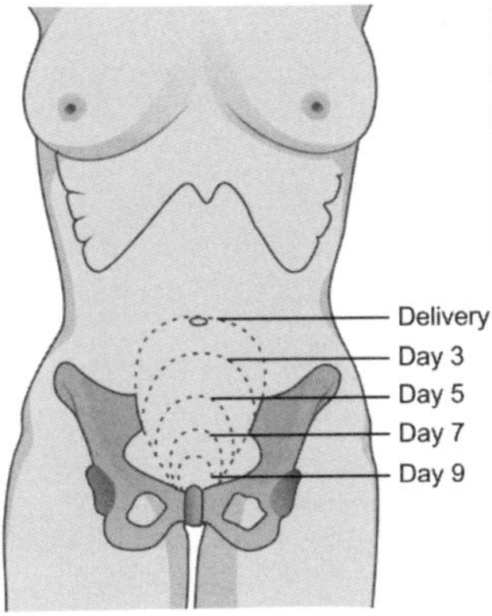

Fundal height and uterine involution pregnancy

isoimmunization immunization of an individual against the blood of another individual of same species

isolation limitation of movement and social contact of patients suffering from or a known carrier of communicable disease

isomer substances having same molecular formula but different chemical and physical properties, e.g. dextrose is an isomer of levulose

isometric contraction contraction without change in muscle length, i.e. tension development without any mechanical work

isoniazid antitubercular agent, bacteriocidal, can cause peripheral neuritis

isopropyl alcohol C_3H_8O, an alcohol used in medical preparations for external use, antifreeze, cosmetics, and as a solvent

isothenuria passage of urine having constant specific gravity; a sign of advanced renal disease

isotonic exercise contraction of a muscle during which the force of resistance to the movement remains constant throughout the range of motion

isotonic solution a solution with osmotic pressure same as that of another solution with which it is compared

isotope elements with nearly identical chemical properties but different atomic weights and electric charges

isoxsuprine hydrochloride a vasodilator and smooth muscle relaxant

isthmus a narrow passage connecting two cavities, a narrow structure connecting two larger parts, a constriction between two larger parts

itch irritation of skin inducing desire to scratch. ***i. barber's*** fungus infection of beard area. ***i. dhobie*** fungus infection of groin and perineum. ***i. ground*** itching in feet due to penetration by hookworm larva. ***i. swimmer's*** dermatitis due to swimming in water containing larvae form of schistosomes

itraconazole antifungal agent

ivy method a method for estimation of bleeding time

J

jacket a bandage usually applied to the trunk to immobilize the spine or correct deformities

Jacquemier's sign blue or purple color of vagina in early pregnancy

jactitation restless to and fro movement of body

jamais vu feeling of being placed in a strange environment or unfamiliarity; a feature of temporal lobe epilepsy

jargon speech or writing that includes unfamiliar terms or abbreviations

jaundice yellow coloration of skin, conjunctiva and mucous membranes due to hyperbilirubinemia. ***j. acholuric*** jaundice with clear urine, i.e. unconjugated hyperbilirubinemia of hemolysis. ***j. cholestatic*** conjugated hyper-bilirubinemia due to stasis of bile excretion, either intrahepatic or extrahepatic. ***j. hemolytic***. jaundice due to hemolysis. ***j. hepatocellular*** jaundice due to hepatitis. ***j. obstructive*** conjugated hyperbilirubinemia with itching due to bile duct stricture, compression or luminal obstruction

jaw Either of the two bones which support the teeth; upper one is known as maxilla and the lower one is mandible

jejunitis Inflammation of jejunum

jejunocolostomy anastomosis of jejunum and ileum as in Crohn's disease

jejunum the second portion of small intestine next to duodenum, about 8 feet in length, making about 2/5 of small intestine

jelly a thick semisolid gelatinous substance. ***j. Wharton's*** soft gelatinous connective tissue that constitutes the matrix of umbilical cord

joint an articulation, between two bones. Joints are grouped according to motion: ball and socket (enarthrosis), hinge (ginglymus); condyloid, pivot (trochoid), gliding (arthrodial) and saddle joint. Joints can move in four ways 1. gliding, in which one bony surface glides on another without angular or rotatory movement. 2. angular 3. circumduction and 4. rotation. Angular movement when occurs forwards or backwards is called flexion and extension and away from the body abduction and towards median plain of body adduction. ***j. ball and socket*** rounded end of one bone fits into cavity of another. ***j. Charcot's*** denervated joint with increased range of movement as in syringomyelia and tabes dorsalis. ***j. condyloid*** joint permitting all forms of angular movements except axial rotation. ***j. hinge*** joint having only forward and backward motion. ***j. pivot*** joint permitting rotation. ***j. saddle*** joint in which the opposing surfaces are reciprocally concavoconvex

joint capsule the sac-like covering enclosing the articulating ends of bones in a diarthrodial joint. It consists of an outer fibrous layer and inner synovial layer

joule work done in one second by current of one ampere against a resistance of one Ohm

jugular foramen opening formed by jugular notches of the occipital and temporal bones

jugular process Projection of occipital bone towards the temporal bone

jugular vein 1. external lies superficial to sternocleidomastoid and joins subclavian vein. 2. internal is direct continuation of transverse sinus and joins subclavian vein to form innominate vein. The vein is more prominent during expiration. The height of pulsating blood column in internal jugular gives an indication of right atrial pressure

junction the place of union of two parts

jurisprudence the scientific study or application of the principles of law and justice ***j. medical*** the application of the principles of law as they relate to the practice of medicine

justo minor pelvis a small gynecoid pelvic in which all diameters are proportionately reduced

juvenile youth or childhood

juxta close proximity

juxtaglomerular apparatus the myoepithelioid cell structure cuffing afferent renal arteriole concerned with production of renin

juxtaposition positioned side-by-side

K

Kahn test a blood test for syphilis diagnosis

kala-azar protozoal tropical disease caused by *Leishmania donovani* manifesting with fever, lymphadenopathy and hepatosplenomegaly with darkening of skin

kalium device for determining alkalinity of a substance

kaliuresis excretion of potassium in urine

kanamycin aminoglycoside antibiotic, used in tuberculosis

kaolin clay powder containing hydrated aluminum silicate used as adsorbent in diarrhea

kaolinosis pneumoconiosis caused by inhalation of kaolin particles

karman catheter catheter used in performing suction curettage of uterus

karyocyte nucleated red blood cell, normoblast

karyotype a photomicrograph of a single cell in the metaphase to show chromosomes in descending order of size

Kawasaki's disease mucocutaneous lymph node syndrome; children are the prime victims and run a risk of coronary arteritis with infarction

kegal exercise an exercise for strengthening the pubococcygeal levator ani muscles in control of urinary and fecal incontinence

keloid hypertrophied, raised, firm, thick scar following trauma or surgical incision

keratin a tough protein substance in hair, nail, horny tissue, produced by keratinocytes

keratinization the process of keratin formation within keratinocytes and its progress upward through the layers of epidermis to the surface stratum corneum

keratitis inflammation of cornea

keratomalacia softening of cornea as in childhood vitamin A deficiency

keratoplasty plastic surgery of cornea. ***k. optic*** replacement of corneal scar with healthy donor corneal tissue. ***k. refractive*** treatment of myopia or hypermetropia by reshaping corneal curvature either by multiple incision or as in keratomileusis

keratoprotein the protein of hair, nail and epidermis

kernicterus bilirubin infiltration of basal ganglia and other areas of brain and spinal cord occurring in erythroblastosis fetalis of newborns when unconjugated hyperbilirubinemia touches 25 mg% or above

Kernig's sign reflex spasm and pain in hamstrings when attempting to extend the knee after flexion of hip; a sign of meningitis

ketamine a nonbarbiturate analgesic-hypnotic substance used IM/IV

ketoacidosis acidosis due to excess of ketone bodies

ketone bodies a group of compounds produced during oxidation of fatty acids and include acetone, beta hydroxy butyric acid and acetoacetic acid

ketosis the accumulation in the body of the ketones causing acidosis commonly occurring in starvation, high fat diet, pregnancy, uncontrolled diabetes mellitus, following ether anesthesia. They impart a fruity odor to the breath

kick chart a chart that records fetal movements; a minimum of 10 fetal movements per day indicates baby's well being else doctor be consulted

kidney paired retroperitoneal structures, one on each side of spinal column, wt—4 to 6 OZ, size 4″ long, 2 to 3″ broad. The kidneys in the newborn are about 3 times as large in proportion to body weight as in the adult. The outer cortex contains the glomeruli, 1 million in number. The inner medulla contains the pyramids 8 to 18 in number made up of collecting tubules being penetrated by cortical substance. Known as columns of Bellini; kidneys are instrumental to the formation of urine which in 95% water and 5% solids (urea, uric acid, cretinine, hippuric acid, sodium and potassium); conversion of vit D into active form and secretion of renin and erythropoietin. ***k. artificial*** hemodialysis device that removes wastes like that of kidney. ***k. contracted*** the small kidneys characteristic of chronic glomerulonephritis or interstitial nephritis. ***k. fatty*** kidney with fatty infiltration causing degeneration of renal substance. ***k. flee bitten*** arteriosclerotic kidney. ***k. floating*** displaceable and movable kidney due to weak fascial support. ***k. granular*** kidney of chronic nephritis where it is small, and of fibrous hard granular texture. ***k. horseshoe*** congenital malformation where the upper or lower poles of both kidneys united by a fibrous isthmus. ***k. polycystic*** kidney with multiple cysts, congenital in origin, can be adult onset type or infantile type. ***k. sacculated*** a condition in which renal parenchyma is absorbed leaving behind the

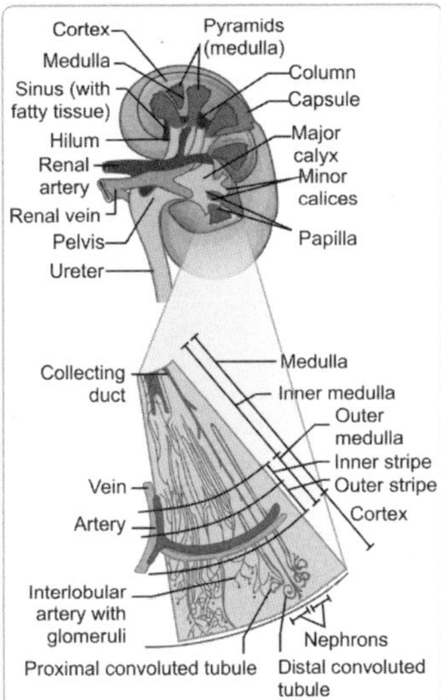

Structure of kidney

K

distended capsule. ***k. sponge*** multiple small cysts in the renal parenchyma. ***k. wandering*** hypermobile kidney

kidney failure Diminished function of the kidneys. This may be acute and temporary or may progress to complete loss of renal function

kidney stone calculus present in renal parenchyma, calyx or renal pelvis, composed principally of calcium, urate, oxalate, phosphates and carbonates, ranging from small granular masses to 5 cm or more in diameter. Most common in patients of hyperparathyroidism, oxaluria, gout and chronic pyelonephritis

Kielland's forcep a forceps for rotation of baby in pelvis as it has no pelvic curve

kinesiology the study of muscles and body movement

Klebsiella short mump gram-negative bacilli, encapsulated, nonspore forming frequently causing respiratory infection. ***K. pneumoniae*** a species causing pneumonia. ***K. rhinoscleromatis*** species causing rhinoscleroma, a destructive granuloma of nose and pharynx

Kleihauer test a microscopic test to detect fetal cells in maternal circulation

kleptomaniac a psychopathic personality suffering from impulsive stealing

Klinefelter's syndrome XXY chromosomal disorder of male manifesting with gynecomastia, tall height, subnormal intelligence, small firm testes

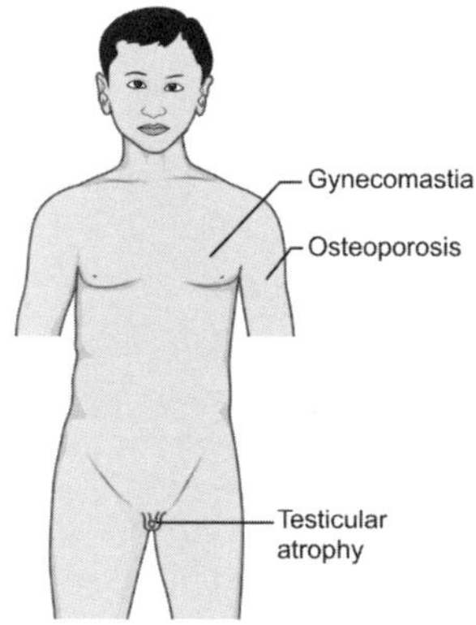

Klinefelter's syndrome

Klumpke's palsy atrophic paralysis of forearm usually due to birth trauma with stretching, avulsion of brachial plexus

knee femerotibial articulation covered anteriorly with patella. ***k. internal derangement*** pertains to a knee with injury to collateral/cruciate ligaments, the menisci, fracture of tibial spine. ***k. housemaid*** bursitis of bursa anterior to patella due to prolonged kneeling. ***k. knock*** outward bending of legs allowing the knees to touch each other. SYN: genu valgum. ***k. locked***. inability to extend the leg due to torn semilunar cartilage

knee chest position position in which patient is on knees with thighs straight, head and upper part of chest resting on table and arms crossed in front of head. Employed for sigmoidoscopic examination of colon and rectum, repositioning of retroverted uterus or displaced ovary

knee presentation a type of breech presentation in which knees lie below the buttocks

knot 1. in surgery, the intertwining of the ends of a suture, ligature, bandage so that the ends will not slip or get loose. 2. An intertwining of a cord or cord-like structure to form a knob or lump

Kocher's forceps artery forcep used to clamp the umbilical cord, also used for rupture

koilonychia dystrophy of finger nails, thinning, spooning as in iron deficiency anemia

Koplik's spot of membrane small red spots with blue white centers on the oral mucosa opposite the molars, a diagnostic sign of measles

Korotkoff's sounds sounds heard in auscultation of blood pressure

kraurosis atrophy and dryness of skin and mucous membrane, esp. of vulva, malignant degeneration may occur

Krukenberg's tumor a malignant tumor of ovary, usually bilateral and frequently secondary to malignancy of GI tract (through peritoneal seedling)

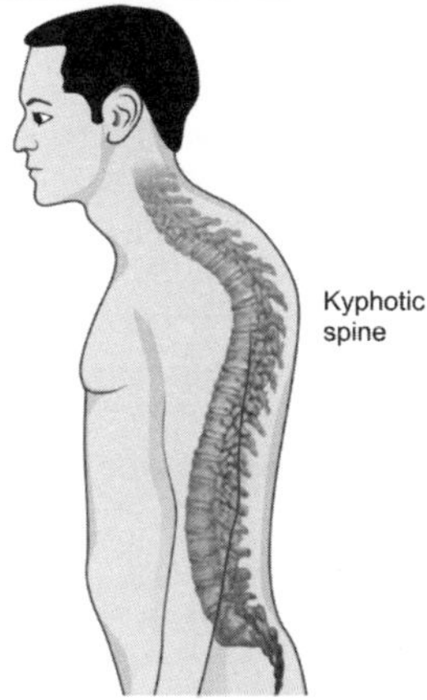

Kyphotic spine

kwashiorkor A severe protein deficiency syndrome in children manifesting with lethargy, dry brittle hair, growth failure, subcutaneous edema, skin changes and hepatomegaly

kyphoscoliosis forward bending of spine along with increased lateral curvature

kyphosis excessive curvature of spine with convexity backwards. May be congenital or secondary to compression fracture, malignancy. SYN: hump back

la 50 the total body surface size of a burn that will kill 50% of victims, used for statistical analysis of mortality figures in burn patients **labetalol** both alpha and beta-blocker used in hypertension

labile unstable, emotions that are easily changeable

labioplasty plastic surgery of labium majus or minus

labium a lip-shaped structure, a fleshy margin or fold

labor the onset of forceful uterine contraction to expel the fetus; divided into three phases, first: from onset of contraction till full dilatation of cervix, second: from full dilatation till delivery of fetus and third: delivery of placenta. ***l. arrested*** failure of progression of labor. ***l. dry*** premature rupture of membranes with escape of liquor. ***l. false*** uterine contractions that do not prog-ress. ***l. induced*** labor precipitated by drugs, (oxytocics) or artificial rupture of membrane. ***l. obstructed*** arrest in progress of labor due to cephalopelvic disproportion, contraction ring, abnormal fetal position, etc. ***l. precipitate*** rapidly progressing labor threatening fetal and maternal injury. ***l. prolonged*** extended duration of labor as first phase exceeding 20 hours in nullipara, 14 hours in multipara or cervical dilatation less than 1.2 cm/hr in nullipara and 1.5 cm in multipara

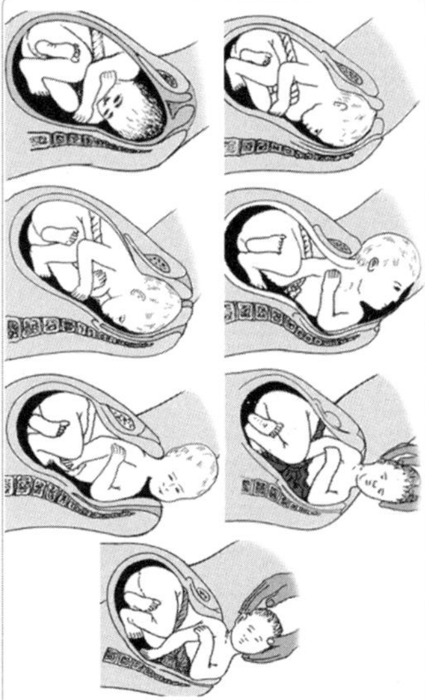

Mechanisms of labor: (A) Engagement descent, flexion; (B) Internal rotation; (C) Extension beginning; (D) Extension complete; (E) Restitution; (F) External rotation; (G) Lateral flexion (expulsion)

laceration tearing of tissues with ragged irregular margins and surrounding contusion. ***l. first degree obstetric*** laceration of perineum involving the fourchette, vaginal mucosa, and skin but not underlying fascia and muscle. ***l. second degree obstetric*** involves underlying fascia and muscle but does not extend to anal sphincter. ***l. third degree obstetric*** laceration extends to involve anal sphincter. ***l. fourth degree obstetric*** laceration involves anal sphincter and rectum with rectovaginal fistula

lacrimation production of tears, weeping

lactalbumin proteins in milk that are not precipitated with ammonium sulfate. They include alpha and beta lactalbumins

lactation secretion of milk by the breast

lactic acid a product of anaerobic glycolysis in muscles and by milk-souring bacteria

lactiferrous capable of producing, transporting or secreting milk

lactobacillus gram positive, anaerobic nonspore forming bacilli producing D or L lactic acid in the milk

lactoferrin iron binding protein of milk

lactogen agent stimulating lactation, like prolactin; human placental lactogen is a polypeptide hormone structurally related to human growth hormone and prolactin secreted by placenta. It is essential in maintenance of growth of fetus

lactoglobulin a milk protein with a concentration of 3g/L in cow's milk, second only to casein among milk proteins

lactose the principal sugar of milk hydrolyzed by β galactosidase to glucose and galactose. Those deficient in this enzyme have discomfort on drinking milk

lactosuria presence of lactose in the urine

lactulose an oral laxative

Lamaze method a method for preparation of childbirth training the body and mind for modifying pain perception during labor

lambda the 11th letter of Greek alphabet; the junction of sagittal and lambdoid sutures

lamivudine (3TC) antiviral, nucleoside analog; inhibition of HIV reverse transcriptase; also inhibits RNA- and DNA-dependent DNA polymerase; used in combination with zidovudine for the treatment of HIV infection

lamotrigene antiepileptic; may be result of blockage of voltage-dependent sodium channels with inhibition of excitatory amino acids; used in adjunctive treatment of refractive partial seizures in adults

Lancefield classification classification of hemolytic streptococci into different groups based on type of hemolysis

lancet a small surgical blade, used for making small drainage incisions

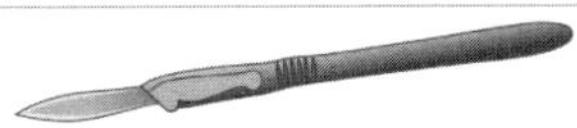

Lancet

L

lancinating Sudden sharp transient pain as if tearing into pieces

Landsteiner's classification classification of blood groups into A, B, AB and O

lanolin a waxy fatty secretion of sebaceous glands of the sheep deposited on wool fibers, used as an ointment base

lansoprazole proton pump inhibitor, used in peptic ulcer

lanugo the fine downy hairs devoid of medulla, covering fetus

laparoscope an endoscope devised for examination of abdominoopelvic organs

laparotomy surgical incision of abdominal wall for access to abdominal organs

laryngitis inflammation of lining of larynx, may be catarrhal, chronic hyperplastic (often precancerous), chronic nonspecific, diphtheritic, membranous (diphtheria, streptococci, pseudomonas)

laryngomalacia a flaccid supraglottic larynx in babies causing inspiratory stridor but with spontaneous cure

laryngoscopy inspection of interior of larynx. l. fiberoptic Indirect (mirror) laryngoscopy

larynx the organ of voice that is part of the air passage connecting the pharynx with the trachea. It accounts for the large bump in the neck called the Adam's apple

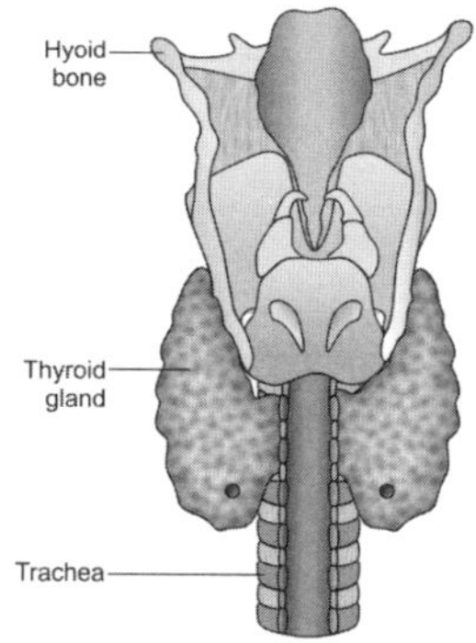

Anatomy of the larynx

laser light amplification by stimulated emission of radiation. ***l. carbon dioxide*** used to remove lesions of skin or other superficial organs. ***l. argon*** its blue green light causes coagulation of bleeding sites in surgery. ***l. neodymium YAG*** laser used for capsulotomy, vitrectomy

last menstrual period (LMP) the first day of last menstrual cycle useful to calculate expected date of delivery (EDD)

Late deceleration a periodic decrease in the fetal heart rate below baseline occurring after the peak of the contraction, due to uteroplacental insufficiency and a sign of fetal distress

latent existing but not apparent, dormant

lateralization the tendency to perform an act predominantly on left or right side of the body

L

lateral on the side of body

lathyrism spastic paraplegia with sensory impairment due to consumption of khesari dal containing fungus Lathyrus sativatus

lavage the washing out of hollow organ, e.g. gastric, peritoneal, intestinal

laxative agent promoting or stimulating bowel movement

lean body mass body weight without fat content

Leboyer method a method of childbirth, child birth in a dark room in serene atmosphere, baby being born gently and quietly

lecithin a fatty substance like phospholipids found in blood, bile, brain, egg yolk, nerves and other animal tissues

Lee-Frankenhauser pledus nerve network of S3-S4 hypogastric and ovarian nerves related cervical supply

Leeds test a test to identify women at higher risk of carrying fetus with Down's syndrome, besides alpha fetoprotein, LCG and unconjugated estril, neutrophil alkaline phosphatase is also estimated

legionnaire's disease an acute bacterial pneumonia caused by infection with ***l. pneumophila*** and characterized by an influenza-like illness followed within a week by high fever, chills, muscle aches, and headache. Contaminated air conditioning cooling towers and stagnant water supplies, including water vaporizers and water sonicators, may be a source of organisms

leiomyoma a low mitotic benign tumor of smooth muscle cell. Can be seen on skin (dermatomyoma) uterus, seminal vesicles, blood vessels (angiomyoma)

leishmaniasis infectious disease caused by flagellate protozoan

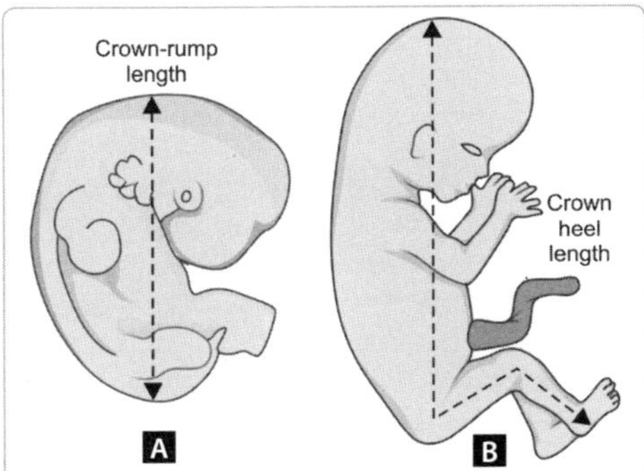

(A) Crown-rump length (B) Crown-heel length;

parasites and transmitted to man by sandflies

length ***l. crown-rump (CR L)*** the length of an embryo from the top of the head to the bottom of the buttocks. ***l. cranial*** skull length between glabella and inion. ***l. crown heel*** fetal or infant length from crown to heel. ***l. foot*** toe to heel length for estimation of age of fetus. ***l. sitting*** distance between vertex and coccyx

lentigo a small brown macule resulting from increased number of melanocyte at dermoepidermal junction, Plural: lentigines

leprosy chronic mycobacterial disease of skin and peripheral nerves caused by *Mycobacterium leprae*; can be divided into borderline, borderline lepromatous, lepromatous, border line tuberculoid and tuberculoid types. ***l. borderline*** affects persons with moderate degree of cell-mediated immunity, can upgrade to tuberculoid or downgrade to lepromatous pole. ***l. lepromatous*** diffuse bilaterally symmetrical lesions in persons with poor cell-mediated immunity. Bacilli are plenty and well-disseminated. ***l. lucio*** a diffuse non-nodular variant of lepromatous leprosy. ***l. tuberculoid*** few hyposthetic macules, enlarged cutaneous nerves, well-developed cellular immunity and few bacteria

lesion a pathological alteration in structure or function of an organ

let down reflex the neurogenic process that stimulates release of milk from breast

lethal deadly, capable of causing death

lethargy a state of excessive fatigue, diminished physical and mental activity

leucine an essential amino acid

leukemia Malignant proliferation of leukocytes and their bone marrow precursors with organ infiltration. Principal types are: acute myeloid, acute lymphoblastic, chronic myeloid, chronic lymphocytic. Acute myeloid has six subtypes: M1 to M6, that includes monocytic, myelomonocytic, promyelocytic and erythroleukemia. ***l. aleukemic*** peripheral blood picture is normal but there is pancytopenia. Bone marrow puncture yields the excess blast cells. ***l. basophilic*** marked increase in basophils of blood and marrow, a variant of chronic myeloid leukemia. ***l. eosinophilic*** peripheral eosinophilia with increased blasts in marrow

leukemoid resembling leukemia with appearance of immature leukocytes in peripheral blood and leukocytosis. Seen in some infectious diseases

leukopenia abnormal decrease in number of blood leukocytes (<4,000/ mm^3)

leukoplakia epithelial hyperplasia with keratosis of mucous membrane appearing as white patch. It chiefly affects gums, lips, cheeks, tongue, larynx, urinary bladder and female genitalia

leukopoiesis Formation, growth and maturation of leukocytes

leukorrhea abnormal white non bloody discharge from vagina

leukotrienes mediators of inflammation derived from arachidonic acid. Leukotriene C4, D4, E4 play roles in anaphylaxis (slow reacting substance) and B4 is a chemoattractant and aggregator of neutrophils

levallorphan tartarate a narcotic antogonist for treatment of respiratory depression caused by narcotics

levamisole the l-form tetramisole, used for treatment of roundworm, hookworm, strongyloides. Also used as an immunopotentiator

levatorani a broad sheet of muscle forming pelvic floor

levonorgestrel a progestin

levothyroxine L thyroxine; yellow crystalline powder for oral supplement in hypothyroid cases

libido sexual desire or appetite

lidocaine a local anesthetic applied as sprays, creams to skin and mucous membrane

lie The relation of long axis of fetus to that of mother; can be longitudinal, transverse or oblique

ligament 1. any band of fibrous tissue connecting bones. 2. any membranous fold sheet or cord-like structure that holds an organ in position. ***l. broad of uterus*** fibrous sheets of peritoneum extending from uterus to lateral pelvic wall. ***l. cruciate of knee*** one anterior and one posterior crossing each other like x that prevent rotation in knee joint. ***l. deltoid***. the medial reinforcing ligament of ankle. ***l. falciform*** a sickle-shaped ligament composed of two layers of peritoneum attaching liver to anterior abdominal wall. ***l. inguinal*** rolled inferior margin of external oblique aponeurosis extending from anterior superior iliac spine of ileum to pubic tubercle. SYN: Poupart's ligament. ***l. lacunar*** a triangular band extending horizontally from the inguinal ligament to iliopectineal line of pubis. ***l. ovarian*** a cord-like bundle of fibers between the folds of broad ligament joining ovary to uterus. ***l. periodontal (PDL)*** the mode of attachment of the tooth to the alveolus. The ligament consists of numerous bundles of collagenous tissue (principal fibers) arranged in groups, between which is loose connective tissue, together with blood vessels, lymph vessels, and nerves. It functions as the investing and supportive mechanism for the tooth. ***l. pectineal*** a strong aponeurotic band extending from pectineal line of pubis to the lacunar ligament. ***l. round of liver*** remnant of umbilical vein extending from umbilicus to anterior border of liver SYN: ligamentum teres hepatis. ***l. round of uterus*** a fibromuscular cord extending from either side of uterus to labium majus passing through inguinal canal

ligation the action to ligate. ***l. tubal*** both Fallopian tubes are tied and cut or crushed for purpose of sterilization

ligator surgical instrument facilitating ligation, superficial or deep

ligature surgical instrument facilitating ligation, superficial or deep

Lightening the descent of fetus deeper into pelvis

linea a long thin mark, ridge, crease or line. ***l. alba***. Midline tendinous band extending from xiphoid process to symphysis pubis, formed by aponeurosis of external oblique, internal oblique and transversalis muscles. **l. nigra**. Pigmented linea alba of pregnancy

lint a loosely woven cotton fabric, one side fluffy other side smooth, used for dressing

lip any projecting labrum, fleshy parts surrounding mouth opening. ***l. cleft***. Notch, furrow or open space in upper lip developmental in origin

lipid any natural compound soluble in apolar but insoluble in polar solvents. Lipids contain fatty acids, one chain alcohols, steroids or sphyngolipids

lipid A the endotoxic component of lipopolysaccharide consisting of glucosamine disaccharide

lipoatrophy atrophy of subcutaneous tissue at sites of insulin injection

lipoma a benign growth of mature adipose tissue cells

lipoprotein compounds of lipid and protein. ***l. high density*** contains 50% protein, 25% phospholipid, 20% cholesterol, and 5% fat, originate both in liver and intestine, function in cholesterol transport, have longer half-life and are cardioprotective. ***l. low density*** contains more of cholesterol and lipids and little triglyceride high blood level is atherogenic. ***l. very low density*** density 1.006 mg/mL. Contains 50% fat, 25% cholesterol and 20% phospholipid

liposuction a method of subcutaneous fat removal

Lippe's loop an intrauterine contraceptive device

liquor amnii the fluid that fills amniotic sac surrounding the fetus, 99% water rest being protein, fat, Na^+, K^+, desquamated epithelial cells, vernix caseosa, etc. It functions as shock absorber, permits free movements of fetus and allows unhindered fetal growth. Volume is nearly 1 liter at 37 to 38 weeks

listeria small gram-positive aerobic rods, e.g. *L. monocytogenes* causing meningitis, septicemia, abscess

lithopedion a retained calcified fetus

lithotomy position the patient lies on her back with thighs and legs flexed, abducted held in place by lithotomy poles. This position is helpful for forceps breech delivery and perinasal suturing

litmus a natural pigment from lichens whose principle is azolitmin. It is used as pH indicator being red at pH and blue at pH 8.3

litter a stretcher for transporting the invalid

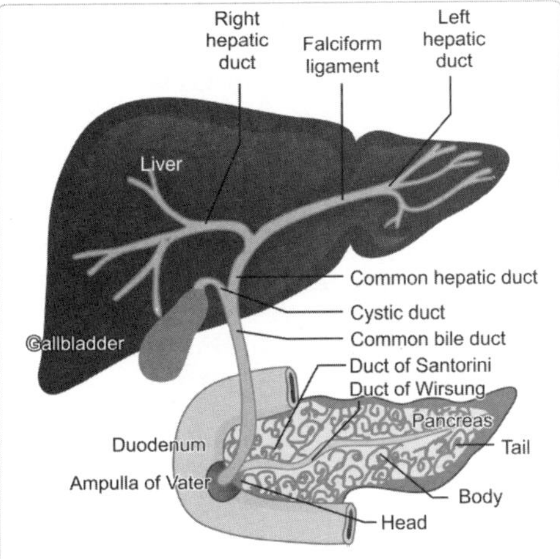

Liver

liver largest glandular organ in the body weighing 1200 to 1600 g. (1/40 of body wt), located in right upper quadrant below right dome of diaphragm; major functions are secretion of bile, synthesis of plasma proteins, fibrinogen, prothrombin; detoxification, metabolism of carbohydrate, fat and protein and storage of glycogen. ***l. amyloid*** large pale gray waxy looking liver due to deposition of amyloid. Amyloid deposits appear as an amorphous eosinophilic substance, in the space of Disse, between hepatocyte and sinusoidal endothelial cells. ***l. cirrhotic biliary*** deeply bile stained nodular liver caused by autoimmune damage to small bile ducts (primary biliary cirrhosis) or obstruction to bile outflow. ***l. cirrhotic*** scarred nodular liver, post hepatitis, alcoholic. ***l. Indian childhood cirrhosis*** enlarged firm liver with a leafy edge. ***l. fatty*** Yellow soft greasy liver with increased cytoplasmic fat within hepatocytes. ***l. nutmeg*** liver affected by chronic vascular congestion as in CHF. **l. polycystic** liver with multiple congenital cysts, often associated with polycystic kidney, usually asymptomatic.

lividity a black and blue discoloration of skin such as caused by contusion

lobe a section of an organ, separated from neighboring parts by fissures

lobule a small lobe

lochia discharge from uterus following child birth. ***l. alba*** light colored uterine discharge consisting of leukocytes. ***l. rubra*** bloody uterine discharge immediately after delivery. ***l. serosa*** the serous, pinkish-brown watery discharge which follows lochia rubra

lochiometra A condition in which lochia is retained inside the uterine cavity

locked twins twins with their bodies and heads so positioned than neither can be born naturally, a cause of obstructed labor

locus a place or spot, as the specific site occupied by a gene in the chromosome. ***l. ceruleus*** a bluish gray area in the floor of fourth ventricle. ***l. histocompatibility*** one of the genes located within major histocompatibility complex that specifies transplantation antigens or immune response functions. ***l. operator*** a regulator locus that governs the transcription of adjacent structural genes of the operon and is the binding site of a repressor protein molecule

lomefloxacin HCl fluoroquinolone antiinfective; a broad-spectrum bactericidal agent that inhibits the enzyme DNA gyrase needed for DNA synthesis; used in lower respiratory tract infections (pneumonia, bronchitis); genitourinary infections (prostatitis); preoperatively to reduce UTIs in transurethral surgical procedures due to susceptible gram-negative organisms

longitudinal study investigations that involves making observations of the some group at sequential time intervals

loperamide a meperidine congener, intestinal smooth muscle relaxant

lorazepam depresses subcortical levels of the central nervous system, including limbic system and reticular formatiŏn; used in anxiety, preoperative sedation, acute alcohol withdrawal symptoms, muscle spasm

lordosis abnormally increased forward curvature of lumbar spine. Also called sway back or saddle back. ***l. compensatory*** lordosis secondary to pelvic obliquity/deformity

losartan angiotensin receptor blocker used in hypertension

Lovset's maneuver a procedure where by fetal shoulders are delivered when arms are extended during breech. It consists in rotating the fetus through a half circle keeping the back uppermost so as to bring posterior arm into anterior position below symphysis pubis and then delivered. The fetus is then rotated in reverse direction half circle and other arm is delivered

low birthweight baby weighing less than 2.5 kg at birth, either being preterm, or small for gestational age

lower uterine segment the part of uterus lying between the vesicouterine peritoneal fold superiorly and uterocervical junction below

lubricant agent used to reduce friction

lumbar pertaining to loins. ***l. puncture*** introduction of needle to subarachnoid space to get CSF samples for cytological and biochemical studies. Also used to introduce drugs, anesthetic agents, or to drain out CSF to reduce pressure

lumbosacral pertaining to lumbar portion of spine and the sacrum

lumen the cavity within tubular structure; the SI unit of luminous flux

lumpectomy surgical excision of breast lump, benign or malignant

lung paired organ of respiration in the chest enveloped by pleura. Subserving the function of oxygen uptake and CO_2 elimination. ***l. farmer's*** extrinsic allergic alveolitis occurring in farmers due to inhalation of moldy hay manifesting with cough, dyspnea and fever. Repeated exposures lead to pulmonary fibrosis. ***l. honeycomb*** small multiple areas of radiolucency with intervening borders of soft tissue density as seen in interstitial pulmonary fibrosis. ***l. post-perfusion*** a condition of atelectasis, pulmonary arteriovenous shunting and consolidation following cardiopulmonary bypass. ***l. uremic*** pulmonary edema with butterfly appearance of lung in X-ray due to circulatory overload and uremic dysfunction of LV

lupus resembling wolf. ***l. discoid*** a disease confined to skin, marked by scaly rash usually in butterfly pattern over nose and cheeks, sometimes extending to scalp but no visceral involvement. ***l. pernio*** sarcoid lesions of the hands and face, especially the ears and nose resembling frost bite. ***l. vulgaris*** redbrown nodular skin lesions of face in tuberculosis. ***l. systemic*** chronic autoimmune disease marked by an erythematous rash on face and other areas exposed to sunlight with vasculitis involving kidneys, brain and arthritis. Antinuclear antibodies to double stranded DNA and native DNA nucleohistone are diagnostic. ***l. drug-induced*** similar to systemic lupus induced by drugs like procainamide and hydralazine but without renal and brain involvement

luteal relating to corpus luteum of ovary

luteinization transformation of granulosa cells into lutein cells in the ovary. Other cells may undergo luteinization including theca cells, celomic cells and cervical cells

luteinizing hormone hormone secreted from anterior pituitary acting in concert with FSH causes ovulation, in males stimulates development of intersitital cells of testes to secrete testosterone

lymph a transparent or slightly opalescent fluid containing lymphocytes, which flows through lymph channels and enters finally into venous system via thoracic ducts

lymphangioma a benign growth composed exclusively of lymph vessels lined by a single layer of endothelial cells. The lesion is often congenital, can be subtyped into capillary, cavernous and cystic. The latter two are most frequent in cervical, mediastinal and retroperitoneal regions of infants (hygroma); capillary lymphangioma is difficult to identify from hemangioma

lymphangitis inflammation of lymphatic vessels. ***l. carcinomatosa*** growth of carcinoma in lymphatics or lymphatic obstruction by carcinoma

lymphedema chronic unilateral or bilateral swelling of extremities caused by obstruction of lymph vessels or disease of lymph nodes, usually congenital, ***type I***: autosomal dominant, associated intestinal protein loss and pleural effusion (Millroy's disease);. ***type II***: slowly progressive form with onset around puberty. ***l. praecox*** lymphedema occurring in girls approaching puberty

lymphocyte a white blood cell derived from lymphoid tissue constituting 25 to 33% of white blood cells in peripheral blood. It has a round nucleus with well-condensed chromatin, no nucleolus, and agranular cytoplasm staining pale blue. ***l. B*** derived from bone marrow, involved in humoral immunity. They recognize antigens irrespective of MCH molecule and transform to plasma cells to secrete antibodies on antigenic stimulation. They are thymus-independent. ***l. T*** thymus derived lymphocyte, that has been exposed to antigen on an antigen presenting cell. They play large role in cellullar immunity. Can be helper cells, killer cells, suppressor cells or null cells

lymphoma malignant disease of lymphoreticular system. ***l. Burkitt's***. malignant lymphoma involving extranodal sites like jaw, orbit, abdominal viscera, and ovaries, the most common childhood tumor of tropical Africa. Possibly caused by EB virus and linked to falciparum malaria. ***l. histiocytic*** lymphoma composed of histiocytes (poorly differentiated lymphocytic lymphomas). ***l. lymphocytic*** a malignant lymphoma composed of lymphocytes. The pattern may be nodulas or diffuse, and the cells may be poorly differentiated, well-differentiated. ***l. prolymphocytic*** the cells are larger and have less condensed nuclear chromatin. ***l. sclerosing*** a lymphoma with prominent stromal component. l. signet ring cell. Cells with a large cytoplasmic vacuole of immunoglobulin which displaces the nucleus to periphery. l. stem cell. Composed of large basket-like cells

lynestrenol a semisynthetic progestin

lysine one of the twenty amino acids. It is an essential amino acid deficient in plant proteins

lysis 1. destruction of cell by specific lysin 2. gradual recovery from an acute disease

lysozyme an antibacterial enzyme present in tear, sweat, saliva and nasal secretion

lytic cocktail a combination of chlorpromazine, promethazine, and pethidine used in treatment of severe preeclampsia and eclampsia

M. mode a motion B mode tracing of ultrasound to visualize moving structures

macerate 1. to soften a solid or tissue by soaking the tissue in enzyme/acid. 2. the autolysis of fetal tissue after fetal death

Mackenrodt's ligaments transverse cervical ligament fixing uterus in pelvic cavity

macrocyte red blood cell 2 micron larger than normal RBC, also called megalocyte

macroencephaly malformation and increase in size and weight of brain due to proliferation of glian with small ventricles and mental retardation

macromelia enlarged limbs

macrophage a large mononuclear cell that ingests degenerated cells, widely distributed in body but greatest accumulation in spleen where they remove senescent RBC. In brain and spinal cord known as microglia and in the blood as it moves on the alveolar surface of lung engulfing airborne particles reaching the alveoli

macropsia condition of seeing objects larger than their actual size

macroscopic visible with naked eye

macrosomia large body size; newborn at term weighing more than 4,000 grams or is large for his or her gestational age

macrostomia abnormally large mouth

macrotia abnormally large ears

macule a nonelevated discolored lesion on the skin

maculopapular spotted and elevated

maculopathy any disease of macula of retina

madarosis loss of eye lashes

magnesium element number 12, the silvery white metal, one of the principal cations governing electrochemical properties of living system. m. carbonate $MgCO_3$, insoluble in water, used as laxative and antacid. ***m. citrate*** used as laxative. ***m. hydroxide*** insoluble in water, used as laxative and antacid. ***m. oxide*** also called magnesia (see above). ***m. sulfate*** $MgSO_4$ effective cathartic, antiarrhythmic and antiepileptic, useful in certain poisonings

magnetic resonance imaging (MRI) also known as nuclear magnetic resonance imaging. MRI is a diagnostic technique in which the phosphorus in cellular tissues is excited by magnetic force. The distribution and alignment of these cellular elements can be captured on phosphorus nuclear magnetic resonance instruments forming a high-resolution tissue image. A higher degree of resolution of soft tissues is possible using this technique than from radiographic techniques. The word nuclear has been dropped from the term because it makes an incorrect inference that radioactivity is involved in the imaging process

malabsorption impaired or incomplete absorption of nutrients by the intestine. ***m. lactose*** lactase deficiency, mostly inherited, commonly manifesting in adults, with pain and diarrhea after lactose ingestion. Unabsorbed lactose is converted to butyric and lactic acid by colonic bacteria, that causes pain. Lactose being hyperosmolar draws fluid to add to stool volume. ***m. syndrome*** manifests with pallor, potbelly, bleeding tendency, weakness due to malabsorption of nutrients, caused by any disease

malacia softening of tissues. ***m. cordis*** morbid softening of heart

malabsorption a disease

malady illness

malaise a vague general discomfort or feeling ill

malaria an infectious disease caused by any of the four plasmodia, transmitted by mosquitoes of the genus anopheles, manifesting with chill and fever, anemia, splenomegaly. ***m. falciparum*** caused by plasmodium falciparum, the parasite develops within small vessels of internal organs frequently blocking them. Fever paroxysm often occurs daily and is often continuous. Patient can have cerebral, gastrointestinal, renal and pulmonary complications. Also known as malignant tertian. ***m. malarae*** caused by *Plasmodium malarae*, Fever paroxysm occurs on every third day. ***m. quotidian*** a form in which paroxysms occur daily, can be caused by combination of *Plasmodium vivax* and *Falciparum* or two generations of *Falciparum*. ***m. relapsing*** a type in which exoerythrocytic cycle persists in liver with relapse, e.g. in *vivax* and ovale infection. ***m. vivax*** caused by *Plasmodium vivax* or *ovale*, the fever paroxysm occurring every other day

malar relating to cheek or cheek bone

male reproductive system consisting of testes, epididymis, vas deferens, seminal vesicles, prostate and penis

malformation a defect or deformity. ***m. Klippel-Feil*** short-webbed neck due to malformation of cervical vertebrae. ***m. Mondini*** congenital deafness due to hypoplasia of latter part of cochlea

malfunction abnormal or inadequate function

malignant denoting any disease resistant to treatment, and of fatal nature. In case of tumor, it denotes uncontrollable undifferentiated growth and dissemination. ***m. hypertension*** the most lethal form of hypertension. Malignant hypertension is a fulminating condition, characterized by severely elevated blood pressure that commonly damages that intima of small vessels, the brain, retina, heart, and kidneys. It affects more African Americans than white Americans and may be caused by a variety of factors such as stress, genetic predisposition, obesity, the use of tobacco, the use of oral contraceptives, high intake of sodium chloride; a sedentary lifestyle, and aging. ***m. hyperthermia*** an autosomal dominant trait characterized by often fatal hyperthermia with rigidity of muscles occurring in affected people exposed to certain anesthetic agents, particularly halothane and succinylcholine

malnutrition faulty nutrition due to inadequate diet, metabolic abnormality, wrong proportions of items, etc.

malpighian body renal corpuscle

malposition misplaced or altered position of an organ in relation to others

malpractice professional misconduct, lack of skill or fidelity in professional duties or illegal immoral conduct

malpresentation any fetal presentation other than vertex

maltase digestive enzyme promoting conversion of maltose to glucose

malt grain, especially barley, containing dextrin, maltose, glucose and some enzymes

maltose $C_{12}H_{22}O_{11}$; a sugar formed by action of a digestive enzyme on starch

mammography a soft tissue X-ray technique for visualization of female breast; used to detect nonpalpable lesions and identify palpable lesions

Manchester operation amputation of cervix with anterior and posterior colporrhaphy

mandelic acid urinary antibacterial agent

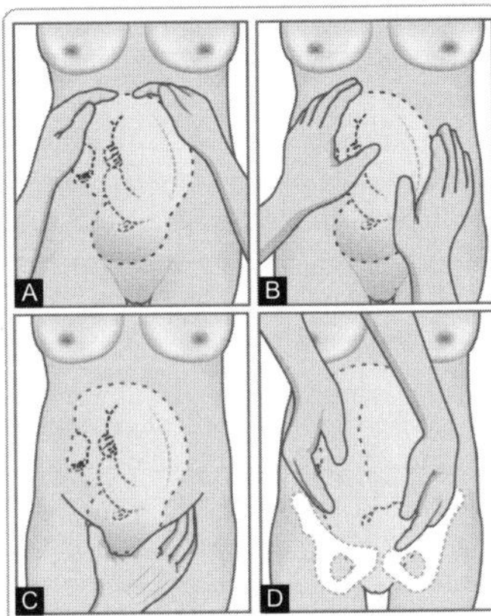

Abdominal palpation: Leopold's maneuver: (A) First maneuver (fundal palpation); (B) Second maneuver (lateral palpation); (C) Third maneuver (Pawlik's grip/second pelvic grip); (D) Fourth maneuver (pelvic palpation/first pelvic grip)

mandible the horseshoe-shaped bone of lower jaw in mammals. Articulating with skull at temporomandibular joint and housing the lower teeth

maneuver a skillful movement. ***m. Bracht's*** in obstetrics, maneuver used in breech extraction whereby breech is allowed to deliver spontaneously upto umbilicus and then the fetal body is held anteriorly toward mother's abdomen to facilitate delivery of vertex. ***m. Credé's*** a method of expressing the placenta in which body of uterus is vigorously squeezed inorder to produce placental separation. ***m. Pinard*** Method of fetal extraction in frank breech presentation; two fingers

M

are passed along fetal thigh to push it away from midline and flex the leg, the foot then easily grasped and brought down and out. ***m. Prague*** a procedure used in breech delivery in which the finger is hooked over shoulder of fetus to exert traction and allow engagement of the head. ***m. Scanzoni's*** rotation of fetal head with mid forceps from posterior to anterior position. ***m. Valsalva*** 1. forced expiration against closed glottis to increase pressure within lungs. 2. forced expiration with mouth closed and nose pinched to open up auditory tubes

mania emotional disorder characterized by excitement, hyperactivity and garrulousness

manic depressive psychosis (MDP) alternating attacks of mania and depression

manipulation treatment by skillful use of hand in reducing dislocation or changing the fetal position

mannitol an alcohol, $C_6H_{14}O_6$, derived from fructose, used in preparation of dietetic sweets and as an osmotic diuretic

manometer an instrument for measuring pressure of liquid and gases

Mantoux test skin test with intradermal injection of tuberculin to determine susceptibility to tuberculosis, the test is positive if wheal exceeds 10 mm in diameter after 72 hours of test

manual with the hand ***m. removal*** of placenta introducing hand into uterus to remove the placenta; better be done under anesthesia

maple syrup urine disease an autosomal recessive disorder marked by deficient oxidative decarboxylation of alpha keto acids; the urine has characteristic maple syrup odor and the symptoms soon after birth are hypoglycemia, hypotonia, convulsion, etc. Also known as branched chain ketonuria

marasmus protein calorie malnutrition in young children with progressive wasting, wizened face, shrunken eyeballs but alerted mind

Marfan's syndrome autosomal dominant trait with defective formation of elastic fibers marked by abnormally long slender extremities, spidery fingers, high arched palate, lax joints, aortic regurgitation, MVP and dislocation of lens

marijuana the dried, chopped leaves, flowers and stems of the common hemp plant canabis sativa, smoked or eaten to induce euphoria

marrow the meshy material filling the medullary cavities of bones. ***m. red*** marrow in the cancellous or spongy bones of sternum, ribs, iliac crest, vertebrae and ends of long bones. Concerned with formation of blood. ***m. yellow*** the fatty marrow in center of long bones

massage rubbing body parts for therapeutic goals. ***m. cardiac*** rhythmic manual compression of heart either by thoracotomy (open cardiac massage) or by pressure applied to sternum (closed cardiac massage). ***m. carotid sinus*** massage of carotid sinus at the angle of jaw for treatment of SVT or identification of tachycardia. ***m. prostatic*** massage of prostate through rectum to express its secretions into prostatic urethra (examination for gonococci)

mastalgia pain in breasts

mast cell a connective tissue cell in bronchi and skin containing histamine, serotonin and heparin release of which cause edema and bronchospasm

mastitis breast infection because of milk in ducts

materia medica the science of the source and preparation of drugs

maternal mortality rate (MMR) the number of maternal deaths due to pregnancy and child birth per 1000 live and still births

maternity care complete care of the pregnant, laboring and newly delivered woman and her newborn; also includes pre-pregnancy counseling, infertility counseling and parenting education.

maternity pertaining to pregnancy, the state of being pregnant

Matthews Duncan expulsion of placenta the placenta is expelled maternal side first at the end of third stage of labor

matrix 1. the intercellular substance in a tissue. 2. the mold for dental restoration in the form of thin steel or plastic strip surrounding tooth. ***m. bone*** the ground substance of bony tissue which is composed of protein and mucopolysaccharide. As the bone matures, the content of collagen fibers and bone salt increases. ***m. cartilaginous*** a basic, homogeneous basophil substance of embryonic skeletal tissue in the center of which articular cartilage develops. ***m. mesangial*** a mesh in the space between the renal glomerular loops, formed from material similar to that of capillary basement membrane. The phagocytic mesangial cells are dispersed in this matrix. The matrix is permeable to substances of higher molecular weight which aggregate to form deposits. **m. retainer** A mechanical device used to secure the ends of metal or plastic bands around a tooth to provide a form into which a restorative material can be condensed to replace a portion of tooth substance removed in cavity preparation

Mauriceau Smellie Veit maneuver a method of delivering the after coming head in breech delivery

McRobert's maneuver maneuver involves helping the woman to lie flat and to bring her knees up to her chest as far as possible. This will rotate the angle of the symphysis pubis superiorly and use the weight of the mother's legs to create gentle pressure on her abdomen releasing the impaction of the anterior shoulder

mean an average of a set of values. ***m. arithmetic*** the ratio of the sum of the terms in a statistical series to their number. ***m. geometric*** a value indicating the central tendency of a statistical series of 'n' terms, equal to the positive 'n'th root of their products. ***m. harmonic*** for a given set of values, the reciprocal of the mean of the reciprocals of the individual values

measles highly contagious disease caused by paramyxovirus occurring in young children with fever, coryza, Koplik spots, erythematous maculopapular rash spreading from head to trunk to limbs, often complicated by meningitis, carditis

meatus an opening to a canal, or passage in the body. ***m. external acoustic*** S-shaped canal of external ear, upto tympanic membrane lined by skin which continues on to the tympanic membrane. **m. internal acoustic** a short canal above the anterior part of jugular foramen in the petrous part of temporal bone transmitting facial, intermediate, and vestibulocochlear nerves and the labyrinthine vessels

mebendazole a benzimidazole given for hookworm, roundworm, trichuriasis and enterobiasis

mebeverine a smooth muscle relaxant used for gastrointestinal motility disorder like IBS

mechanism of labor the sequence of fetal movements where by it adopts for safe passage through maternal pelvis during birth

meconium the odorless, sticky, greenish black semisolid intestinal content of fetus. It is replaced by feces within 2 days of birth

median in statistics denoting the middle value in a distribution, i.e. the point in a series at which half of the plotted values are on one side and half on the other

mediastinum 1. The central space in chest bounded anteriorly by sternum, posteriorly by vertebral column and laterally by pleural sacs. 2. Any septum or partition between two parts of an organ. ***m. anterior*** that portion of lower mediastinum located in front of heart behind the sternum. It contains thymus gland, few lymph nodes and loose areolar tissue. ***m. lower*** the part of mediastinum below the plane of manubriosternal joint in front and lower border of 4th thoracic vertebra behind. It is divided into anterior, middle and posterior. ***m. middle*** it contains the heart, pericardium and the emerging great vessels. ***m. posterior*** it contains esophagus, thoracic duct, thoracic aorta, vagus and lymph nodes ***m. superior*** it lies above the pane of manubriosternal articulation and contains aortic arch and its branches, superior vena cava, brachiocephalic veins, left recurrent laryngeal nerve, thoracic duct, thymus, vagus nerve and some lymph nodes

medical termination of pregnancy It is the deliberate induction of abortion prior to 20 weeks gestation by a registered medical practitioner in the interest of mother's health and life

medicine a drug: the art and science dealing with the maintenance and restoration of health. ***m. adolescent*** the branch of medicine dealing with care and treatment of individuals from onset of puberty to the age of 19. ***m. aviation*** a specialized branch of medicine dealing with physiologic, pathologic, psychologic conditions which occur in fliers, and people transported in air. It helps in selection of aircraft personnel, air transport of sick and wounded. ***m. behavioral*** the applications of the principles of learning and learning theory to treat those disorders caused at least in part by psychologic factors as if they were behavioral. Specific techniques are applied to reverse the expressions of maladaptive functioning whether purely psychologic as in phobias or partly physiologic as in faulty patterns of learned autonomic nervous system response leading to cardiovascular disease. ***m. clinical*** the study and practice of medicine at bed side, as opposed to theoretical and laboratory investigations. ***m. community*** medicine dealing with community healthcare and their solution as a whole rather than individual health problem, e.g. preventive medicine, public health services. ***m. family*** Medical speciality dealing with first patient contact, long-term care, and a broad responsibility to all members of the family irrespective of age. ***m. folk*** treatment of disease at home with remedies and techniques passed from generation to generation. ***m. emergency*** a branch of medicine that specializes in providing immediate diagnosis and treatment of those who are acutely or often suddenly ill or severely injured. ***m. environmental*** the study of environmental aspects related to health and their modification for better health. ***m. experimental*** Study of disease process and various therapies in animal models. ***m. forensic*** the application of medical knowledge and skill to the solution of problems encountered in administration of justice. ***m. geriatric*** medicine dealing with diagnosis, treatment and prevention of disease in elderly. ***m. holistic*** an approach to healthcare based on theory that health is the result of harmony between body, mind and spirits and that stress of any kind including physical, psychological and social pressure is inimical to health. m. internal. The branch of medicine which deals with the diagnosis and nonsurgical treatment of diseases. ***m. nuclear*** application of nuclear energy in the diagnosis and treatment of disease, e.g. use of radioisotopes. ***m. occupational*** a branch of medicine dealing with prevention of disease and injury among people at work. It has two functions: to ensure suitability of an individual for particular work and to identify and control health and safety hazards in the work. ***m. oral*** the study and treatment of diseases of soft tissues of mouth. ***m. perinatal*** a specialized branch of medicine dealing with the management of mother and fetus during pregnancy and the infant immediately after delivery. ***m. physical and rehabilitation*** the branch of medicine concerned with use of physical agents and modalities including electricity light, heat, sound, mechanical devices and physical activity, in the diagnosis, treatment and prevention of disease. ***m. space*** a special branch of aviation medicine which deals with the stresses imposed on man by projection through and beyond the earth's atmosphere, flight in interplanetary space and return to earth. Such stresses include the agravic state, exposure to radiation and isolation. ***m. tropical*** the medical specialty concerned with diseases and disorders contracted in tropic or which exhibit unique characteristics in tropical countries

medium 1. a material in which a substance, an impulse, or information is transported. 2. a material in which interaction takes place. 3. culture medium. ***m. contrast***. In radiology, a substance of different radiopacity from that of the organ or tissue studied, to allow X-ray demonstration of contour or lumen. When the substance is more radiopaque than tissue is positive contrast, e.g. barium sulfate, iodine, when the substance is less radiopaque than tissue—negative contrast, e.g. air. ***m. Neal and Nicolle*** a saline rabbit's blood medium suitable for culture of *Leishmania donovani*

medroxyprogesterone a progesterone widely used as contraceptive and to treat precocious puberty in female, functional uterine bleeding, dysmenorrhea, endometriosis, threatened and habitual abortion and to suppress postpartum lactation

medulla the innermost or middle part of an organ. ***m. oblongata*** the caudal portion of brainstem that extends between pons and most rostral part of cervical spinal cord. Its upper posterior part forms the floor of fourth ventricle. It contains central nuclei of glossopharyngeal, vagus, accessory and hypoglossal nerves and regulates life sustaining cardiovascular and respiratory reflexes

mefenamic acid an agent with analgesic, anti-inflammatory and antipyretic properties

mefexamide a CNS stimulant, used to treat fatigue and depression

mefloquine antimalarial agent, schizonticide

megacolon abnormally large colon, either segmental or total, manifesting with constipation

megaesophagus abnormal enlargement of lower esophagus

megaloblastic anemia anemia due to vit B12 folic acid deficiency

megaloblast large nucleated erythrocyte precursor seen in bone marrow in vit B12 and folic acid deficiency

megaloureter abnormally dilated ureter in absence of obstruction

megavitamin a vitamin dose far in excess of daily recommended dose

megestrol acetate a synthetic progestin used as antineoplastic agent in palliation of metastatic endometrial cancer

meglitinide antidiabetic agent

Meig's syndrome polyserositis associated with ovarian fibroma

meiosis the reduction cell division during maturation of sex cells in which two nuclear cell divisions occur in quick succession thus forming four gametes each containing half the number of chromosomes

Meissner's corpuscle endorgan for touch present in epidermis

Meissner's plexus autonomic plexus in submucosa of alimentary tract regulating intestinal secretions

melalgia pain in the lower extremity melanin the natural pigment of hair and skin formed by oxidation of tyrosine via dopa and dopaquinone to a complex polymeric material

Melanoblast a derivative of neural crest which differentiates in an embryo into a melanocyte

melanocyte a cell capable of forming melanin, mature pigment cell

melanocyte stimulating hormone (MSH) a hormone from anterior pituitary that controls melanin formation and deposition

melanoma any benign or malignant melanocytic tumor

melasma cloasma affecting cheeks, forehead and lips

melena black tarry stool due to GI bleed. ***m. spuria*** melena in breastfed babies where blood originates from fissures in mother's nipple

membrane a thin tissue covering the surface of certain organs and lining the cavities of the body ***m. mucous*** contains mucous secreting cells and limes tubular structures, has four layers—epithelium, basement membrane, lamina propria, and lamina muscularis

menacme the height of menstrual activity in a woman life

menarche appearance of first menstrual period

Mendelson's syndrome aspiration of acid gastric juice into respiratory tract with severe bronchospasm and pulmonary edema

Mendel's law the law of inheritance, some being dominant and others recessive

meninges the three membranes that cover the brain and spinal cord; consisting of dense fibrous outer dura mater, thin innermost pia mater and trabeculated middle arachnoid mater. The last two are grouped as leptomeninges

meningioma tumor of meninges, specially from dura where arachnoid villi are numerous. Usually benign, producing symptoms due to compression or bone erosion, can undergo sarcomatous changes

meningitis Inflammation of meninges; can be cerebral, spinal or cerebrospinal. Pachymeningitis involves dura mater while leptomeningitis involves pia arachnoid but the latter is more common. ***m. mollarets*** acute meningitis with CSF pleocytosis and presence of abundant large endothelial cells in CSF; rapid spontaneous remission. ***m. tuberculous*** occurs due to hematogenous spread or rupture of cortical tuberculoma into CSF. Subacute onset with chronic course, often with encephalomyelopathy, cerebral arteritis, subarachnoid adhesions

meningocele a congenital sac-like skin covered protrusion of meninges through a defect in skull or vertebral column. Common to mid-occipital area or lumbosacral area

meningocyte a mesenchymal epithelial cell of subarachnoid space

Meningomyelitis Inflammation of spinal cord and its covering membranes

meningomyelocele a protrusion of spinal cord and associated meninges through a developmental defect in spinal canal

menometrorrhagia abnormal bleeding during or between menstrual periods.

menopause the normal physiologic cessation of menstruation commonly between 45 to 50 years of age. Frequent symptoms include hot flushes, headache, vulvar dyscomfort, painful sexual intercourse and mental depression. ***m. artificial*** cessation of menopause by irradiation or surgical removal of ovaries. ***m. premature*** early menopause, idiopathic or secondary to pituitary disease, systemic illness

menorrhagia excessive or prolonged menstruation, SYN: hypermenorrhea

menoschesis suppression of menses

menses periodic bloody discharge from uterus, called menstruation

menstruation the periodic discharge from uterus of a non-clotting bloody fluid at 4 to 5 weeks interval. ***m. anovulatory*** menstruation not preceded by ovulation. ***m. vicarious*** bleeding from sites other than uterus occurring at the time of normal menstruation

menthol peppermint camphor, an organic compound derived from peppermint oil or prepared synthetically. It provides a sensation of coolness in mucosal membranes by stimulation of cold receptors

mentoanterior in a face presentation, having the fetal chin pointing anteriorly in relation to maternal pelvis

mentoposterior in face presentation, having fetal chin pointing posteriorly in relation to maternal pelvis

mentotransverse in face presentation, having the fetal chin pointing laterally in relation to maternal pelvis

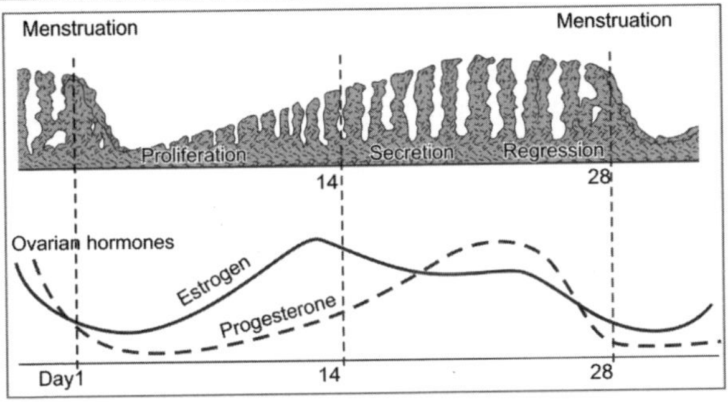

Endometrial changes related to ovulation and menstruation

mentum the anterior prominence of mandible produced by mental protuberance; the chin

meptazinol a narcotic analgesic, with less respiratory depression

mercury a heavy, silvery poisonous metallic element liquid at room temperature, atomic no. 80, used in thermometer

meridian a line surrounding a spherical body passing through both poles or half of such circle containing both poles

merocrine denoting secretory cells that remain intact during discharge of secretory products as those in the salivary glands

mesentery a double layer of peritoneum attaching various organs to body wall and conveying to them their blood vessels and nerves; commonly referred to peritoneal fold attaching small intestine to the posterior body wall

mesoderm the middle of primary germ layers, in between outer ectoderm and inner entoderm. From this layer are derived the majority of skeletal system, the circulatory system, the musculature, the excretory system and most of the reproductive system in vertebrates

mesosalpinx the upper free portion of broad ligament investing the Fallopian tube

mesovarium a short thick peritoneal fold that attaches ovary to posterior layer of broad ligament and permits passage of blood vessels and nerves to ovary

mestranol an estrogen used in preparation of oral contraceptive

metabiosis the dependence of an organism upon the preexistence of another for its development

metabolism a general term applied to chemical processes taking place in the living tissues for maintenance of life. ***m. acid-base*** the processes influencing hydrogen ion concentration in the body. ***m. aerobic*** metabolic activity dependent upon oxygen. ***m. intermediary*** the chemical changes associated with the synthesis of cellular components from food materials and their degradation

metabolite a substance taking part in or produced by metabolic activity

metacarpus the five bones of hand between the carpus and the phalanges

metafemale a female with 3X chromosomes (trisomy X) usually short-statured, mentally retarded and obese

metalloenzyme an enzyme having a metal ion as an integral part of its active form

metalloprotein a protein with metal ion bound to it. Many enzymes are metalloproteins

metamale a male with one X chromosome but two Y chromosomes; usually tall, lean, often having tendency toward aggressive behavior

metaphase the second stage of cell division by mitosis during which the chromatids are aligned along the equatorial plate of cell and attached by spindle fibers to centromere

metaplasia the abnormal transformation from one differentiated adult tissue to another type adult tissue within a given organ

metastasis transfer of a disease from its primary site to a distant location either by blood, lymphatic channel, CSF flow, etc.

metatarsus the anterior portion of foot between the toes and the instep. Composed of 5 cylindrical bones

metformin a structural analogue of phenformin, hypoglycemic agent

methadone a synthetic narcotic analgesic with morphine-like effect. It is used in opium withdrawal and as a maintenance treatment in heroin addicts

methanol methyl alcohol, prepared synthetically or from distillation of wood. Toxic and causes blindness when drunk

methemoglobin a derivative of hemoglobin with oxidized iron, hence incapable of carrying oxygen

methotrexate a potent folic acid antagonist used as cytotoxic agent and immunosuppressant

methotrimeprazine a phenothiazine with potent analgesic properties used in obstetric analgesia, and as a preanesthetic medication

methoxyflurane a colorless nonexplosive liquid used as a slow anesthetic

methyldopa sympathetic activity inhibitor used in treatment of hypertension

metoclopramide HCl central dopamine receptor antagonist; enhances response to acetylcholine of tissue in upper GI tract, which causes contraction of gastric muscle, relaxes pyloric and duodenal segments, increases peristalsis without stimulating secretions; antiemetic action occurs centrally; used in prevention of nausea, vomiting induced by chemotherapy, radiation, delayed gastric emptying, gastroesophageal reflux

metrectomy hysterectomy

metritis inflammation of uterus

metronidazole a nitroimidazole compound used for treatment of amebiasis, trichomoniasis, anaerobic infections

metropathia hemorrhagica excessive prolonged bleeding from uterus associated with cyst formation in the endometrium

metrorrhagia it is defined as irregular, acyclic bleeding from the uterus

metyrapone an inhibitor of adrenocortical steroid C-11 betahydroxylation, administered orally or IV as a diagnostic test to determine the capability of pituitary to increase production of corticotropin

miconazole antifungal, topically used 2%

microorganism any single celled organism

microbe a microorganism, a one-celled plant

microcephaly abnormally small hand hence always mentally subnormal

micrognathia abnormal smallness of jaw, specially the lower jaw producing bird-like profile

micronutrient any essential dietary constituent like vitamins and minerals required by body in small quantities

micturition the act of urination

midforceps application of forceps when the head is engaged but the leading part of the fetal head is above +2 station

midpelvis the area of pelvis extending from the posterior inferior aspect of symphysis in a line through ischial spines to sacrum intersecting it at S2 or S3 vertebra

midwife a woman who attends women during delivery

midwifery practical obstetrics

migraine a recurrent hemicranial intense headache associated with nausea, vomiting and visual disturbances. ***m. abdominal***. episodic abdominal pain, nausea, vomiting in migraine sufferers. ***m. complicated*** an attack of migraine accompanied by prolonged aphasia, hemi-plegia, hemianopia, epilepsy. etc. ***m. hemiplegic*** migraine in which recurrent attacks of hemiplegia occur. ***m. ophthalmoplegic*** oculomotor palsy occurring during an attack of migraine. ***m. equivalent*** symptoms produced by migraine-like mechanism but without an associated headache, e.g. transient partial loss of vision

milia distended sebaceous glands, which produce tiny pinpoint papules on the skin of newborn infants, commonly found over the bridge of the nose, chin and cheeks

miliaria skin eruption due to retention of sweat in sweat follicles. SYN: sweat fever, summer eruption; can be m.

papulosa, profunda, rubra and even pustular types

miliary of the size of a millet (2 mm diameter)

milk the secretion of mammary glands. ***m. witch's*** a few drops of milk expressed from newborn's nipple during first few days of life

milli the prefix indicating one thousandth

mineral any naturally occurring homogeneous inorganic substance, having a characteristic crystalline structure and chemical composition

miscarriage spontaneous abortion

miscarry to give birth to a nonviable fetus

misdiagnosis wrong diagnosis

missed abortion the product of conception fails to grow and is retained within uterus

mitochondria a double membrane cytoplasmic organelle, self-reproducing, present in cell cytoplasm of all living cells; responsible for energy production (ATP), each cell has several hundreds of mitochondria, each of 15.00 Å length

mitosis multiplication or division of a cell that results in formation of two daughter cells normally receiving the same chromosome and DNA as that of original cell

mitral left atrioventricular valve

mittelschmerz intermenstrual pain specially at the time of ovulation

mobilization a process or an operation whereby an object or a substance is freed or made mobile

molding the process of shaping. The changes in shape of fetal head as it passes through the birth canal

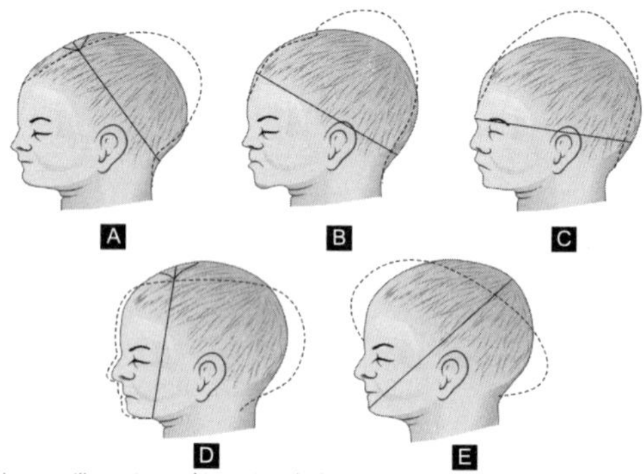

Diagrams illustrating molding when the head presents in varying degrees of flexion: (A) Vertex presentation; head well-flexed; (B) Vertex presentation; head partially flexed; (C) Vertex presentation; head deflexed; (D) Face presentation; (E) Brow presentation

M

mole 1. intrauterine mass. 2. pigmented cellular nevus; circumscribed pigmented growth on skin. 3. Gram molecule. ***m. carneous*** a spontaneous abortion in which the ovum is surrounded by a capsule of clotted blood. ***m. hydatidiform*** a developmental anomaly of placenta consisting of a nonmalignant mass of clear vesicles resembling bunch of grapes formed from cystic swellings of chorionic villi. The moles may cause uterine enlargement disproportionate to period of gestation

molecule the smallest unit of a substance which can exist in a free state and still retain the chemical properties of the substance

Mongolian blue spot a smooth brown to gray blue nerves in the sacral region of newborn

Mongolism Down syndrome due to trisomy 21

Mongoloid having characteristics or resembling mongolism

monilia a genus of molds or fungi, commonly known as fruit molds, now called candida

monitor 1. to keep close watch over. 2. an apparatus used to record or display data. ***m. apnea*** an alarm

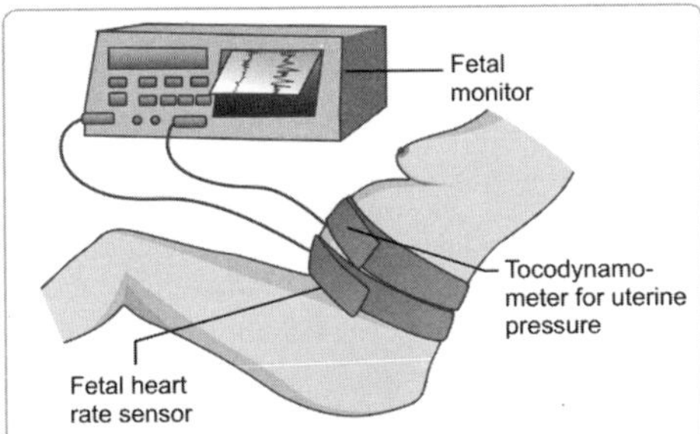

External fetal monitoring

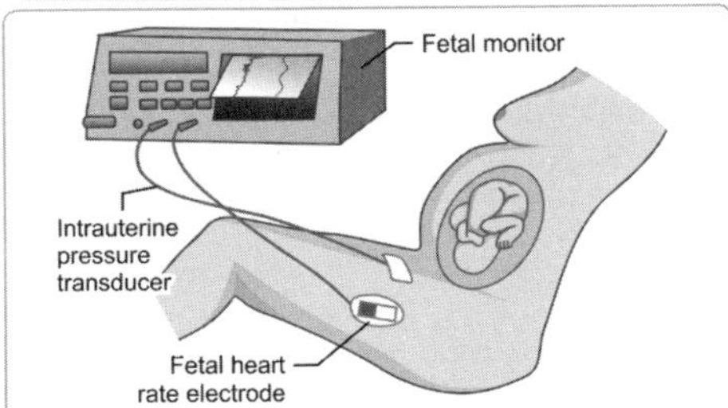

Internal fetal monitoring

system for alarming attendants to the occurrence of apnea commonly in a premature infant. ***m. cardiac*** continuous display of cardiac rhythm in a screen to detect irregularities in the heart rhythm. ***m. electronic fetal*** an electronic instrument monitoring fetal heart rate and patterns of uterine contraction

monoamine compound containing only one amine group. ***m. oxidase*** an enzyme that catalyzes the oxidation of a wide variety of physiologic amines into aldehydes and ammonia. It is important for catabolism of epinephrine and tyramine

monolclonal derived from a single cell or clone of single cell. ***m. antibody*** being derived from single clone of cells the antibody molecules are identical and will react with same antigenic site

monosaccharide a carbohydrate which cannot be further broken down, simple sugar

monosomy condition in which one chromosome of a pair of homologous chromosomes is missing

monozygotic denoting identical twins, or twins formed by division into two of the embryo derived from a single fertilized egg

mons in anatomy, a slight prominence, or elevation. ***m. pubis*** the fleshy prominence formed by a pad of fatty tissue over the symphysis pubis in female

montelukast leukotriene antagonist for asthma

Montgomery's glands or tubercles sebaceous glands around nipple

mood A prevailing emotional state of mind

morbid diseased, pathologic, pertaining to or affected by disease

morbidity the condition of being diseased; within a given population, the number of sick persons or cases of disease recorded as of a stated point in time or over a stated period. Thus morbidity can be expressed as the number of new cases arising (incidence) or the number of cases existing whether old or new (prevalence)

more reflex a neonatal reflex in which the baby extends the arms to any sudden movement or noise sick and premature babies lack this reflex

morgue a place where dead bodies are kept pending identification, autopsy or burial/cremation

Moro reflex a normal reflex of young infants in which there is a sudden loud noise causing the child to stretch out the arms and flex the legs

morphine the principal alkaloid of opium; white, crystalline, insoluble in water, alcohol and ether; potent narcotic analgesic, can cause respiratory depression. Repeated use causes physical dependence and addiction. Used as morphine sulfate or tartarate

morphology the study of configuration or structure of living organism

mortality the quality of being mortal. The death rate. **m. neonatal** death during first month or four weeks of life. **m. perinatal** the combined mortality from stillbirths and deaths in first week of life

morula a cluster of cleaving blastomeres resulting from early division of zygote; a stage in the development of the embryo prior to the blastula

mosaic 1. in genetics, an individual whose cells consist of at least two genotypically distinct populations that arose after fertilization through somatic mutation or somatic nondisjunction

mother surrogate one who replaces an individual's mother in emotional feelings. A mother who bears offspring of another

motilin a gastrointestinal peptide of 22 amino acids located in enterochromaffin cells, chiefly of duodenum and upper jejunum that stimulates gastric and colonic motility

motion sickness a condition marked by nausea, dizziness, and often vomiting and headache, induced by some movement as in travelled by airplane, train, bus or ship

motor 1. carrying or transmitting an impulse to a peripheral effector organ of the nervous system, either to elicit a response or to inhibit it. 2. producing movement

moulding the process of overriding of cranial bones at the sutures and fontanelles where by the fetus adopts itself to the pelvis. Moulding if abnormal in direction excessive or extremely rapid can tear the falx cerebri and tentorium cerebelli causing intracranial hemorrhage

moxibustion a technique used in traditional Chinese medicine that uses moxa sticks that acts as a heat source when held over acupuncture points. It is used to turn breech to apholic presentation

mucoid resembling mucus

mucopolysaccharidoses (MPS) a group of inherited disorders with accumulation of mucopolysaccharides in reticuloendothelial system, intimal smooth muscle cells and fibroblasts within body; manifesting with coarse facies, mental retardation, corneal clouding, skeletal dysplasia, joint stiffness, etc. ***MPS IH*** is known as Hurler syndrome. It is due to deficiency of the enzyme alpha-L-iduronidase with accumulation of heparan sulfate and dermatan sulphate. ***MPS IS Scheie's syndrome*** it is a variant of ***MPS IH*** but without mental retardation. ***MPS IHS*** it is intermediate between MPSIH and MPSIS. ***MPS II Hunter syndrome*** it is due to deficiency of L-iduronosulfate sulfatase. Unlike MPS IH there is no corneal clouding. ***MPS III sanfilippo syndrome*** corneal clouding is absent and skeletal growth is normal. ***MPS IV Morquio's syndrome*** the deficient enzyme is N-acetyl galactosamine-6-sulfatase. Distinguishing features, are dwarfism, kyphoscoliosis, cardiac lesions and joint hypermobility. *MPS VI*

Maroteaux-Lamy syndrome. Deficient enzyme is N-acetyl galactosamine-4-sulfatase. Clinically it is similar to *MPS IH* but there is no mental retardation. ***MPS VII*** the deficient enzyme is beta-glucuronidase

mucopurulent containing mucus and pus

mucosa a mucous membrane with epithelial lining, basement membrane, and often lamina propria. It may contain goblet cells, may be keratinized and the covering epithelium may be stratified squamous, columnar or pseudostratified columnar depending upon location

mucus-trap suction apparatus a type of suction apparatus used in aspirating the nasopharyx and trachea of a newborn infant. It consists of a catheter with a mucus trap, which prevents mucus from the baby from being drawn into the operator's mouth

mucus a viscid secretion containing mucin, leukocytes, epithelial cells, etc. secreted by mucous membrane

multigravida a woman who has been pregnant two or more times. SYN: multipara

multipara a woman who has given birth to two or more babies live or still excluding abortions

multiple gestation pregnancy with more than one fetus, e.g. twins

multiple pregnancy a pregnancy of more than one fetus

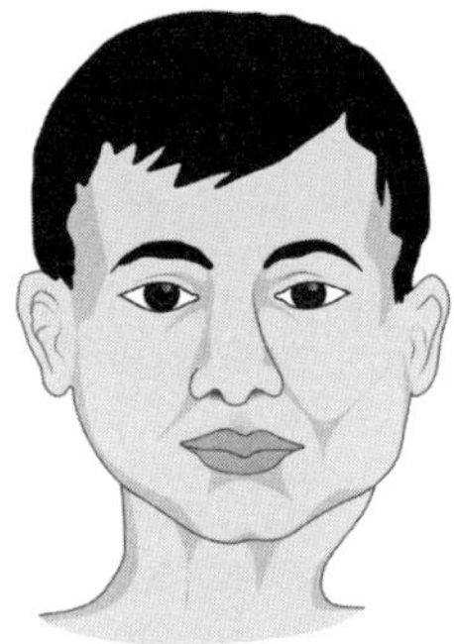

Mumps

multiple sclerosis (MS) an autoimmune demyelinating disorder due to decrease in suppressor T lymphocyte function, manifesting with visual loss, gait disorder, motor dysfunction and bladder bowel disturbance. Multiple sites of involvement in brain and spinal cord common

mumps a febrile viral disease characterized by inflammation of salivary and parotid glands

murmur a soft blowing or rasping sound heard during cardiac auscultation; produced due to excess blood flow through normal valves or normal flow through diseased valves. ***m. Austin Flint*** a mid or late mitral diastolic murmur heard in aortic regurgitation due to partial closure of mitral valve due to aortic regurgitant jet. ***m. Carey Coomb*** diastolic murmur of mitral valvulitis in rheumatic fever. ***m. Durozeiz*** systolic and diastolic murmurs heard over femoral artery in aortic insufficiency. ***m. Graham Steell's*** early diastolic murmur of pulmonary insufficiency in pulmonary hypertension

muscle contractile tissue of mesodermal origin with properties like irritability, conductivity, and elasticity. Can be smooth, striated and cardiac. Smooth muscles (involuntary muscle) are found to line GI tract, bronchi, urinary and genital ducts, gall bladder, urinary bladder. The cells are fusiform or spindle-shaped with one central nucleus. Striated (skeletal) muscles are under conscious control. The muscle fibers are grouped into bundles called fasciculi and each cell or fiber has multiple nuclei. Denervation causes complete paralysis of striated muscle but not of cardiac or smooth muscle

muscle cramp painful contraction of muscle, idiopathic or due to electrolyte imbalance

muscular dystrophy a group of genetically determined painless degenerative myopathies that progressively cripple. ***MD Duchenne*** sex-linked recessive developing in childhood with pseudomuscular hypertrophy causing early death

mutation change in genetic structure; can be natural or induced by drugs, chemicals and radiation

mutism unable to speak. ***m. akinetic*** condition in which patient can neither speak nor can move body parts

myalgia pain in the muscles often with tenderness

myasthenia weakness of muscles. ***m. gravis*** an autoimmune disease with extreme muscle weakness due to presence of acetylcholine receptor antibodies

Mycobacterium a genus of acid-fast organism causing leprosy and tuberculosis. They are gram-positive, nonspore-forming and nonmotile rods. ***m. atypical*** forms of mycobacteria causing mild but resistant form of tuberculosis in man. They are *M. avium*-intracellulare, *M. kansasii*, *M. chelonei*, *M. marinum*, *M. xenopi*, etc.

mycoplasma organisms in between bacteria and viruses, responsible for atypical pneumonia, urethritis; common forms are — *M. hominis*, *M. orale*, *M. salivarium*

myelocele protrusion of spinal cord through a defect in spinal arch—usually spina bifida

myeloma a tumor originating from marrow element. ***m. multiple*** a plasma cell tumor with multiple lytic bone lesions and increased paraprotein in blood and urine

myelomeningocele a condition where spinal cord along with meningeal covering protrudes through the spinal defect

myocardial infarction death of myocardium usually due to coronary thrombosis or spasm

myocarditis inflammation of myocardium, mostly viral, due to coxsackie group of viruses

myocardium the thick middle muscle layer of heart

myoepithelial cells spindle-shaped contractile cells found between glandular elements and basement membrane of sweat, mammary and salivary glands

myoma a tumor containing muscle tissue

myometrium the muscular layer of uterus

myxedema a condition resulting from hypofunction of thyroid; commonly autoimmune or due to iodine lack, dyshormonogenesis

myxoma tumor composed of mucous connective tissue similar to that present in embryo or umbilical cord. It is soft, gray, lobulated, translucent and incompletely encapsulated

Müllerian duct the paired embryonic ducts developing into uterus, uterine tubes and vagina in female

nabothian cyst retention cysts of the nabothian glands in the cervical canal, usually associated with ectropion

Naegele German obstetrician (1777-1851). ***n. obliquity*** anterior parietal presentation of fetal head in labor. ***n. pelvis*** an obliquely contracted pelvis. ***n. rule*** the method of counting expected date of delivery by counting 90 days backwards from LMP and adding 7 days to that date

naevus a circumscribed area of dilated superficial vessels; a birth mark

nalmefene HCl opioid antagonist; reverses the effects of opioids by competitive antagonism of opioid receptors; used in management of opioid overdose and complete or partial reversal of opioid drug effects, including respiratory depression

nalorphine narcotic antagonist

naltrexone narcotic antagonist

nandrolone anabolic steroid

nape back of neck

napkin rash rash in the area covered by napkins in neonate

naproxen/naproxen sodium non-steroidal anti-inflammatory; inhibits prostaglandin synthesis by interfering with cyclo-oxygenase needed for biosynthesis; possesses analgesic, anti-inflammatory, antipyretic properties; used in mild-to-moderate pain, osteoarthritis, rheumatoid, gouty arthritis, primary dysmenorrhea

narcissism sexual pleasure sought by observing one's own naked body; self-admiration

narcolepsy recurrent attacks of uncontrollable desire to sleep but easily awakenable

narcotic an agent that in moderate doses relieves pain but in higher doses causes coma and respiratory paralysis

nares the nostrils ***n. posterior*** the opening of nose into nasopharynx

nasal flarings A sign of respiratory distress; the edges of the nostrils fan outward as the baby inhales

nasogastric tube tube inserted through nose into the stomach for feeding or stomach wash

nasopharynx part of pharynx situated above the level of soft palate

naturopathy a therapeutic system that employs natural forces as light, heat, air and water to cure ailments rather than drugs

nausea unpleasant epigastric sensation preceding vomiting. ***n. gravidarum*** morning sickness of pregnancy

nebulizer an apparatus for producing fine spray or mist

Necator a genus of nematode hookworms, includes ***n. americanus***

necrobiosis degeneration and swelling of collagen in the dermis, common to diabetics

necrosis death of tissue following cut-off in blood supply, physical or chemical injury, infection, etc. ***n. coagulation*** necrosis where the necrosed area is converted to a homogeneous mass

N

necrotizing enterocolitis inflammatory disease of bowel in neonate with edema, ation and hemorrhage that may progress to perforation and peritonitis

negligence in low, the failure to do something that a reasonable person of ordinary prudence would or would not do in a given situation

Neisseria gram-negative bacteria, lie in pairs, e.g. *N. gonorrhoeae*, *N. meningitidis*, *N. sicca* and *N. catarrhalis* (last two cause respiratory infection and often endocarditis)

neomycin an aminoglycoside antibiotic isolated from *Streptomyces*, toxic to kidney and eighth cranial nerve but effective against many gram +ve and -ve bacteria, particularly resistant tubercle bacilli

neonatal pertaining to first 4 weeks after birth

neonate child upto 4 weeks old

neonatologist a pediatrician who specializes in caring for newborn infants, particularly at risk and sick babies

neonatology a branch of pediatrics dealing with disorders of newborn infant

neoplasm a tumor or new growth. ***n. benign*** growth having a definite capsule and noninfiltrating. ***n. malignant*** growth that lacks a capsule, infiltrates surrounding structures or has distant metastasis, or recurs after surgery

nephritis inflammation of kidneys involving glomeruli, tubules and interstitial tissue singly or combinedly, can be acute/chronic; interstitial, salt losing

nephron the glomerulus, Bowman's capsule and the tubule system which act as functioning unit of kidney and number one million in each kidney

nephropathy any diseased condition of kidney including inflammatory, degenerative, arteriosclerotic lesions, e.g. analgesic nephropathy, hypokalemic nephropathy, membranous nephropathy, etc.

nephrosis noninflammatory degenerative disease of kidney, e.g. lipoid nephrosis manifesting as nephrotic syndrome

nephrotic syndrome a symptom complex with leakage of protein in urine due to damage to capillary wall of glomeruli

nerve block a block by local analgesic agents in nerve conduction

nerve bundles of nerve fibers connecting CNS or spinal cord with various parts of body. ***n. adrenergic*** sympathetic nerves that liberate noradrenaline at the neuroeffector synapse. ***n. afferent*** any nerve that transmits impulses from periphery towards centre. ***n. cholinergic*** parasympathetic nerve liberating acetylcholine for impulse transmission. ***n. efferent*** nerves that transmit impulses from center towards periphery. ***n. mixed*** nerve contains both motor (efferent) and sensory (afferent) fibers. ***n. secretory*** nerve that stimulates secretion from glands. ***n. spinal*** 31 pairs of peripheral nerves, 8 cervical, 12 thoracic, 5 lumbar, 5 sacral, 1 coccygeal

neuralgia sharp pain along the course of nerve. ***n. glossopharyngeal*** severe pain in the back of throat, tonsils and middle ear along the distribution of glossopharyngeal nerve. ***n. trigeminal*** neuralgia involving the gasserian ganglion or one or more branches of trigeminal nerve

neural tube defect defective closure of neural tube during embryogenesis leading to defects like spina bifida, anencephaly, meningocele, meningomyelocele

neuritis inflammation of a nerve

neuroblastoma a malignant tumor of neuroblasts in children giving rise to cells of sympathetic nervous system; specially adrenal medulla

neuron a nerve cell; consisting of cell body and its processes, i.e. axons and dendrites. ***n. afferent*** neuron conducting impulses to the brain and spinal cord. ***n. associative*** neuron coordinating impulses between sensory and motor neurons. ***n. efferent*** neurons conducting impulses away from brain and spinal cord. ***n. lower motor*** neuron with cell body in anterior gray column. ***n. upper motor*** neuron with cell body in motor cortex. ***n. preganglionic*** neuron of autonomic nervous system whose cell body lies in central nervous system and axon terminates in peripheral ganglia. ***n. postganglionic*** neurone whose cell body lies in an autonomic ganglion and its axon terminates in effector organ

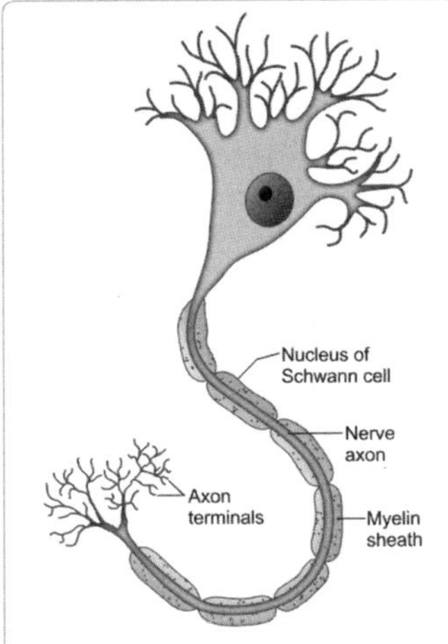

Neuron

neurosis a minor mental disease where person's insight is maintained. ***n. anxiety*** neurosis where vague anxiety or apprehension interferes with effective functioning. ***n. obsessional*** neurosis where obsession dominates

neurosyphilis syphilis affecting the nervous system. ***n. meningovascular*** the meninges and the cerebral blood vessels are affected the most with ischemia, infarction, hydrocephalus

N

neurotransmitter chemical substance released by stimulation of presynaptic neuron that excites or inhibits target cell, e.g. acetylcholine, dopamine, norepinephrine

neutron electrically neutral particle equal in mass to proton

nevus congenitally discolored localized area of skin; vascular skin tumor due to hyperplastic blood vessels. ***n. junctional*** nevus in the basal layer of epidermis appearing as a nonhairy pigmented area, with high malignancy potential

newborn period from birth through the first 28 days of life

niacin a water-soluble vitamin of B complex group present in animal and plant tissues, required for synthesis of enzymes

nicotine alkaloid of tobacco, a vasoconstrictor, stimulant and addictive agent

nifedipine calcium channel blocker; Inhibits calcium ion influx across cell membrane during cardiac depolarization; produces relaxation of coronary vascular smooth muscle, dilates coronary arteries; increases myocardial oxygen delivery in patients with vasospastic angina; dilates peripheral arteries; used in chronic stable angina pectoris, vasospastic angina, hypertension

night blindness (nyctalopia) inability to see in dark due to deficient rhodopsin or its slow regeneration after exposure to light, a feature of retinal pigmentary degeneration or vitamin A deficiency

nipple the conical protuberance at center of breast containing erectile tissue and pierced by milk ducts

nitrazepam benzodiazepine, anxiolytic

nitrofurantoin urinary antibacterial agent

nitroglycerine any nitrate of glycerol used for vasodilatation in angina pectoris as 2% ointment or tablets; be kept in tinted glass (not plastic) container without cotton plug

nitrous oxide inhalation anesthetic used in conjunction with oxygen. SYN: laughing gas

node a small swelling or constriction. ***n. AV*** the mass of Purkinje fibers at lower end of interatrlal septum giving origin to ***bundle of His***. **n. Bouchard's** bony enlargement of proxymal interphalangeal joint in osteoarthritis. ***n. Heberden's*** nodes in terminal interphalangeal joints of hand in osteoarthritis. ***n's of Ranvier*** constriction of myelin sheath along the course of medulated nerve fiber. ***n's Osler*** tender nodes in pulp of finger and toes in subacute bacterial endocarditis. ***n's of Parrot*** osteophytes around anterior fontanel in congenital syphilis. ***n. Schmorl's*** prolapse of nucleus pulposus into vertebral body. ***n. singer's*** small white nodes on vocal cords due to vocal abuse. ***n. sinoatrial*** node in the wall of right atrium near entry of SVC acting as the pacemaker of heart

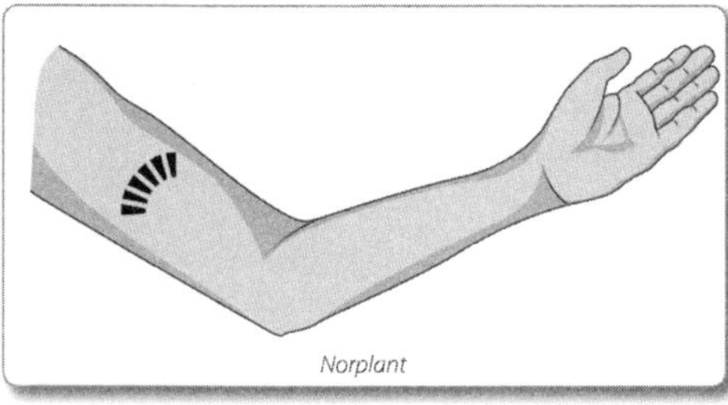

Norplant

nodule a small node; collection of cells. ***n. Aschoff's*** myocardial nodule with central fibrinoid necrosis with surrounding epithelioid cells, a feature of rheumatic carditis

nonmaleficence the concept in the healthcare services of the duty to avoid harm to the interests of others

nonspecific urethritis a sexually transmitted disease caused by Chlamydia

nonstress test a noninvasive test used to determine fetal well-being, involves external fetal monitoring of the fetal heart rate and observing the response of the heart rate to fetal movement; interpreted as reactive or nonreactive

norepinephrine (norafrenaline) vasopressor hormone secreted by adrenal medulla

norethandrolone an anabolic steroid

norethindrone progestational agent

norethisterone a progesterone only contraceptive pill, useful for breastfeeding mothers

norfloxacin a quinolone with broad spectrum antibacterial activity

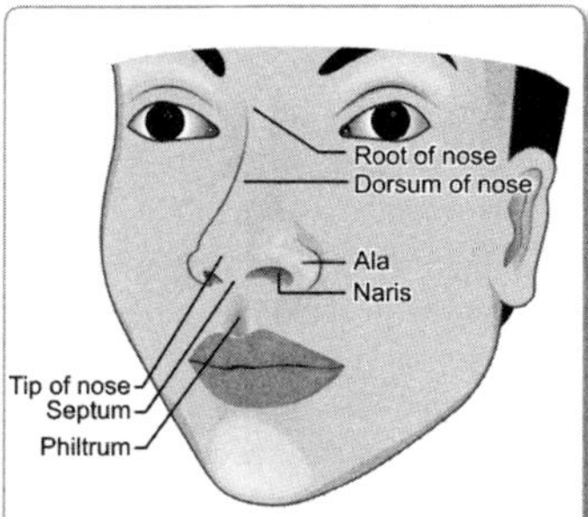

Nose

norgestrel a progestational agent used for hormonal contraception

normoblast type of nucleated red blood cell during erythropoiesis

norplant a subdermal implant used for long-term contraception. It consists of six silastic (silicone rubber) capsules containing 35 mg (each) of levonorgestrel (100)

nose the organ of olfaction that bears the nostrils and envelopes the anterior part of the nasal cavity

nosocomial relating to or occurring in a hospital

nosophilia an unusual desire to be sick

notifiable diseases all communicable and contagious diseases to be notified to local health authorities under the statutes of law

notochord a flexible supporting rod of cells that forms the supporting axis of the body in chordates and in the embryos of higher vertebrates

nuchal back of neck, US measurement of skin thickness at back of neck at 11–13 weeks can be helpful in diagnosis of Down's syndrome

nuchal displacement a complication of breech delivery when arm is displaced behind child's neck

nuclear family family of husband, wife and children, without grandparents, auncles and aunts

nuclear magnetic resonance when certain atomic nuclei with odd number of protons or neutrons or both are subjected to strong magnetic field they absorb and reemit electromagnetic energy. Application of a radio frequency pulse causes deflection in the net magnetization vector and image production. The technique is useful for imaging of brain, soft tissue and heart

nuclear medicine medicine dealing with diagnostic, therapeutic and investigative aspects of radionuclides

nucleic acid a complex product consisting of pentose, phosphoric acid, purines and pyrimidines

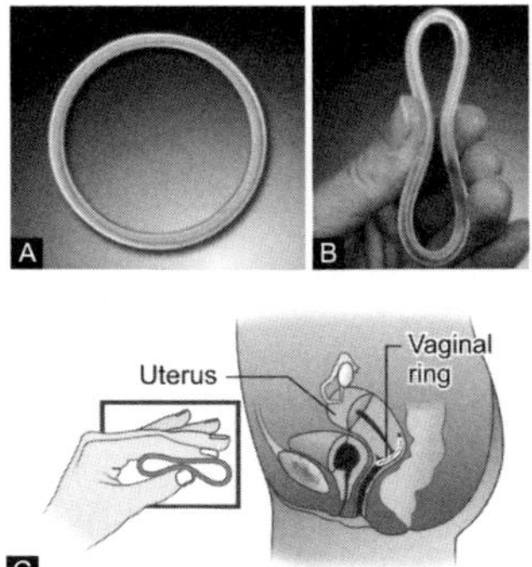

NuvaRing

nucleolus a spherical body within the nucleus

nullipara a woman who has not produced a viable child

nurse person providing healthcare

nursery newborn care center

nursery school school for children of 2½–5 years

nutrition the process involved in assimilation and utilization of food

NuvaRing a vaginal ring containing female hormones, ethinyl estradiol and etonogestrel that prevent ovulation (release of an egg from an ovary)

nylon a synthetic material of exceptional strength used for sutures

nystagmus involuntary to and fro movement of eye ball

nystatin antifungal agent

obese fatty

oblique slanting or diagonal

obliquity the state of slanting. ***o. Litzmann's*** inclining of fetal head with posterior parietal bone presenting. ***o. Naegele's*** inclining fetal head with oblique biparietal diameter in relation to pelvic brim

oblongata oblong, e.g. medulla oblongata

obstetric branch of medicine dealing with childbirth, puerperium and management of pregnancy

obstetric conjugate the pelvic diameter measured from sacral promontory to upper inner border of symphysis pubis

obstetrician doctor skilled in art of obstetrics

obstructed labor a state in which it is mechanically impossible for the child to be born often requiring cesarean delivery common factors are cephalopelvic disproportion, Bandl's ring placenta previa

obturator anything that closes a cavity or opening

obturator foramen an opening in the membrane

occipito anterior the fetal occiput is the lowest and presenting pase as in well-flexed fetus presenting anteriorly in maintenance pelvis

occipito posterior the fetal occiput directed towards right or left of sacroiliac joint of mother's pelvis

occlusion the state of being closed

occlusive cap rubber cap to cover cervix to prevent conception

occult blood test examination of stool for microscopic hemorrhage

oedema excessive accumulation of fluid with weight gain 50% of women develop mild ankle oedema towards term

oestrogen see estrogen

ointment a semisolid medicinal preparation used as a vehicle for external medication, as an emollient, or as a cosmetic agent

olfaction the act of smelling

oligohydramnios less than normal amniotic fluid, a feature of postmaturity

oligomenorrhea scanty or infrequent menstruation

oliguria decreased formation of urine

ombudsman a person appointed to receive complaints about unfair administration

omentum a double fold of peritoneum attached to stomach, the portion attached to greater curvature of stomach extending to envelop the intestines is called greater omentum and the portion extending from lesser curvature of stomach to transverse fissure of liver is called lesser omentum

omnivorous eating both meat and vegetables

omphalitis inflammation of umbilicus

omphalocele congenital umbilical hernia

O

oncogene genes that can cause tumor formation

oncogenesis tumor initiation and growth

oncology the branch of medicine dealing with tumors

onychomycosis fungal infection of nails

oocyte encysted form of zygote in certain sporozoa

oogenesis growth and maturation of ovum

oogonium the primordial cell from which an oocyte originates

ookinesis the mitotic phenomenon taking place with an ovum during maturation and fertilization

oophorectomy removal of an ovary

oophoritis inflammation of ovary

oophorrhaphy suture of displaced ovary to pelvic wall

operant conditioning conditioning or influencing behavior by rewarding for certain desired acts

operculum the plus of mucus that fills the cervical canal during pregnancy and is shed at beginning of labor

ophthalmia inflammation of the eye. ***o. gonococcal*** severe purulent conjunctivitis. ***o. neonatorum*** severe purulent conjunctivitis of newborn, usually gonococcal. ***o. sympathetic*** uveitis of healthy eye following trauma to other eye

ophthalmoscope instrument for examination of fundus and retina

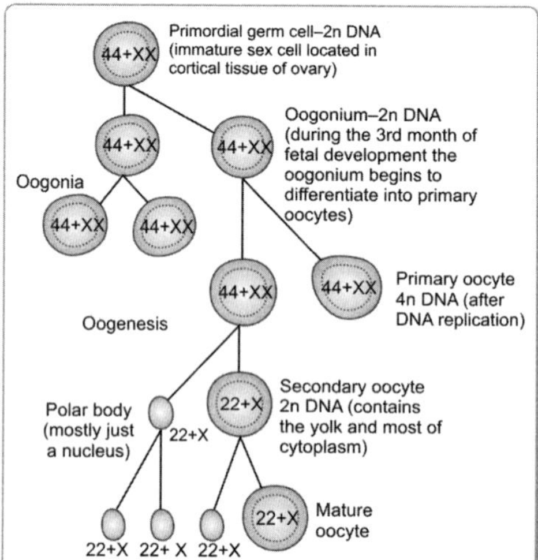

Oogonium

opiate receptor specific receptors on cell surfaces to which combine the opiates, endorphins and encephalins for mediating their effects

opioid synthetic narcotics or endogenous substances with opium-like activity, e.g. encephalins and endorphins

opisthotomus a form of tetanic spasm where the body bends backwards

opium substance derived from juice of unripe capsules of poppy

opportunistic a microorganism which does not ordinarily cause disease but becomes pathogenic under certain circumstances

opsonin a substance present in blood that prepares bacteria for phagocytosis

opsonization the process through which an antibody and/or complement modifies an antigen (e.g. bacteria and other cells) so as to make them more readily engulfed and destroyed by white blood cells

optic pertaining to vision

oral contraceptive pill 1. combined estrogen progesterone pill with failure rate of 0.1–1 per 100 women years 2. posterone only pill prescribed to breastfeeding mothers or those of 35 years with failure rate of 0.3–5 per 100 women year

orbit the bony socket containing the eye formed by frontal, sphenoid, ethmoid, maxillary and palatal bone

orchiopexy surgical fixation of testis

orchitis inflammation of testis

organic 1. pertains to living organisms. 2. in chemistry pertaining to compounds of carbon. 3. physical not mental or psychogenic

organism any living entity capable of carrying on life process

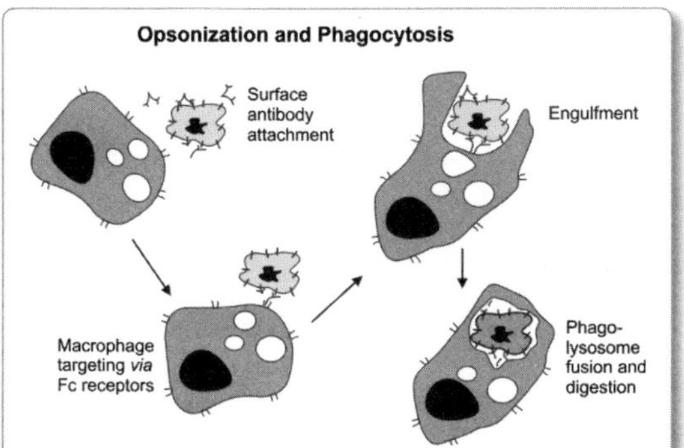

Opsonization

O

organogenesis development of organs

orgasm the intense pleasure of sexual intercourse at climax with pelvic throbbing, contraction of levator ani and anal sphincters to culminate in seminal ejaculation

orifice an opening or entrance to a cavity

oropharynx portion of pharynx below the level of soft palate

orthostatic standing upright. ***o. albuminuria***. Albuminuria when assuming erect position. ***o. hypotension***. Fall in blood pressure while assuming erect position

Ortolani's test a method of diagnosing congenital dislocation of hip

os 1 bone. ***o. calcis*** the heel bone or calcaneus; ***o. innominate*** nameless bone right and left, articulate with sacrum to firm pelvic girdle 2. a mouth or opening ***o. external*** Opening of cervix to vagina, ***o. internal*** Cervical canal opening into cavity of uterus

Osiander's sign Increased pulsation felt in the lateral vaginal fornices

osmol the quantity of a solute existing in solution as molecules, commonly stated in grams, that is osmotically equivalent to one mole of an ideally behaving electrolyte

osmosis the passage of solvent through a membrane from a dilute solution into a more concentrated one

osmotic pressure the pressure developed when two solutions of different concentrations of some solute are separated by a semipermeable membrane

ossification the formation of bone

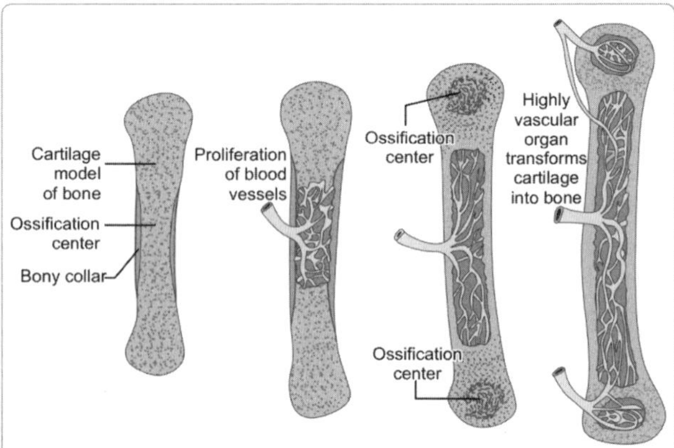

Ossification

osteoblast cells of mesenchymal origin concerned in the formation of bony tissue

osteogenesis imperfecta autosomal dominant disease characterized by hypoplasia of bone and cartilage leading to fracture with minimal trauma, hypermobility, blue sclera

osteomalacia failure of ossification due to fall in serum calcium, possibly resulting from vitamin D deficiency, inadequate calcium in the diet, renal disease, and/or steatorrhea. Manifestations include incomplete fractures and gradual resorption of cortical and cancellous bone

osteomyelitis inflammation of marrow and hard tissue of bone

osteopathy a school of healing art which teaches that the body is a vital mechanical organism whose structural and functional integrity are coordinated and interdependent

osteopetrosis a familial disease characterized by excessive radiographic density with a tendency towards fracture and obliteration of marrow cavity

osteoporosis absolute decrease in quantity of bone tissue with enlarging marrow cavity and Haversian spaces

osteosclerosis abnormal increase in density of bone

otitis media inflammation of the ear

otolith calcareous concretions within membranous labyrinth

otosclerosis a disease characterized by new bone formation around oval window with immobilization of foot plate of stapes and hence conductive hearing loss

otoscope instrument for visualization of external ear and the tympanic membrane

out growth growth or development from a preexisting structure or state

outlet route of exit or egress **o. pelvic**. The lower opening of pelvis bounded ischial spines

output yield ***o. cardiac*** volume of blood expelled from left ventricle per minute. ***o. urine*** when <400 mL/day urine passed in 24 hours; it is oliguria

ovarian agenesis failure of development of ovaries. SYN: Turner's syndrome

ovarian follicle an ovum and the granulosa cell surrounding it occupying the cortex of ovary

ovarian hormones 1. follicular hormones—estradiol, estrone, and estriol 2. luteal hormone-progesterone

ovarian pregnancy fertilized ovum implanted on ovary

ovarian vein syndrome ureteric obstruction by large dilated ovarian vein, commonly right, during pregnancy causing urinary stasis and infection

ovary the glandular female reproductive organ giving rise to ova

ovotestis ovarian and testicular tissue combined in the same gonad

ovulation the maturation and discharge of ovum

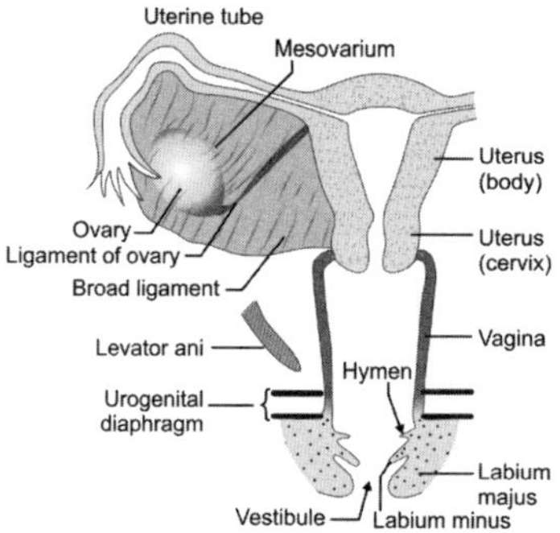

Ovary

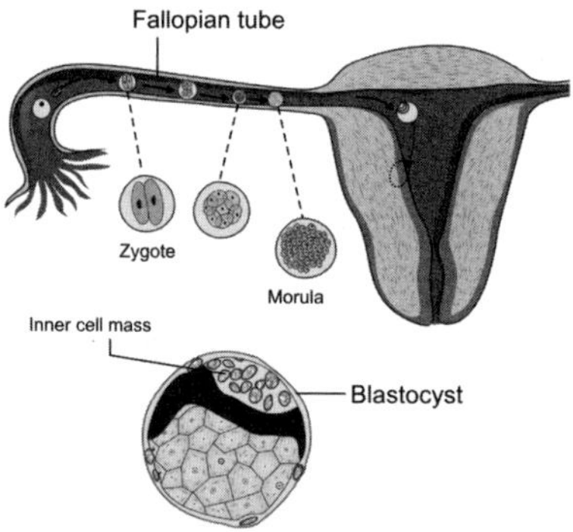

Development of the fertilized ovum

ovum the female germ cell

oxazepam a benzodiazepine, tranquilizer

oxidase enzyme that promotes an oxidation reaction

oxidation an increase in positive valence of an element or decrease in negative valence occurring due to loss of electrons; the process of combining with oxygen

oxygen the colorless and odorless gas that supports combustion and essential to animal life. It constitutes one-fifth of the atmosphere, eight-ninth of water and one-half of the earth's crust

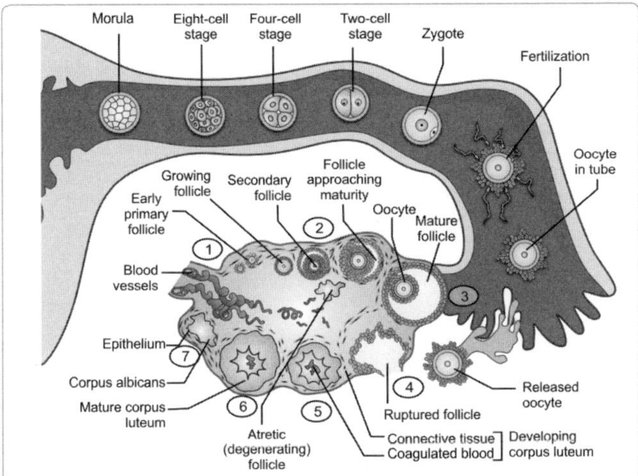

Ovulation

oxyhemoglobin hemoglobin combined with oxygen

oxytetracycline an antibiotic of tetracycline group from *Streptomyces rimosus*. Where the hydrogen atom of tetracycline is replaced by a hydroxyl group

oxytocin an octapeptide secreted by posterior pituitary, causes uterine contraction and promotes lactation

oxytocin challenge test a test to assess fetal wellbeing by administering oxytocin via intravenous infusion to induce uterine contractions and assessing the fetus's response; can be interpreted as positive (abnormal), negative (normal) or suspicious (inconclusive)

ozone O_3 an allotropic form of oxygen, a powerful oxidizing agent, used as disinfectant

P

pack a dry or moist; hot or cold blanket or sheet used for therapeutic purpose

packed cell blood containing cellular elements only, devoid of plasma

Paget's disease skeletal disease of elderly with thickening, softening and bending of bones

pain sensory and emotional experience associated with irritation/ inflammation of tissue

palate roof of the mouth separating it from nasal cavity

palliative an agent which relieves but does not cure a disease

palmar erythema reddening of the palms seen in pregnant women

palpation examination by application of hand or fingers

palpitation rapid throbbing pulsation of heart

palsy paralysis/loss of ability to act. **p. Bell's** lower motor facial palsy. **p. bulbar** paralysis of lower cranial nerves. **p. cerebral** nonprogressive palsy of childhood from developmental defect of brain, or birth asphyxia or trauma. **p. Erb's** palsy of C5–C6 due to lesion of brachial plexus. ***p. shaking*** paralysis agitans

pancreas a compound acinotubular gland in front of L1–L2 vertebra behind the stomach, secretes hormones like insulin, glucagon and digestive enzymes. ***p. annular*** a portion of pancreas encircles duodenum

pancreatitis inflammation of pancreas. ***p. calcareous*** pancreatitis accom-

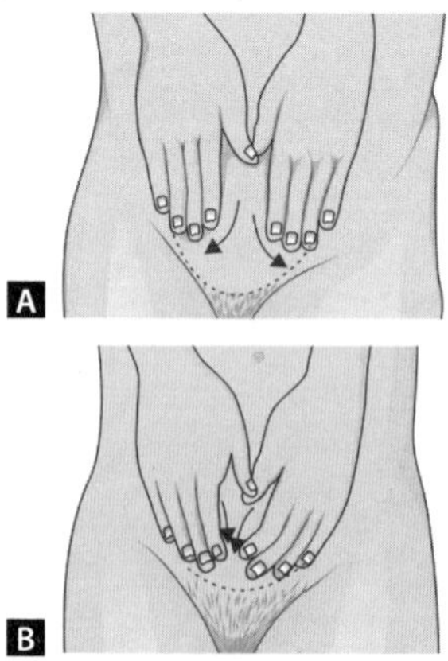

Pelvic palpation: (A) Fingers diverge when head is engaged; (B) Fingers converge when head is not engaged

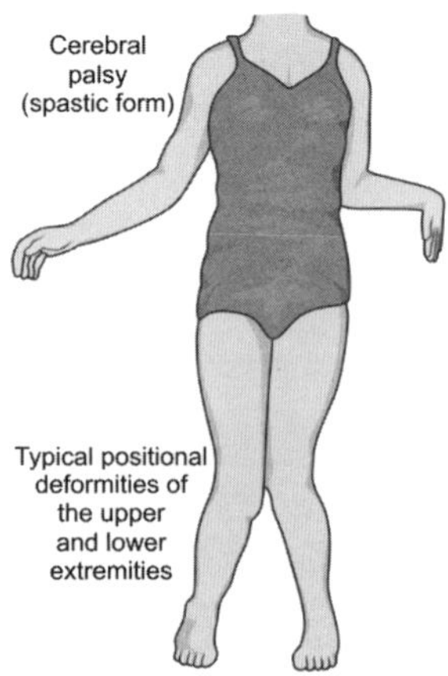

Cerebral palsy

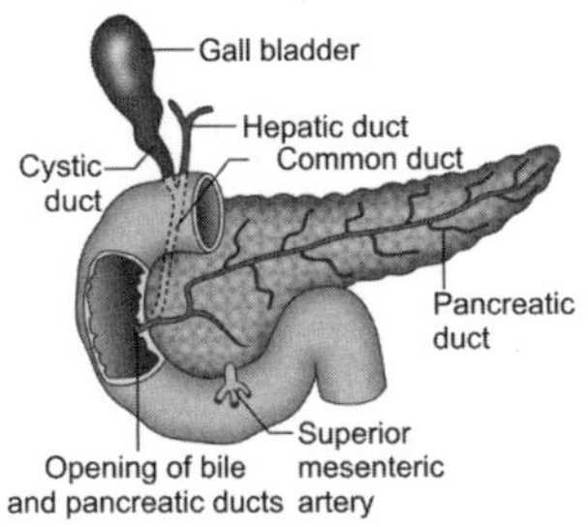

Pancreas

panied by pancreatic calcification. ***p. chronic*** scarred pancreas due to chronic inflammation

pancuronium a neuromuscular blocking agent used as muscle relaxant in surgery and in mechanical ventilation

pancytopenia reduction in all cellular elements, i.e. RBC, WBC, platelets in blood

pandemic disease widely prevalent in population

panhysterectomy removal body and cervix of uterus

panic attack acute intense anxiety with sweating, palpitation, nausea, chest pain and feeling of approaching death

Papanicolaou test a study for detection of cancer from examination of cells shed from **abnormal mucosal** growths

papilla small elevation, *nipple-like*. ***p. circumvallate*** large papilla near base of tongue. ***p. filiform*** small papilla at tip of tongue. ***p. interdental*** triangular shaped gingiva between the teeth. ***p. interproximal*** the cone-shaped projection of the gingiva filling the interdental spaces up to the contact areas when viewed from the labial, buccal, and lingual aspects. When viewed buccolingually or labiolingually, the crest of the interproximal papilla appears as a rounded concavity at an area below the contact point of the teeth. If recession has occurred, this concavity may become an area of pathology, and the entire papilla may require reshaping to restore health. ***p. lacrimal*** small elevation at inner end of eyelid through which lacrimal duct opens. ***p. of hair*** a conical portion of dermis through which capillaries enter into hair root. ***p. of Vater*** elevation in medial wall of second part of duodenum through which pancreatic and common bile duct open. ***p. renal*** apex of renal pyramids

papilloma benign epithelial tumors including wart, condyloma and polyp

papule solid circumscribed elevation of skin

papyraceous like paper. ***p. fetus*** often in twin pregnancy one fetus dies and becomes flattened

para prefix meaning near, e.g. parametrium connectine tissue near uterus

para woman who has given birth to viable fetus—dead or alive ***p. nulli*** para o

P

paracentesis cavity puncture for draining fluid

paracervical block block of cervical plexus by injection through lateral fornix to relieve pain of cervical dilatation but inadvertent injection into uterine artery may cause fetal body candida and even fetal death

paracetamol oral antipyretic analgesic but overdose can cause liver failure

paradoxical respiration 1. seen in open pneumothorax where lungs fill during expiration. 2. moving up of diaphragm during inspiration in diaphragmatic palsy

paraldehyde colorless liquid polymer of acetaldehyde used as a hypnotic, analgesic and anticonvulsant

paralysis loss of muscular function usually due to nerve dysfunction; may be spastic or flaccid. ***p. agitans*** Parkinson's disease characterized by rigidity, akinesia, tremor and gait disorder. ***p. Bell's*** lower motor facial palsy. ***p. crossed*** paralysis of one side of body and opposite side of face, a feature of lesion in brainstem. ***p. familial periodic*** flaccid palsy usually on awakening due to disturbances in serum potassium. ***p. hysteric*** apparent paralysis due to psychiatric conflict. ***p. Erb's*** paralysis of muscles of upper arm due to C5 C6 root lesion. ***p. Klumpke's*** birth injury causing paralysis of arm and hand muscles (Policeman's hand in bribe). ***p. Pott's*** tuberculosis of spine causing paraplegia. ***p. pseudobulbar*** upper motor palsy of cranial nerves due to central lesion. ***p. Saturday night*** compression of radial nerve in spiral groove (usually due to alcoholic binge on Saturday night). ***p. Todd's*** transient muscular palsy (upto 24 hours) following epilepsy, due to neuronal exertion

paralytic ileus intestinal palsy with distention of abdomen, vomiting and obstipation

paramedic a trained person to assist doctor

paramedical supplementary to medical profession like occupational, speech and physiotherapy

parametritis inflammation of parametrium

paranasal sinuses frontal, maxillary, ethmoidal and sphenoidal sinuses

paranoia paranoid schizophrenia

paranoid ideas of persecution, suspicious thinking

paraphilia a psychosexual disorder that includes fetishism, transvestism, pedophilia, voyeurism which mean bizarre acts for sexual excitation

paraphimosis inflamed or narrowed prepuce unable to be retracted over glans and strangulating it

paraphrasia unintelligible speech due to incorrect and jumbling up of words used

paraplegia paralysis of both legs. ***p. dolorosa*** extremely painful paraplegia due to pressure of a neoplasm on nerve roots and spinal cord. ***p. Pott's*** tuberculosis of spine with paraplegia

parasite organism living at expense of another organism. ***p. external*** parasite living on outer surface of host, e.g. lice, fleas, ticks, etc. ***p. facultative*** parasite capable of living independent of the host at times

parasympathetic nervous system the preganglionic fibers arise from midbrain, medulla and sacral portion of spinal cord through 3rd, 7th, 9th and 10th cranial nerves and S2-S4 somatic nerves to synapse with postganglionic neurones located in autonomic ganglia. Parasympathetic stimulation causes smooth muscle contraction, increased glandular secretion (except that of sweat) and slowing of heart

parathyroids 4 small glands lying in neck adjacent to thyroid whose extirpation leads to hypocalcemia, carpopedal spasm, and tetany

parenteral any route other than alimentary canal

paresis partial or incomplete paralysis

paresthesia sensation of numbness, pricking, needling, tingling due to irritation of a nerve or its central connections

parietal forming wall of a cavity or outer shell. ***p. cells*** large cells or oxyntic cells secreting HCl in stomach

parity carrying pregnancy up to viability (28 weeks gestation)

paronychia infection of nail margin soft tissue

paroophoron vestigial structure consisting of minute tubules, the remains of caudal group of mesonephric tubules, homologous to paradidymis of male

parotid duct the duct of parotid gland 2" long opening into mouth opposite 2nd upper molar

parotid gland one of the salivary glands near angle of mouth secreting saliva

parotitis inflammation of parotid gland

paroxysm periodic recurrence of symptoms

partogram graphical record of progress of labor, particularly the dilatation of cervix descent of fetal head

parturient concerning childbirth

parturition delivery or childbirth

passive exercise exercise to muscle given by an assistant or machine

passive smoking inhaling smoke by persons around the smoke

passivity dependence upon others, not willing to take responsibility

pasteurization the process of sterilizing a fluid without changing its chemical composition

Patau's syndrome trisomy 13 affecting hand, face and feet with mental retardation

patent ductus arteriosus persistent communication between aorta and pulmonary artery after birth

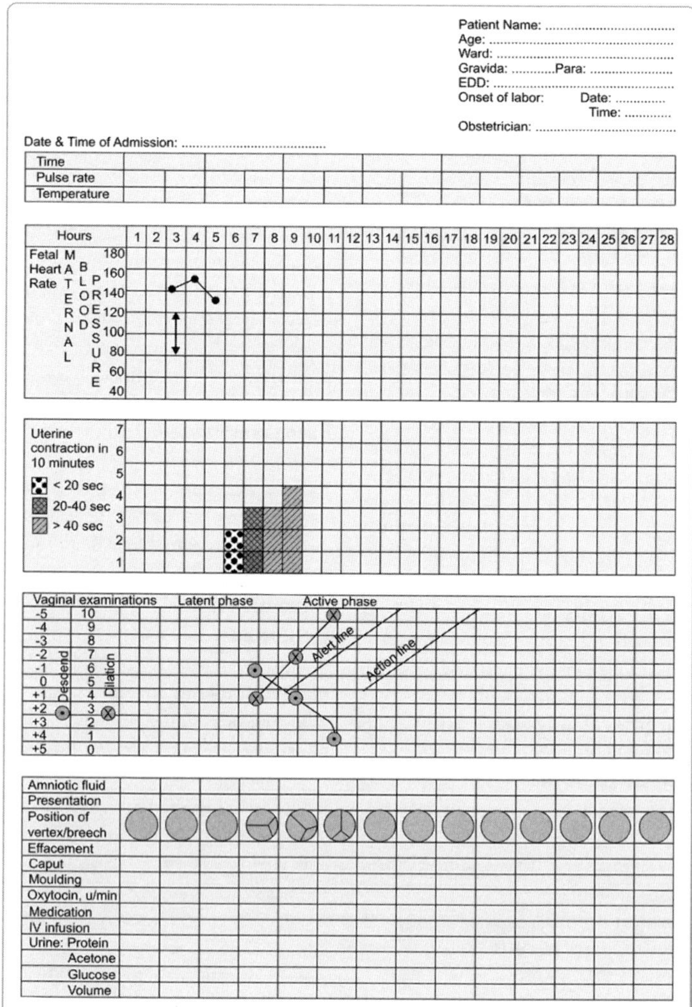
Patient Name:
Age:
Ward:
Gravida: Para:
EDD:
Onset of labor: Date:
Time:
Obstetrician:
Date & Time of Admission:
Time
Pulse rate
Temperature
Hours
1 2 3 4 5 6 7 8 9 10 11 12 13 14 15 16 17 18 19 20 21 22 23 24 25 26 27 28
Fetal Heart Rate
MATERNAL BLOOD PRESSURE
180 160 140 120 100 80 60 40
Uterine contraction in 10 minutes
7 6 5 4 3 2 1
< 20 sec
20-40 sec
> 40 sec
Vaginal examinations
Latent phase
Active phase
Alert line
Action line
Descend
Dilation
-5 -4 -3 -2 -1 0 +1 +2 +3 +4 +5
10 9 8 7 6 5 4 3 2 1 0
Amniotic fluid
Presentation
Position of vertex/breech
Effacement
Caput
Moulding
Oxytocin, u/min
Medication
IV infusion
Urine: Protein
Acetone
Glucose
Volume

Partogram

paternity test group of tests (blood group, HLA) done to determine if a particular individual has fathered the specific child in question

pathogen any microorganism capable of causing disease

pathology branch of medical science dealing with nature and cause of disease and the functional/structural changes caused by the disease

patulous open, spread apart

Paul-Bunnell test test for heterophil antibody in patients of infectious mononucleosis

Pawlik's grip a method of estimating the mobility and engagement of the presenting part by palpation of lower pole of uterus

pediatrics medical science dealing with children below 14 years of age

pedicle the stem that attaches the tumor to the organ

pedigree the tree or chart involving one's ancestors as used for genetic analysis

peduncle a connecting band of nervous tissue. ***p. cerebellar inferior*** connects spinal cord and medulla with cerebellum. ***p. cerebellar middle*** channel for pontocerebellar fibers. ***p. cerebellar superior*** connects cerebellum with midbrain. ***p. cerebral*** a pair of white bundle connecting cerebrum to midbrain; the pathway for descending corticospinal and corticonuclear projection

pellagra avitaminosis due to want of nicotinic acid manifesting with diarrhea, dermatitis and dementia

pelvic inflammatory disease infection of fallopian tubes, broad ligament and supporting tissues of uterus

pelvic inlet upper pelvic entry, i.e. space between sacral promontory and upper aspect of symphysis pubis

pelvic outlet lower pelvic outlet outlined by tip of coccyx, ischial tuberosities and lower margin of symphysis pubis

pelvimetry measurement of pelvic dimension manually or by X-ray

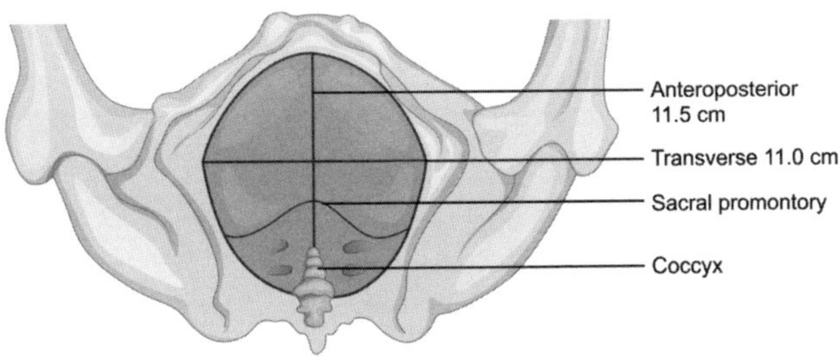

Diameters of pelvic outlet

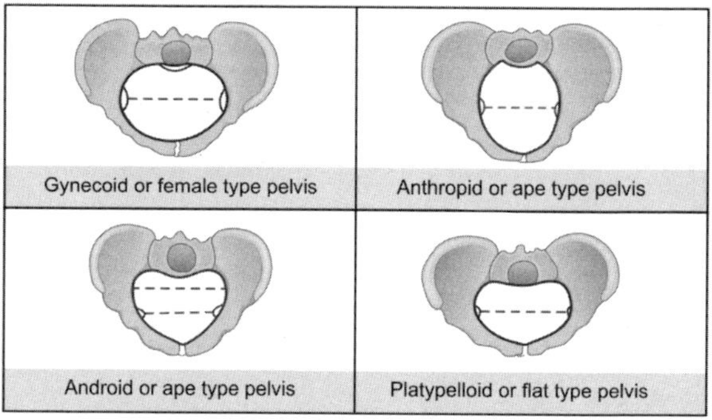

Types of pelvis

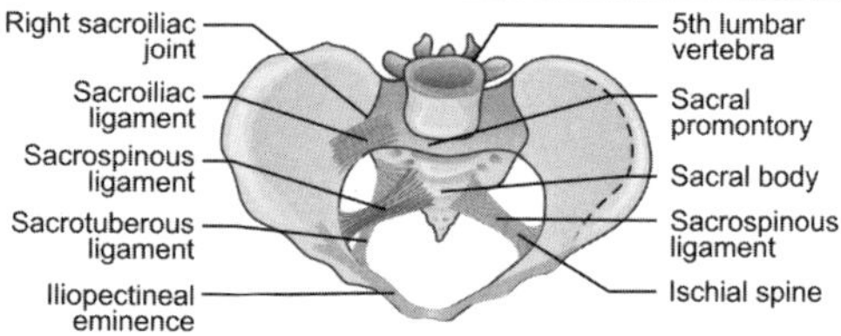

Normal female pelvis

pelvis the structure formed by iliac bones, sacrum and coccyx. Inlet A-P diameter = 11 cm. Diagonal conjugate = 13 cm. True conjugate = 11 cm. Transverse diameter = 11 cm. Outlet AP diameter = 11 cm. ***p. android*** male type pelvis with shallow sacral hollow. ***p. anthropoid*** long narrow pelvis. ***p. contracted*** pelvis in which one or more diameters are less so as to impede birth of fetus.

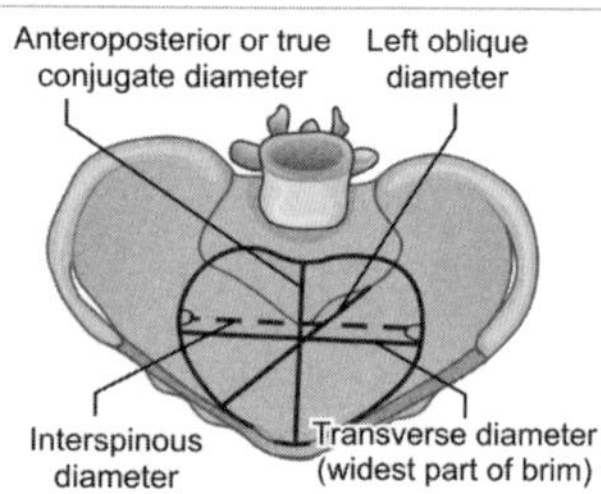

Brim of pelvis showing diameters

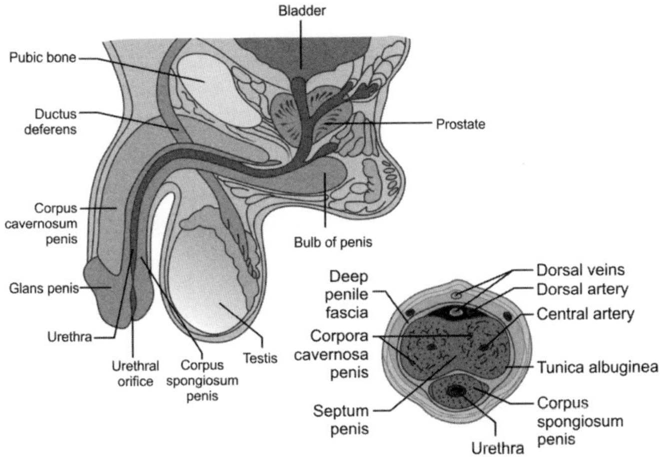

Penis

p. funnel-shaped pelvis with normal inlet but markedly contracted outlet. ***p. Naegeles*** obliquely contracted pelvis. ***p. Otto*** pelvis in which head of femur extends into pelvic cavity due to depressed acetabulum

pemphigus a bullous disease that appears suddenly on normal skin and disappears leaving pigmented spots. ***p. erythematous*** erythematous macules and blebs resembling lupus erythematosus and perphigus vulgaris. ***p. foliaceus*** pemphigus with a chronic course and purulent bulous fluid from beginning. ***p. vegetans*** pemphigus with pustules instead of bullae followed by warty vegetations. ***p. vulgaris*** common form of bullous pemphigus with bilateral distribution

pendulous bulging down

penicillamine a derivative of penicillin used to treat rheumatoid arthritis and heavy metal poisoning

penicillin antibiotic synthesized by various molds, bactericidal to gram-positive cocci, *Spirochaetes* and *Rickettsiae* by inhibition of cell wall synthesis

penis the male organ of copulation consisting of root, body and glans penis. The body contains paired corpora cavernosa and corpus spongiosum through which passes the urethra

P

pentazocine an analgesic with strong addictive potential

pepsin proteolytic enzyme of gastric juice which converts proteins into proteoses and peptones

peptide compound formed by combination of 2 or more amino acids

percentile a term used in statistics to show how common some characteristic is. The chart is used in midwifery for birth weight of babies in different period of gestation.

percussion the use of finger tips to tap the body directly or indirectly to determine position, size and consistency of underlying structure

perforation a hole

pericarditis inflammation of pericardium often with serofibrinous effusion and rarely constriction. ***p. constrictive*** pericarditis leading to restriction in ventricular filling with equalization in diastolic pressure in both ventricles and atria

pericardium a bilayer fibroserous sac enclosing heart

perinatal around the time of birth, the first week of life

perineorrhaphy repair of perineum and perineal body following injury sustained during childbirth

perineum the structures occupying the pelvic outlet and constituting pelvic floor. ***p. tears of*** first degree tear involves vaginal mucosa, second degree involves the musculature in addition and in third degree tear the anal sphincter is also torn

periosteum a fibrous membrane covering the bone, supporting the blood vessels supplying bone and giving attachment to ligaments and muscles. Its inner cellular layer forms new bone

peristalsis successive waves of contraction and relaxation of the walls of a hollow muscular structure (e.g. intestinal tract, ureter) and moving the contents onward

peritoneum a serous membrane reflected over abdominal viscera and lining the abdominal cavity

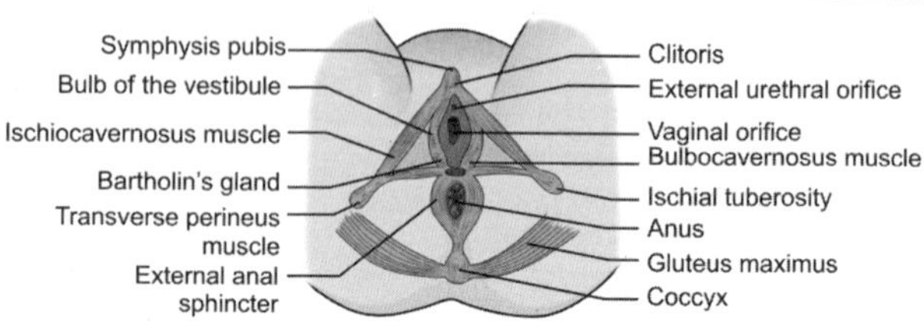

Perineum

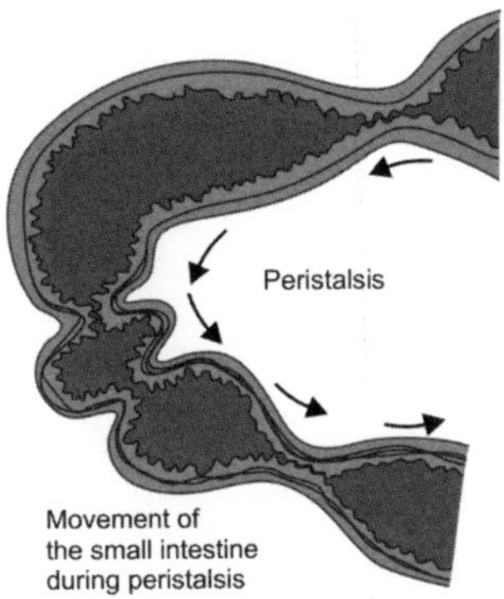

Peristalsis

peritonitis inflamed peritoneum manifesting with board-like rigidity of abdomen and aperistalsis, commonly follows rupture of follow organ, pelvic inflammation, or is primary can be localized or generalized; acute or chronic, adhesive and aseptic

periventricular leukomalacia cystic ischemic lesion in periventricular region, a consequence hemorrhage into germinal matrix, associated with spastic cerebral palsy

pernicious anemia vitamin B12 deficient anemia due to antibodies to gastric parietal cells leading to deficient intrinsic factor secretion

peroxidase an enzyme essential for oxygen transfer, hence important in cellular respiration

persistent mentoposterior face presentation with chin towards sacrum causing obstructed labor

persistent occipitoposterior a deflexed vertex with occiput facing the sacrum causing delayed labor but spontaneous face-to-pubes delivery is possible

personality the composition of one's characteristics, behavior, grooming, etc. ***p. compulsive***. a type of personality where individual's perfectionism, indecisiveness hampers with social adjustment and interpersonal relationship. ***p. extroverted*** individual's activities and libido are directed to other individuals or environment. ***p. histrionic*** personality with self exaggeration, dramatization, irrational and angry outbursts. ***p. introverted*** person's activities and libido are directed towards himself. ***p. paranoid*** undue suspiciousness, mistrust and hypersensitiveness. ***p. schizoid*** shyness, seclusiveness, eccentricity

perspiration waterloss from skin via evaporation of sweat; 1 liter of sweat evaporation removes 580 calories of heat from the body

pertussis acute infectious respiratory disease caused by *B. pertussis*. SYN: whooping cough

pessary device inserted into vagina to support pelvic structures like uterus, urethra

petechiae hemorrhagic spots on the skin

pethidine meperidine hydrochloride

petit mal little illness. A form of epilepsy

Pfannenstiel incision a transverse abdominal incision given just above symphysis pubis

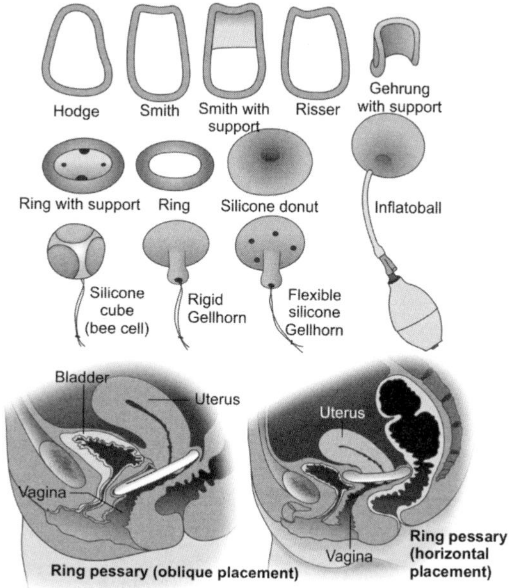

Pessary and its placement

pH the symbol for hydrogen ion concentration ranging from 0–14, 7 is neutral, above 7 is alkaline and below 7 acidic normal blood pH 7.4, i.e. alkaline

phage typing a method of identifying particular strains of bacteria that are lysed by only strain specific bacteriophages

phage viruses that can lyse bacteria

phagocyte a cell capable of ingesting and digesting cell debris, protozoa, bacteria, etc.

phagocytosis the process of ingestion and digestion of bacteria by phagocytes

phalanx bones on finger and toes; proximal, middle and distal

phallus penis

phantom an appearance or illusion of body part. ***p. limb*** following amputation, patient feels as if the limb exists. ***p. tumor*** muscular contraction or abdominal fat mistaken as tumor

pharmaceutics science of dispensing medicines

pharmacodynamics study of drugs and their action on living organisms

pharmacognosy the science of natural drugs and their properties

pharmacokinetics study of metabolism and action of drugs including absorption, distribution metabolism, elimination

pharmacopeia publication depicting standard formula and preparation of drugs

pharmacy the practice of compounding and dispensing medicines; a drug store

pharynx the common gateway in throat for food and air extending from base of skull to 6th cervical vertebra. Nasopharynx is the portion above palate; oropharynx lies between palate and hyoid bone and laryngopharynx below the hyoid bone

phenergan promethazine hydrochloride

phenindione an anticoagulant

phenobarbital phenylethyl barbituric acid used as a hypnotic and anticonvulsant

phenol a coal tar derivative effective as a bacteriostatic agent. SYN: carbolic acid

phenomenon a change perceivable by senses. ***p. Bell's*** rolling of eyeball upward and outward on attempting to close the affected eye in lower motor neurone facial palsy

phenothiazine the basic compound used for manufacture of tranquilizers, anthelmintics, dyes and some insecticides

phenotype the physical appearance or the sum total of visible traits which characterize the members of a group

phenylalanine an essential aminoacid, normally converted to tyrosine in liver

phenylbutazone an analgesic anti-inflammatory agent sparingly used for adverse effects on marrow

phenylephrine adrenergic agent used as nasal decongestant

phenylketonuria an autosomal recessive disease where due to defective enzyme system phenylalanine is not converted to tyrosine and there is likelihood of brain damage

phenylpyruvic acid a metabolic derivative of phenylalanine

phenytoin anticonvulsant drug, also antiarrhythmic

pheochromocytoma a benign chromaffin cell tumor of adrenal medulla producing adrenaline and noradrenaline

philadelphia chromosome dislocation of long arm of chromosome 21 to chromosome 9, seen in 90% patients of chronic myelocytic leukemia

phimosis narrowing of prepucial orifice so that it cannot be retracted over glans penis

phlebitis inflammation of a vein

phlebolith a concretion in a vein

phlebothrombosis clotting of blood inside vein without any infection

phlegmasia inflammation. ***p. alba dolens*** edema of leg due to thrombophlebitis

phobia irrational fear resulting in desire to avoid the feared object/situation

phocomelia congenital malformation where proximal part of a limb is ill-developed

phosphatase enzymes that catalyze hydrolysis of phosphoric acid esters. ***p. acid*** present in semen, prostatic secretion, osteoclasts and odontoclasts. ***p. alkaline*** present in developing bone, plasma, and teeth; excreted by liver, increase in obstructive jaundice, bone metastasis and osteomalacia

phosphate salt of phosphoric acid (PO_4). Monosodium and disodium phosphates help to maintain acid-base balance of blood. ***p. acid*** phosphate in which one or two atoms of hydrogen in phosphoric acid are replaced by a metal. ***p. triple*** calcium-ammonium and magnesium phosphate

phospholipids lipid containing phosphorus e.g. sphingomyelin, the principal lipid cell membrane

phosphorus a mineral essential for bone formation and cellular metabolism

photophobia intolerance to light, a feature of keratitis, uveitis, etc.

photoretinitis macular burn on exposure to intense light

photosensitizer substance that compounds abnormal reaction of skin to light

phototherapy therapeutic use of sunlight or artificial blue light to reduce serum bilirubin in newborn

phrenic concerning diaphragm

phthisic concerning pulmonary tuberculosis

physical therapy rehabilitation for restoration of function and prevention of disability by using exercise, heat, massage, ultraviolet, etc.

physiology the branch of science dealing with functions of living organisms

physique the body organization development and structure

phytonadione synthetic vitamin K

phytotherapy treatment using plant substances such as aromatherapy and herbal medicine

pia mater the innermost membrane enveloping spinal cord

pica perverted appetite with eating of uneatables like plastic, clay, plaster, etc.

pie chart a circular diagram divided into segments showing the proportional distribution of observations of particular event

Pierre-Robin syndrome small jaw, cleft palate and absent gag reflex

pigment any organic coloring material in the body. ***p. bile*** bilirubin and biliverdin, the hemoglobin degradation products in blood secreted in bile, urobilin and bilifuscin excreted in stool and urine. ***p. blood*** hematin, hemin, methemoglobin and hemosiderin, all derivatives of hemoglobin

pile hemorrhoid. ***p. sentinel*** thickened anal mucous membrane at the lower end of an anal fissure

pilonidal cyst sacrococcygeal cyst from the entrapped epithelial tissue beneath the skin, a developmental defect

pilonidal sinus a small sinus opening near coccyx, a remnant of neural canal

Pinard's stethoscope a trumpet shoped instrument to hear fetal heart sound

pineal body a gland-like structure near splenium of corpus callosum secreting melatonin

pinna the auricle or external ear

piperazine drug used for enterobiosis and ascariasis

pitressin vasopressin secreted from posterior pituitary (contains ADH + pressor agent)

pituitary endocrine gland of size 1.3 cm × 1 cm × 0.5 cm at base of brain secreting various hormones like TSH, GH, ACTH, LH, oxytocin and vasopressin

placebo an inactive substance, used in controlled studies of drugs

placenta the oval structure in pregnant uterus through which fetus derives its nutrition. ***p. accreta*** placenta

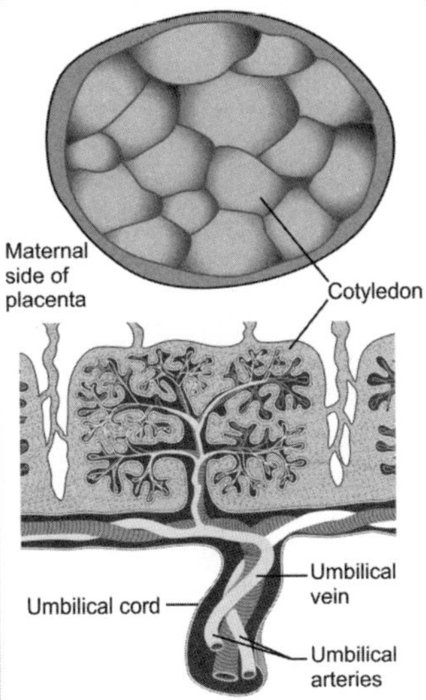

Placenta

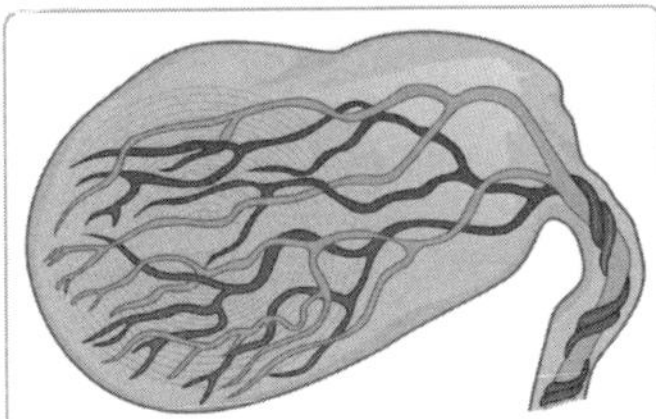

Velamentous insertion of the cord

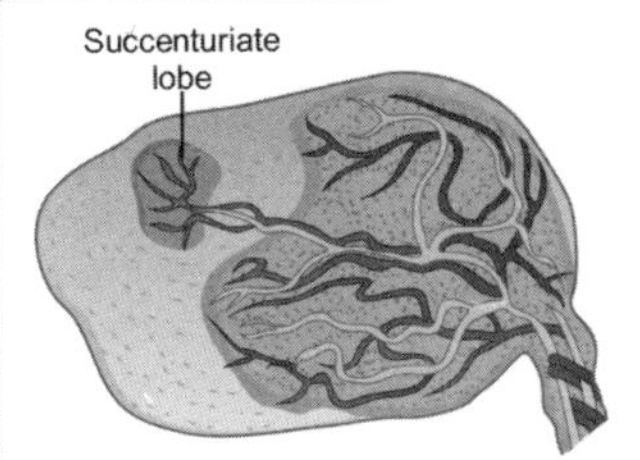

Succenturiate lobe of placenta

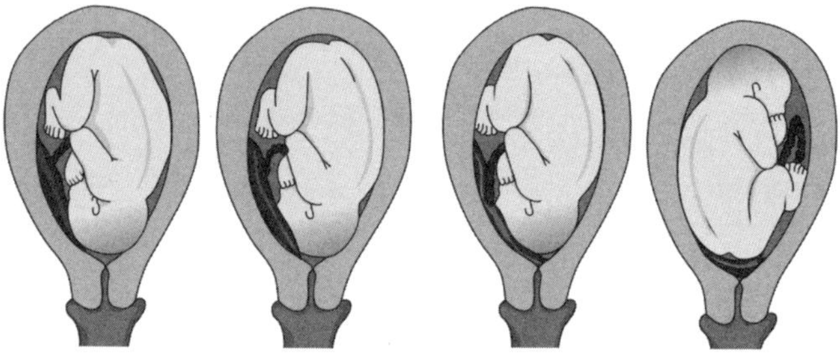

Types of placenta previa

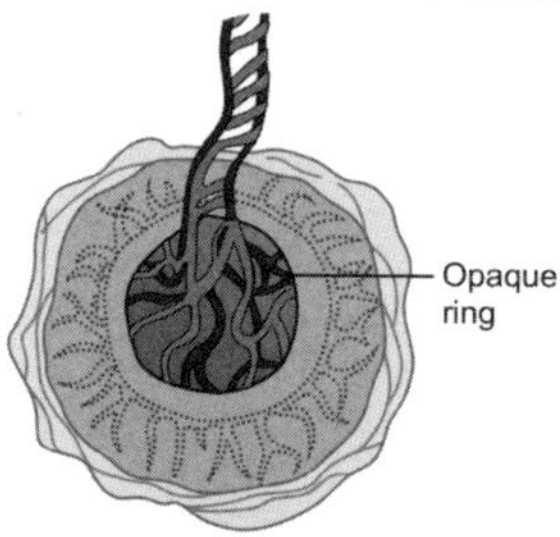

Circumvallate placenta

whose cotyledons have invaded the uterine musculature so that placental separation after delivery is difficult. ***p. circumvallate*** cup-shaped placenta with raised edges. ***p. percreta*** placental cotyledons invade uterus right up to serosal lining threatening rupture of uterus. ***p. previa*** placenta implanted to lower uterine segment, often causing painless profuse third trimester bleeding. ***p. retained*** placenta not expelled even 2 hours after fetal delivery. ***p. succenturiate*** an accessory placenta having vascular connection with main placenta. ***p. velamentous*** placenta where the umbilical cord is attached to membranes, so that the umbilical vessels enter placenta at its margins

placental dysfunction a placenta that is failing to meet fetal requirements.

placental souffle auscultatory sound of placental blood flow

placenta previa a placenta, which is abnormally implanted in the lower uterine segment so that it partially or fully covers the internal os of the cervix

plagiocephaly irregular closure of cranial sutures resulting in deformed skull

plague disease caused by *Pasteurella pestis*. **p. bubonic** common form of plague with suppurative lymphadenitis. ***p. hemorrhagic*** rare form of plague with prominent hemorrhagic manifestations particularly into skin. ***p. pneumonic*** virulent form of plague with extensive involvement of lungs

planned parenthood birth control

plaque a patch on skin or mucous membrane ***p. dental*** a gummy mesh harboring microorganism growing on the crowns of teeth, a forerunner of dental caries

plasma exchange removal of patient's, plasma with replacement by colloid solution. This removes the immune complexes, excess antibodies or drugs and poisons

plasmapheresis similar to plasma exchange

plasma the liquid portion of blood, the medium for transporting nutrients and suspending the corpuscles

plasmid extranuclear cell inclusion having genetic function; commonly seen in bacteria and used in DNA cloning and recombinant DNA technology

plasmin fibrinolytic enzyme derived from plasminogen

plasmodium a genus of protozoa that includes causative agents of various types of malaria

plaster 1. plaster of Paris used to immobilize a part or make an impression. 2. medicinal agents formed into a tenaceous mass, e.g. belladonna plaster

plastibel a sterilized plastic device used for non-operative circumcision. The bell is slipped into penile foreskin and sting is tied. The foreskin becomes gangrenous and drops off

platelet concentrate platelets prepared from few units of blood and suspended in plasma

platelet round or oval disk-like cells in blood which help in blood coagulation and hemostasis

plegia suffix meaning paralysis

pleocytosis increased number of lymphocytes in CSF

plethora congestion with fluid

plethysmography the method of measuring volume of blood flow through a part from change in volume

pleura a bilayered membrane that encloses the lungs

pleurisy inflammation of pleura; may be primary or secondary, acute or chronic, serous or serosanguinous. ***p. diaphragmatic*** inflammation of diaphragmatic pleura causing intense pain under margin of the ribs, hiccough, and often dyspnea. ***p. dry*** pleurisy where a fibrinous exudate covers the pleural surface causing pain during respiration. ***p. encysted*** pleurisy with effusion encysted by adhesion

pleurodesis production of adhesion between visceral and parietal pleura

plexus a network of nerves, lymphatics or blood vessels. ***p. enteric*** one of the two plexuses of nerve fibers and ganglion cells lying in the wall of alimentary canal namely Auerbach's plexus and submucosal Meissner's plexus. ***p. pampiniform*** a network of veins draining the testis in male or ovary in the female

P

pneumonia inflammation of lung tissue. ***p. alba*** pneumonia of newborn due to congenital syphilis. ***p. aspiration*** pneumonia following aspiration of purulent matter from throat/mouth or gastric content. ***p. caseous*** pneumonia associated with tuberculosis. ***p. interstitial*** pneumonia with infiltration of pulmonary interstitium. ***p. eosinophilic*** pneumonia with eosinophilia as during migration of round worm larva, microfilaria or due to drugs like nitrofurantoin, penicillin. ***p. Friedlander's*** lobar pneumonia caused by *Klebsiella pneumoniae*. ***p. giant cell*** an interstitial pneumonia of childhood with infiltration of lung by multinucleated giant cells, e.g. post-measles. ***p. hypostatic*** pneumonia of aged and debilitated patients due to congestion of one part of lung at all times. ***p. atypical*** mild pneumonia but with radiological evidence of extensive lung infiltration as caused by *Mycoplasma pneumoniae*. ***p. Woolsorter's*** pulmonary anthrax

pneumonitis hypersensitive diffuse granulomatous disease due to inhalation of organic dusts

pneumothorax presence of air in pleural cavity. ***p. artificial*** intentionally induced pneumothorax to cause pulmonary collapse as a treatment option in pulmonary tuberculosis ***p. tension*** a type of pneumothorax where air enters pleural space with each act of respiation but without an exit leading to high pleural pressure and collapse of lung

pO_2 partial pressure of oxygen in blood, about 100 mm Hg in adult, 60 to 90 mm Hg in babies

podalic version rotating the fetus to bring feet to the lower pole

polarity the gradient of the strength of uterine contraction being highest in fundus and minimal in lower segment thus bringing about dilatation of cervix

pole one extremity or end of an organ of the body, e.g. uterus or of the fetus

poliomyelitis acute viral disease that causes destruction of anterior horn cells in spinal cord and often cranial nerve nuclei with ensuing palsy. ***p. ascending*** the paralysis begins in lower extremity and then ascends up-trunk often to involve respiratory muscles. ***p. bulbar*** paralysis of cranial nerves and the respiratory center. ***p. nonparalytic*** pain and stiffness in muscles but no paralysis

polycystic having many cysts

polycystic ovary an endocrine disorder with anovulation and multiple cysts in the ovaries

polycythemia an excess of red blood cells. ***p. rubra vera*** a malignant disorder of marrow with increase in RBC mass, WBC and platelets

polydactylism having supernumerary fingers or toes

polydipsia excess thirst

polygraph an apparatus for simultaneous recording of BP, pulse, respiration, electrical resistance of skin

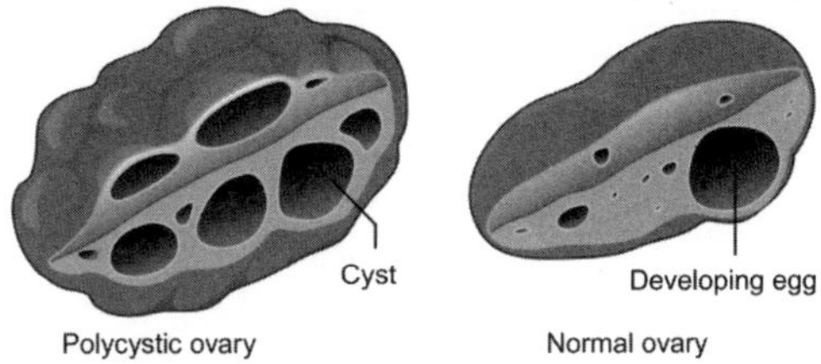

Polycystic ovary

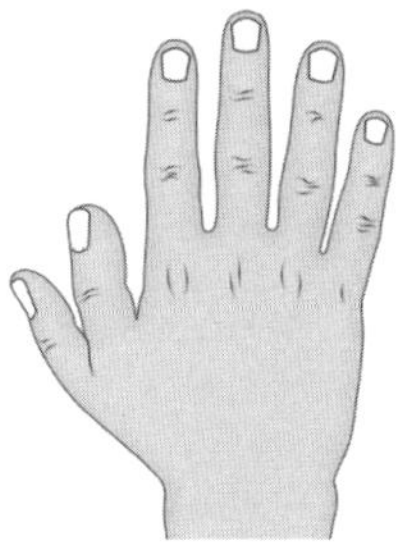

Polydactyly

polyhydramnios excess of amniotic fluid

polymenorrhea menses occurring at rapid frequency

polymerase chain reaction (PCR) A process whereby a strand of DNA can be cloned millions of times within a few hours. The process can be used to make prenatal diagnoses of genetic diseases and to identify an individual by analysis of a single tissue cell

polymorph a polymorphonuclear leukocyte

polymyositis a connective tissue disorder characterized by inflammation and degeneration of muscles and dermatitis

polyneuropathy involvement of many peripheral nerves

polyp a tumor with a pedicle

polyposis presence of many polyps. ***p. familial*** multiple polyps in colon with rectal bleeding and chances of malignant changes

polysaccharide complex sugars which on hydrolysis yield more than 2 molecules of simple sugar

polyuria excessive passage of urine of low specific gravity

pons a structure dorsal to the medulla and intimately related to the pathways to the cerebrum. The cranial nerves whose nuclei lie in the pons are the trigeminal, abducens, and facial nerves, and part of the acoustic nerve. The pons is intimately related to the medulla, has the same blood vessel supply, and is involved in many lesions that affect the medulla. It is specially involved with the cerebellar manifestations of disease and may cause serious muscular incoordination in motor function of the head, neck, and facial structures

popliteal concerning back of knee

pore a small opening

porphyrin nitrogen-containing organic compounds obtained from hemoglobin and chlorophyll

portal system the portal vein and its branches which drain the abdominal viscera and carry the blood to liver to be drained to inferior vena cava via hepatic vein

portal vein the vein formed from union of superior and inferior mesenteric, splenic, gastric and cystic veins

position end expiratory pressure a method to prevent collapse of alveoli at end expiration

position manner in which the body of patient is put. ***p. Fowler's*** the position where head end of bed is elevated by 11/2 feet and knees are elevated. ***p. left lateral recumbent*** patient lies on left side; right knee and thigh drawn up. ***p. lithotomy*** patient lies on back with thighs drawn on abdomen and abducted. ***p. Trendelenburg*** dorsal position with patient supine on a bed tilted to about 45° with head low

posseting regurgitation of small amount of milk after feed

postcoital contraception oral contraceptive, usually levonor-gestrel tab to be taken within 72 hours of unprotected intercourse

posterior situated at back or behind; dorsal

posthumous occurring after death

postmature infant born after 42 weeks of gestation

postmortem after death

postnasal located behind the nose

postpartum after child birth

postpartum depression depression occurring in puerperium

postpartum hemorrhage bleeding after childbirth in excess of 500 mL usually due to uterine atony, or cervical laceration

postpartum psychosis psychosis occurring within the six months following childbirth. The symptoms and signs are hallucination, delusion, preoccupation with death, etc.

post-term pregnancy when the pregnancy continues past 42 weeks gestation

posture attitude or position of body

potassium mineral element found in combination with other elements in the body. ***p. bicarbonate*** used to neutralize acid in stomach. ***p. chloride*** used in IV solutions and as oral preparation to supplement during digoxin and diuretic therapy. ***p. citrate*** used as alkalizer. ***p. iodide*** Used in expectorant preparations. ***p. permanganate*** topical astringent and antiseptic, antidote for phosphorus poisoning. ***p. tartarate*** a cathartic

potency strength, power, ability to perform sexual intercourse in case of male

Potter's syndrome congenital renal agenesis with pulmonary hypoplasia umbilical cord has two vessels and face had low set ears with furrows below eye (potter facies)

pouch any pocket or sac. ***p. Rathke's*** an embryonic outpocketing that forms anterior lobe of pituitary

Poupart's ligament the rolled up lower end of external oblique aponeurosis stretching between anterior superior iliac spine and pubic tubercle. SYN: inguinal ligament

povidone iodine a complex of povidone and iodine used for skin preparation prior to surgery, as vaginal tablets, as lotions and ointments for antiseptic purposes

previa going before in time or place

prandial related to meal

prazosin alpha-adrenergic receptor blocker; antihypertensive agent

precipitate labor childbirth occurring with undue rapidity with feat of severe perineal laceration and fetal intracranial trauma

precipitate the process of deposition of substances from solutions

precocious development, physical or mental earlier than expected

preconception prior to conception ***p. cane*** health education and regular medical examination aimed at promoting optimum health during pregnancy and exclusion of diseases like diabetes, syphilis, HIV, toxoplasma, rubella, HSV etc, cardiovascular, pulmonary and renal compromise

precursor a substance that precedes another substance, e.g. angiotensinogen is a precursor substance of angiotensin

prediabetes the stage or condition prior to development of clinical diabetes

preeclampsia toxemia of pregnancy with albuminuria, hypertension and edema

pregnancy-induced hypertension a hypertensive disorder during pregnancy including conditions preeclampsia and eclampsia; characterized by hypertension, proteinuria and edema

pregnancy test tests employed to confirm pregnancy by using patient's urine or blood which assess the chorionic gonadotrophins. The test is positive beginning 40th day from the last menstrual period. Radio-immunoassay is better and more accurate

pregnancy the condition of development of embryo in the uterus. ***p. abdominal*** development of embryo in the abdominal cavity drawing its blood supply from omentum. ***p. ampullar*** implantation of ovum in the ampulla of Fallopian tube. ***p. cornual*** pregnancy in one of the horns in a bicornuate uterus. ***p. ectopic*** condition where ovum develops outside the uterus. ***p. molar*** pregnancy where ovum degenerates into moles. ***p. gingivitis*** an enlargement or hyperplasia of the gingivae caused by hormonal imbalance during pregnancy. It is usually limited to the interdental papillae. Incomplete cleaning of the interproximal space with dental floss is the initiating factor. The hormonal change is a precipitating factor

pregnanediol progesterone metabolite (end product) in urine

pregnenolone a synthetic corticosteroid

preleukemia some blood changes that may be forewarners of leukemic process, i.e. unexplained anemia, purpura, mucositis

premature ejaculation ejaculation shortly after the onset of sexual excitement

premature infant infant with birth weight below 5 lb or born prior to 37 weeks of gestation

premedication drugs given prior to general anesthesia like atropine, opiates

premenstrual tension syndrome the syndrome of irritability, anxiety, depression, rage, edema and breast tenderness prior to the onset of menstruation

prenatal diagnosis diagnosis of developmental defects and diseases while the baby is in utero by use of chemical tests, ultrasound, amnioscopy and amniocentesis

prenatal period the time of pregnancy from the first day of last menstrual period (LMP) to the start of true labor

prepuce the foreskin or skinfold over glans penis

presbycusis sensory neural deafness of old age

presbyopia recession of near point of eye with advancing age due to loss of elasticity of crystalline lens

prescription a written order or direction for using a drug. A prescription consists of four main parts, i.e. superscription, inscription, subscription and signature

presentation in obstetrics, the fetal part presenting at the pelvic inlet; can be breech, vertex, face, brow

pressure compression, force exerted on any body tissue, e.g. blood vessel. ***p. blood*** pressure exerted by moving column of blood against arterial wall. ***p. central venous*** pressure in the right atrium. ***p. end diastolic*** pressure in the ventricles at the end of diastole. ***p. intracranial*** pressure to which CSF is subjected in subarachnoid space. ***p. intraocular*** pressure within the eyeball, maintained by vitreous and aqueous humor, usually 10 to 20 mm Hg. ***p. negative*** pressure less than atmospheric pressure. ***p. oncotic*** osmotic pressure exerted by colloids in a solution. ***p. osmotic*** the force at which solvent like water passes through a semipermeable membrane separating solutions of different concentrations. ***p. wedge*** pressure obtained by wedging a fluid filled catheter in a distal branch of pulmonary artery which is equivalent to left atrial pressure

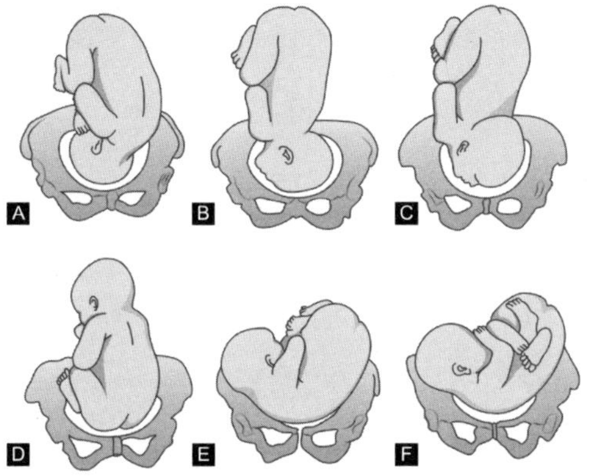

Fetal presentation: (A) Vertex; (B) Brow; (C) Face; (D) Breech; (E) Shoulder--dorsoanterior; (F) Shoulder--dorsoposterior

preterm in obstetrics labor occurring before 37th week of gestation

prevalence the number of cases of a disease present in a specified population at a given time

preventive medicine the branch of medicine concerned with prevention of mental and physical illness and disease

priapism painful sustained penile erection without any sexual desire

primigravida woman conceiving for first time

primipara woman who has delivered a viable baby

probe an instrument for knowing depth and direction of sinus and wound. ***p. lacrimal*** an instrument useful in probing the lumen of duct structures, such as the nasolacrimal or salivary gland ducts. ***p. periodontal*** a fine calibrated instrument designed and used for measuring the depth and topography of gingival and periodontal pockets. Also used to determine the degree of attachment and adaptation of the gingival tissues to the tooth

probenecid a benzoic acid derivative, uricosuric and delays excretion of penicillin and its derivatives

procaine a local anesthetic used in infiltration anesthesia, nerve block, and spinal anesthesia

prochlorperazine a phenothiazine derivative for treating nausea and vomiting

procidentia complete prolapse of uterus where it completely protrudes outside the introitus

P

procreate to give birth

proctalgia pain in and around anus and rectum

proctitis inflammation of anus and rectum

proctoscopy instrument for examination of rectum

prodrome a symptom heralding an approaching ailment

prodrug chemicals which exhibit their pharmacologic property after biotransformation in the body

progesterone hormone secreted by placenta, corpus luteum and adrenal cortex; essential for secretory phase of endometrium, mammary growth and development and growth of placenta

progestin group of synthetic drugs having progesterone-like effect on uterus

prognathism abnormally forward projecting lower jaw

prolactin hormone of anterior pituitary that helps in milk production

prolapse falling down of a body part or organ ***p. of cord*** the umbilical cord lies in front of presenting part and prolapses after rupture of membrance causing fetal anoxi. ***p. rectum***. protrurion of rectal mucosa and often the muscle coat through anus p of arm the fetal arm prolapses in shoulder presentation p of uterus the uterus protrudes into lower part of vagina due to weakness of its support

proliferate to increase by reproduction of similar forms as to the parent source

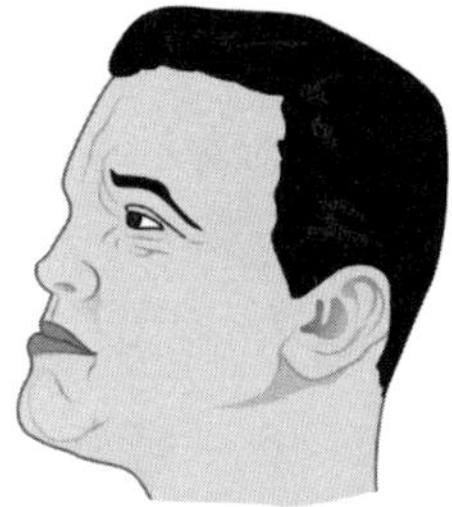

Prognathism

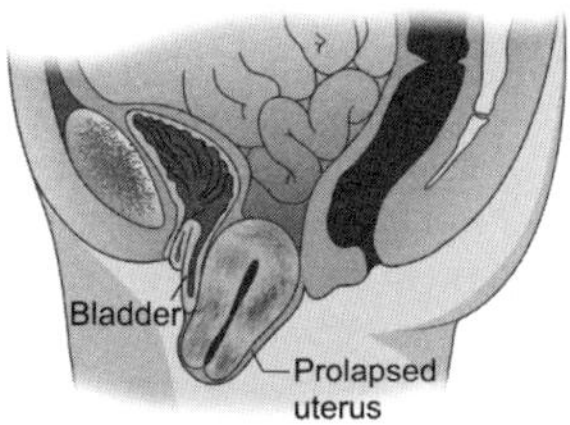

Prolapse of uterus

prolonged labor labor lasting more than 24 hours due to poor uterine contraction, cephalopelvic disproportion, malpresentation or malposition

prolonged pregnancy pregnancy beyond 42 week (294 days)

promethazine an antihistaminic agent

promontory a projecting surface or part. ***p. of sacrum*** the anterior projecting surface of sacrum

pronation the position of face downwards or palm facing downwards

P

pronucleus the laploid nucleus of a sex cell

prophylaxis prevention of disease

propofol general anesthetic; action: produces dose-dependent central nervous system depression; mechanism of action is unknown; used in induction or maintenance of anesthesia as part of a balanced anesthetic technique

propranolol betaadrenergic blocking agent used for hypertension, arrhythmias, angina pectoris, portal hypertension, etc.

proprioceptor receptors responsible for body position and equilibrium, e.g. muscle spindles, pacinian corpuscles and labyrinthine receptors

proptosis protrusion of eyeball as in exophthalmic goiter, retro-orbital mass or cavernous sinus thrombosis

propylthiouracil antithyroid drug for hyperthyroidism

prostacyclin the precursor intermediate of prostaglandins; vasodilator

prostaglandin a large group of biologically active 20-carbon unsaturated fatty acids produced by the metabolism of arachidonic acid, e.g. PGA1, PGD2, PGE2, PGI2

prostate the musculoglandular organ of the size of 2 × 4 × 3 cm that surrounds neck of urinary bladder and urethra in male

prosthesis an artificial part or organ. ***p. periodontal*** any restorative and replacement device that, by its intent and nature, is used as a therapeutic aid in the treatment of periodontal disease; it is an adjunct to other forms of periodontal therapy and does not cure periodontal disease by itself

protamin a simple strongly basic protein used to neutralize excess heparin or to slow down absorption of insulin

protean variable

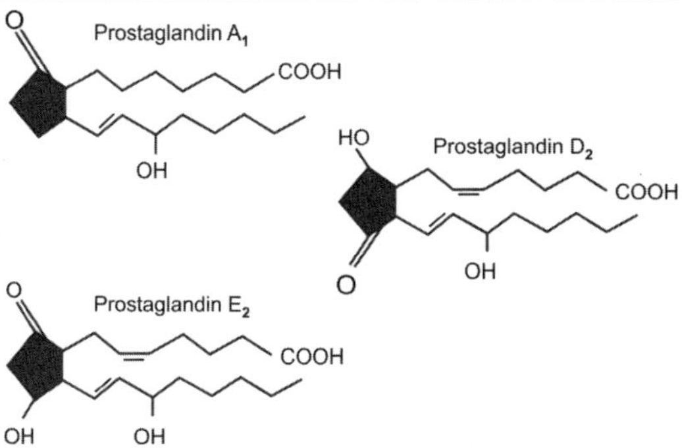

Prostaglandin

P

proteinuria loss of protein usually albumin in urine. ***p. orthostatic*** proteinuria occurring on assuming erect posture but not during recumbency. Hence morning urine is protein-free but urine of daytime contains albumin

proteous an intermediate product of proteolysis

proteus a genus of enteric bacillus, ***P. vulgaris*** causes urinary infection while ***P. morgagni*** in addition causes enteritis, ***P. mirabilis*** is usually saprophytic

prothrombin a blood coagulation factor synthesized in liver which is converted to thrombin

prothrombin time the time taken for decalcified plasma to clot on addition of thromboplastin and calcium. Usually employed to evaluate effects of anticoagulants

protocol description of steps to be taken in an experiment

proton a positively charged particle in the atom

protoplasm a thick viscous colloid, the physical basis of all living organisms

proximal nearest to center of a system

pruritus itching. ***p. senilis*** pruritus in aged due to degeneration of skin. ***p. vulvae*** itching around vulva, a feature of diabetes

pseudo prefix meaning false

pseudocyesis symptoms of pregnancy like amenorrhea, abdominal enlargement, morning sickness, etc. in absence of uterine enlargement as occurring in women who are too keen to have pregnancy

pseudodementia social withdrawal but without mental deterioration

pseudohermaphrodite individual with sex chromatin and sex organs of one sex but with some of the physical appearance of opposite sex. ***p. male*** genetically male with a small rudimentary penis and a scrotum without testes resembling labia; usually occurs due to disease of adrenals or feminizing tumors of undescended testis. ***p. female*** a genetically female with large clitoris resembling penis and hypertrophied labia mimicking scrotum

pseudohypertrophy increase in size of tissue but with diminished function

pseudomenstruation vaginal spotting in newborn girls on third day of birth due to organ withdrawal

pseudomonas a genus of motile gramnegative bacilli some of which produce yellow and blue pigments. ***p. aeruginosa*** causes urinary tract infection and wound infection. ***p. pseudomallei*** causes melioidosis

psoas a muscle in the loin, inserted to lesser trochanter of femur. It flexes the thigh, adducts and rotates it medially

psoriasis a chronic itchy disorder of skin marked by lesions on extensor surfaces with silvery yellow white scales. A psoriatic skin produces nearly 2700 cells/cm^2 in comparison to 1250/cm^2 per day in normal person and cell cycle is reduced to 36 hours in comparison to the normal of 311 hours

psyche mind

psychiatry the branch of medicine dealing with diagnosis, treatment and prevention of mental illness

psychologist person trained in methods of psychological analysis, therapy and research

psychometry the measurement of psychological variables like intelligence, aptitude, behavior and emotion

psychomotor epilepsy temporal lobe epilepsy

psychomotor retardation generalized slowing of physical and mental reactions

psychoneurosis emotional maladaptation due to unresolved emotional conflicts

psychopath antisocial personality

psychosexual pertains to mental and emotional aspects of sexuality

psychosis an impairment of mental function to the extent of interfering with individual's adaptation to family, society, self-care and ordinary demands of life. There is personality disintegration and loss of contact with reality; hallucinations and delusions

psychosomatic pertains to body and mind, i.e. a disease producing physical symptoms due to some disturbance in emotional state

psychotherapy a method of treating disease by mental means like suggestion, hypnotism rather than physical means

ptosis drooping of an organ or eyelid

ptyalin a salivary enzyme that hydrolyzes starch and glycogen to maltose and glucose

puberty the period of sexual maturity between 13 to 15 years in boys and 9 to 16 years in girls, probably related to decrease in secretion of pineal gland. **p. precocious** onset of puberty earlier than normal

pubescence puberty

pudenda external genitalia especially of female

puerperal sepsis infection of genital tract in the puerperium

puerperium period of six weeks following childbirth

pulmonary arterial webs web-like deformities in pulmonary angiogram at the site of previous thromboembolism

pulmonary embolism see embolism pulmonary

pulmonary infarction consequence of blockage of a branch of pulmonary artery by embolus from calf or pelvic veins common on puerperium

pulse the waveform of blood passing through an artery as a consequence to cardiac contraction. ***p. alternating*** pulse with weak and strong beats. ***p. anacrotic*** pulse with a secondary wave on ascending limb. ***p. bigeminal*** pulse where every third beat is irregular. ***p. collapsing*** pulse

P

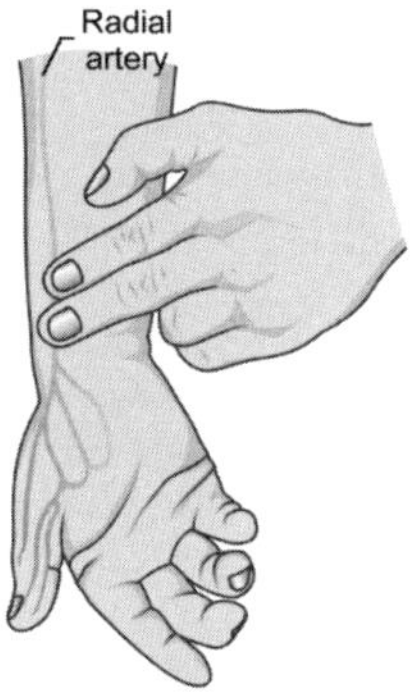

Common site for pulse taking

striking the finger with force but then abruptly subsiding. ***p. corrigans*** bounding and forceful pulse of aortic regurgitation. ***p. deficit*** pulse rate counted from wrist and cardiac rate auscultated over chest differ as in atrial fibrillation. ***p. paradoxical*** pulse disappearing at the end of inspiration as in pericardial tamponade. ***p. thready*** barely perceptible pulse. ***p. waterhammer*** sudden jerky pulse with immediate collapse.

pulseless disease aorto-arteritis causing absence of brachial and radial pulse

pulse pressure difference between systolic and diastolic pressure. Pulse pressure above 50 and below 30 are considered abnormal

puncture to make a hole, or wound by a sharp pointed instrument. ***p. cisternal*** puncture of cerebromedullary cisterns through suboccipital space to obtain CSF. ***p. lumbar*** puncture of subarachnoid space between L3–L4 vertebrae to obtain CSF for analysis, or to do myelogram. ***p. sternal*** aspiration of bone marrow from sternum

pupil the opening at the center of iris. ***p. Argyl Robertson*** pupil that reacts to accommodation but with loss of light reflex. ***p. Hutchinson's*** one side dilatation of pupil with contraction on other side due to intracranial space occupying lesion. ***p. pinpoint*** excessively constricted pupil in opium poisoning, myopias and in pontine hemorrhage

purgative drug stimulating bowel movement

purine end products of nucleoprotein digestion consisting of adenine, guanine and uric acid

purulent containing pus, suppurative

pus liquid product of inflammation containing albuminous substances, leukocytes and organisms. Blue or green pus is due to infection by pseudomonas group and fetid pus is due to growth of anaerobes

pustule small elevated skin lesion containing pus, may be flat, round or umbilicated

putative supposed. ***p father*** the man believed to be father of the illegitimate child

pyelites inflammation of renal pelvis

pyelogram X-ray of ureter and renal pelvis

pyelonephritis inflammation of kidney substance and pelvis, in 85% caused by *E. coli*

pyemia presence of pus forming organisms in blood, a form of septicemia, causing metastatic abscess

pyloric stenosis narrowing of pyloric orifice due to peptic ulcer or postpyloric duodenal ulcer or congenital hyperplasia of pyloric circular muscles

pylorus the lower orifice of stomach which opens intermittently to allow partly digested food to enter into duodenum

pyogenic pus-producing

pyometra pus in the uterus

pyosalpinx pus in Fallopian tube

pyoureter pus in the ureter

pyrantel pamoate drug used in helminthiasis, specially ascariasis and enterobiasis

pyrazinamide bactericidal antitubercular drug, very effective in killing intracellular slowly growing bacilli

pyrexia fever

pyridoxine vitamin B6 that includes pyridoxal and pyridoxamine

pyrimethamine antimalarial agent (Daraprim)

pyrogen agent that produces fever

pyruvic acid an intermediate product in metabolism of carbohydrates and fats. Its blood level increases in thiamine deficiency

pyuria pus in the urine

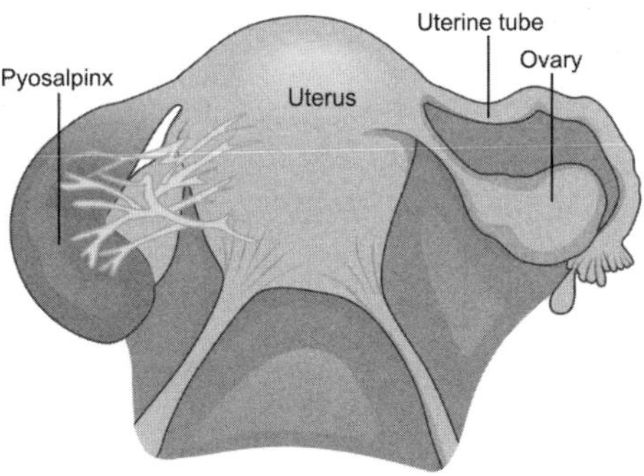

Pyosalpinx

Q

Q fever acute infectious disease caused by *Coxiella burnetii*, a rickettsial organism, characterized by fever, sweating, myalgia

QRS complex a group of waves depicted on an electrocardiogram; called also the QRS wave. It actually consists of three distinct waves created by the passage of the cardiac electrical impulse through the ventricles and occurs at the beginning of each contraction of the ventricles. In a normal electrocardiogram, the R wave is the most prominent of the three; the Q and S waves may be extremely weak and are sometimes absent

quack person who pretends to have knowledge and skill of medicine

quadrangular lobe a region on superior surface of each cerebellar hemisphere

quadrant one fourth of circumference of a circle

quadruplet four fetuses born in same labor

quarantine the period of isolation when one is exposed to infectious disease which is the longest incubation period of disease

quartan occurring every fourth day

quickening feeling of first movements of fetus in utero usually between 18 to 20 weeks of pregnancy

quinine an antimalarial alkaloid from cinchona bark used orally as sulfate, bisulfate and hydrochloride and parenterally as dihydrochloride. Quinine tannate is tasteless, best for giving to young children, used for falciparum malaria

quinolone a class of compounds whose well known derivatives are norfloxacin, ciprofloxacin, pfloxacin and ofloxacin

quintuplet birth of 5 children at same time to a mother

quotidian occurring daily

quotient number of times a number is contained in another. ***q. intelligence*** division of one's mental age by actual age. ***q. respiratory*** division of amount of CO_2 in expired air by the oxygen. Normal value is 0.9

Q wave the downward deflection before R wave in ECG. Prominent Q waves indicate myocardial necrosis

rabies an acute infectious CNS disease with fatal outcome; transmitted to humans by bite of rabid animals like dogs, foxes and cats. Bats, foxes and raccoons serve as reservoir of infection

racemose grape-like ***r. glands*** compound and lobulated in structure

rachitic pelvis flat pelvic brim similar to that of platypeloid pelvis

radial relating to radius ***r. palsy*** paralysis of radial nerve with wrist drop. ***r. keratotomy*** a form of surgery with radial incisions on cornea for correction of myopia

radical dealing with root or cause of a disease. ***r. cure*** cure that completely removes the cause. ***r. free*** a molecule containing odd number of electrons and an open bond causing cell membrane damage

radiculitis inflammation of spinal nerve roots

radioactive capable of emitting radiant energy

radioactivity the ability of a substance to emit rays of particles (alpha, beta or gamma) from its nucleus

radiograph(s) an image or picture produced on a radiation sensitive film emulsion by exposure to ionizing radiation directed through an area, region, or substance of interest, followed by chemical processing of the film. It is basically dependent on the differential absorption of radiation directed through heterogeneous media. ***r. bite-wing*** a form of dental radiograph that reveals approximately the coronal halves of the maxillary and mandibular teeth and portions of the interdental alveolar septa on the same film

radioimmunoassay a method for determining concentration of substances particularly protein bound hormones to the range of picograms

radioisotope a radioactive form of an element

radiopaque impermeable to X-ray or other form of radiation

radiopelvimetry measurement of pelvis by use of X-rays

radiopharmaceuticals radioactive chemicals or their combination with carriers. Used for determining size and function of body organs

radioresistant tumors that cannot be destroyed by radiation, and hence are radioresistant

radiotelemetry transmission of data via radio from a patient to a remote monitor for analysis

radiotherapy the treatment of disease by application of X-rays, radium, ultraviolet or other forms of radiations

radium a radioactive and fluorescent metallic element with half-life of 1622 years

ramipril ACE inhibitor

Ramstedt's operation division of hypertrophic pyloric sphincter to relieve obstruction

ramus a branch or division of a forked structure

R

random controlled trial a study plan for a proposed new treatment in which subjects are assigned on a random basis to participate in either an experimental group receiving the new treatment or a control group that does not

random sample the selection of samples from population where each individual in the group has same opportunity of being selected

ranitidine H_2 receptor blocker, used in peptic ulcer

rape intercourse, homosexual or heterosexual, against consent or with consent which is obtained by force. The age of victim for consent varies from countries to countries. In India, it is 16 years

raphe a ridge, crease or point of joining of two halves of a part

rash any eruption of skin usually associated with communicable disease. ***r. butterfly*** skin rash on cheeks and over the bridge of nose as seen in systemic lupus erythematosus. ***r. diaperdiaper*** skin inflammation in diaper areas in infants. ***r. drug*** rash due to drugs like ampicillin, sulphas, iodides and bromides. ***r. macular*** flat rash not protruding above the skin surface. ***r. mulbery*** dusky rash in typhus fever. ***r. nettle*** smooth, elevated itchy rash SYN: urticaria

rate the frequency of occurrence of an event expressed with respect to time or some other standard. ***r. birth*** the number of live births per 1000 in a given population per year. ***r. case fatality*** the ratio of the number of deaths caused by a disease to the total number of people who contracted the disease. ***r. death*** the number of deaths in a year per a specified population. ***r. glomerular filtration*** rate of filtrate formation in glomeruli of the kidneys; normal 120 mL/min. ***r. heart*** the number of heartbeats per minute

ratio relationship between two substances. ***r. albumin globulin*** ratio of albumin to globulin in blood; usually 1.3:1 or 1.4:1. ***r. arm*** in chromosome the ratio of long arm to short arm. ***r. lecithin-sphingomyelin*** the ratio of lecithin to sphingomyelin in amniotic fluid, an indicator of fetal maturity, usually at term. ***r. Odd's*** in epidemiological and case control studies a relative measure of disease occurrence. ***r. therapeutic*** a ratio of effective therapeutic dose to minimum lethal dose

Raynaud's disease intermittent pallor and cyanosis of digits on exposure to cold in females due to abnormal vascular response

reaction response of an organism to a stimulus

reagent a substance that reacts in a chemical reaction to detect presence of another substance

receptor in pharmacology, a cell component that combines with a drug or hormone to alter the function of the cell

recessive gene gene that does not express itself in presence of its dominant allele

recidivity tendency to relapse or to return to a former position/condition

recipient one who receives, e.g. blood, kidney, heart, lungs, etc.

recombination in genetics, the joining together of gene combinations in the offspring that were not present in the parents

recovery room the room where patients are kept to recover from effects of anesthesia after the surgery

rectal crisis rectal pain and tenesmus in CNS disorders

rectal reflex desire to defecate when rectum is filled with stool

rectocele prolapse of posterior vaginal wall along with anterior wall of rectum

rectourethral concerning rectum and urethra

rectouterine concerning rectum and uterus

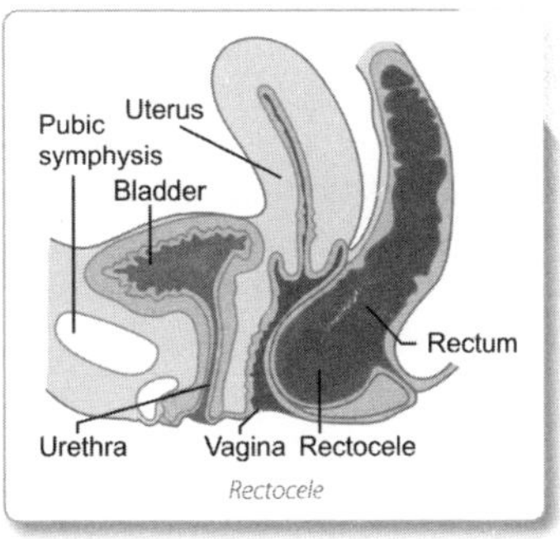

Rectocele

rectovaginal concerning rectum and vagina

rectovesical concerning rectum and bladder

rectum the lower 5" of large intestine, responsible for initiation of defecation reflex through S1S2S3 sacral segments of spinal cord

red cross internationally recognized sign of medical installation or a medical personnel bearing immunity against attack in war

referred pain pain felt at a point remote from point of origin due to similar segmental inervation

reflection 1. the condition of being turned back on itself, e.g. peritoneum. 2. in psychology, mental consideration of something already considered

reflex involuntary instantaneous response to a stimulus; usually purposeful and adaptive. In a simple reflex, the reflex circuit consists of a sensory receptor, afferent neuron, reflex center in brain or spinal cord, efferent neuron supplying the organ (muscle or gland) ***r. Babinski*** flexion of great toe and fanning out of other toes on stroking the lateral aspect of sole of foot in healthy persons. ***r. Bainbridge*** acceleration of heart rate with ventricular distention. ***r. grasp*** grasping reaction of finger on stimulation of hollow of palm, its presence in adults is evidence of diffuse cerebral disease, e.g. GPI., dementia, etc. ***r. hung up*** abnormal slowness of relaxation phase of deep tendon reflex e.g. hung up ankle jerk in hypothyroidism. ***r. light*** contraction of pupil on focussing a bright light on it. ***r. mass*** a condition following complete transection of cord where a weak stimulus brings about widespread responses (muscle contraction, defecation, urination etc.), due to release from inhibition of higher cortical centers. ***r. neck righting*** turning of the body in the direction of head rotation in supine infants elicited between 4 months to 2 years of age. ***r. parachute*** extension of arms, hands and fingers when the infant is suspended in prone position and dropped a short distance to a soft surface. Asymmetrical response indicates motor abnormality in children above 9 months of age. ***r. rooting*** stroking the cheek of the infant causes turning of mouth towards the stimulus. It is present upto 7th month of age. ***r. stepping*** leg movements simulating walking when the infant is held erect, inclined forward with sole of feet touching a flat surface. The reflex is present at birth and is gone by 6 weeks of age. ***r. tonic neck*** in the infant forcibly turning the head causes extension of extremities on the side to which head is turned with flexion of extremities on the other side

reflexology a system of complementary therapy where feet represent the whole body and massage to different parts of feet can relieve hypertension constipation

regional anesthesia a nerve block with an anesthetic agent which ranges from local infiltration to spinal block anesthesia, the most commonly used regional anesthesia in childbirth is the epidural

regurgitation backward flow. ***r. aortic*** backflow of blood from aorta to left ventricle during diastole due to incompetent aortic valve. ***r. duodenal*** reflux of duodenal secretions and bile into stomach. ***r. mitral*** backflow of blood from left ventricle into left atrium during ventricular systole due to incompetent mitral valve. ***r. pulmonary*** backflow of blood from pulmonary artery into right ventricle. ***r. tricuspid*** regurgitation of blood from right ventricle into right atrium

rehabilitation the processes of treatment and education for a disabled patient to achieve maximum function and independent living. ***r. cardiac*** a combination of psychological support, progressive exercise and patient education to achieve maximum functional ability after one has had myocardial infarction

relapse reappearance of symptoms after apparent cure

relapsing fever infectious disease caused by *B. recurrentis*

relaxant an agent decreasing tension, tone of a muscle

relax to diminish anxiety, tension, nervousness

renal failure failure of kidneys to perform excretory and metabolic functions resulting in anuria/ metabolic changes

renal threshold the level of substances in blood beyond which they are excreted in urine

renal transplant surgical implantation of donor kidney to replace a diseased host kidney

reproduction the process by which plants and animals give rise to offsprings. ***r. asexual*** reproduction by fission or budding without involvement of sex cells

research scientific and diligent study, investigation and experimentation to establish facts and intelligently analyze them to derive conclusion

resection partial excision. ***r. wedge*** resection of a piece of tissue in form of a wedge as in polycystic ovary

residual relates to that left as a residue

residual urine urine left in bladder after urination; commonly it is less than 50 mL

resistance 1. power of resisting. 2. in psychology, the force which prevents repressed thoughts from entering conscious mind from the unconscious. 3. the power of body to withstand infection

respiration the act of breathing for interchange of gases, i.e. O_2 and CO_2 ***r. abdominal*** use of diaphragm and abdominal muscles for respiration as in rib fracture, pleurisy. ***r. paradoxical*** a condition seen in paralysis of diaphragm whereby the affected side diaphragm moves up during inspiration and moves down during expiration. ***r. Cheyne-stokes*** abnormal bizarre breathing with periods of apnea followed by gradually increasing depth of respiration followed by a slow decline to end in apnea; seen in diencephalic dysfunction. ***r. Kussmaul's*** deep gasping respiration of diabetic ketoacidosis. ***r. thoracic*** respiration performed entirely by expansion of chest as in peritonitis, diaphragmatic inflammation

respiratory distress syndrome dyspnea in newborn due to deficient pulmonary surfactant, causing atelectasis, commonly seen in prematures. SYN: hyaline membrane disease

respiratory failure inability of lungs to perform ventilatory function with PaO_2 of <60 mm Hg and PCO_2 >50 mm Hg

respiratory quotient the relationship between CO_2 produced and oxygen consumed

restitution restoration putting right a corrective movement of fetal head

resuscitation revival after apparent death

retained placenta placenta fails to be delivered after childbirth due to lack of uterine contraction or morbid adhesious of placenta

retardation slowing down, delayed mental or physical response

retch to make an involuntary attempt to vomit

retention 1. keeping within body of substances like urine, stool. 2. holding back

R

retention of urine inability to pass urine due to obstruction in urinary passage, during labor it is due to stretching of urethra and trigone by presenting part

reticuloendothelial system the phagocytic cell system of body capable of ingesting particulate matter like bacteria, colloid particles. It includes macrophages (both fixed and wandering), reticular cells, Kuffer cells of liver and spleen, microglia of CNS, adventitial cells of blood vessels and dust cells of lungs

retina the innermost light sensitive layer of eye extending from optic disk to margin of pupil. The various layers of retina from without inward are: pigment epithelium, rods and cones, external limiting membrane, external nuclear layer, external plexiform layer, internal nuclear layer, internal plexiform layer, layer of ganglion cells, layer of nerve fibers, internal limiting membrane

retinopathy any disorder of retina; may be arteriosclerotic, diabetic, hypertensive, syphilitic, etc.

retraction shortening, state of being drawn back

retraction ring a ridge of uterus separating upper contractile segment from lower dilating segment

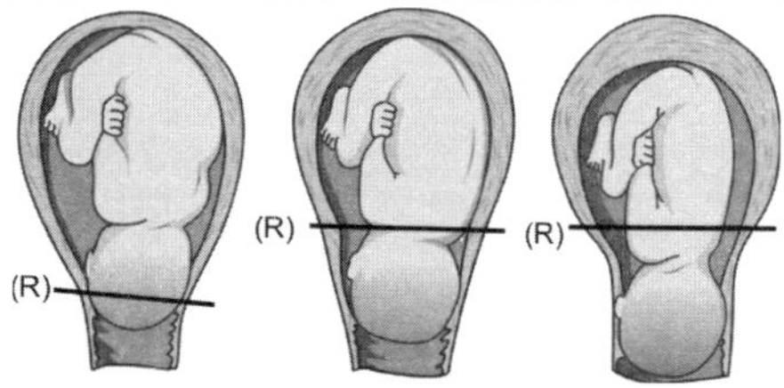

Formation of retraction ring

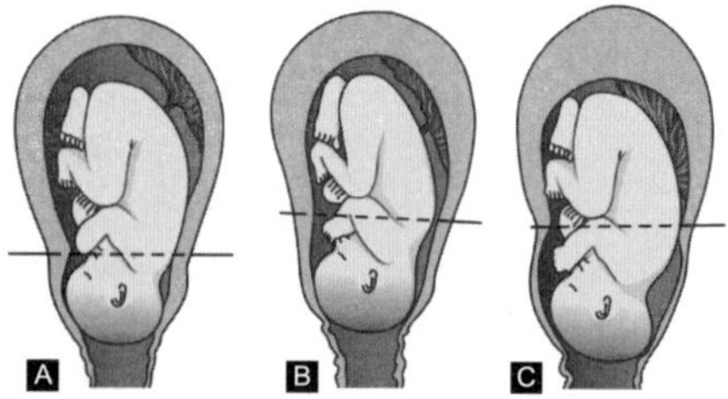

Pathogenesis of retraction ring (Bandl's ring); (A) Normal labor; (B) Early obstruction; (C) Late obstruction

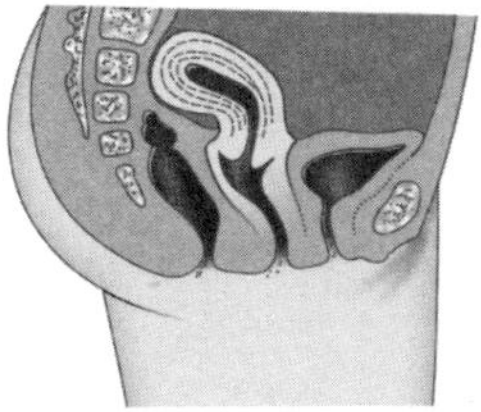

Retroflexion of uterus

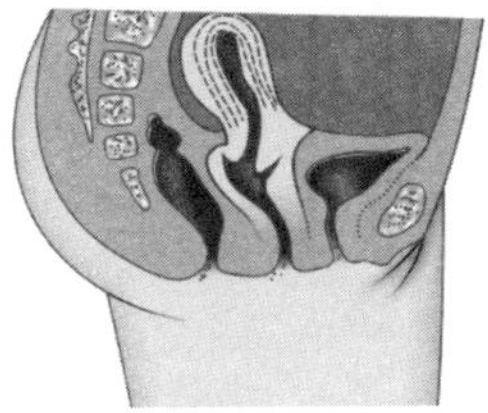

Retroversion of uterus

retractor instrument for holding back a tissue

retro situated behind or backward in position e.g., retroocular, retrobulbar, retrocecal, etc.

retroflexed bent backwards, a retroflexed uterus is the state where uterine body is bent backwards on cervix

retrograde amnesia memory loss for events just preceding the time of patient's illness

retrograde ejaculation semen discharge into bladder rather than through urethral meatus as in diabetic neuropathy

retrograde moving backward

retrolental fibroplasia bilateral retinal vessel occlusion followed by fibrous proliferation often involving the vitreous in premature newborns exposed to high concentration of oxygen

retroperitoneal fibrosis fibrotic tissue growth in retroperitoneal space often compressing ureters, venacava and aorta, a sequel to mathysergide treatment of migraine. SYN: Ormond's syndrome

retroposition backward displacement of an organ

retrospective study a study where patient's records are analyzed after they have experienced the disease

retroversion of uterus backward tilting of entire uterus including cervix so that the latter points towards symphysis pubis

retroviruses a group of viruses containing reverse transcriptase, e.g. RNA-containing tumor viruses causing leukemia, lymphoma, in lower animals and AIDS infection in human

Rey syndrome a syndrome characterized by encephalopathy, and hepatic failure in children in consequence to viral infection, aspirin use

Rh-blood group a blood group antigen on human RBCs, in common with rhesus monkeys. A Rh-ve mother if bears a Rh+ve fetus, Rh antibodies produced in mother may cross the placenta to destroy the fetal RBCs

rheumatic fever a systemic illness that follows streptococcal sore throat manifesting with carditis, fleeting polyarthritis, chorea, erythema marginatum, subcutaneous nodules, etc. believed to be an autoimmune phenomenon

rheumatism a generic term to denote inflammation of muscle, joint pain. ***r. palindromic*** a disease of unknown etiology manifesting with joint pain, joint swelling lasting from few hours to days with periods of complete normalcy. ***r. soft tissue*** pain around a joint not related to any joint pathology, e.g. bursitis, tendinitis, perichondritis, Tietz syndrome, etc.

rheumatoid arthritis bilaterally symmetrical polyarthritis involving the fingers and toes with bony erosion, joint deformity and involvement of great vessels, vertebra, etc.

rheumatoid factor an IgM autoantibody present in up to 75% of patients suffering from rheumatoid arthritis

rheumatoid resembling rheumatism

rhinitis inflammation of nasal mucosa, can be allergic, atrophic (rusting and bad odor), hyperplastic, etc.

rhythm regularity of occurrence of an action or movement or impulse. ***r. alpha*** in EEG a rhythm of 8 to 12 per second. r. beta. Rhythm frequency of 15 to 30 per second in EEG, predominantly in frontomotor leads. ***r. cicardian*** the recurrence of biological activities every 24 hours not being influenced by environment. r. delta A slow EEG rhythm of 4 or less per second with relatively high voltage, usually recorded over tumor or hematoma. ***r. ectopic*** impulse originating outside SA node. ***r. escape*** an impulse originating from a site other than SA node when the latter fails to initiate the impulse. ***r. gallop*** three heart sounds heard (S1S2S3) in sequence in each cardiac contraction resembling gallop of horse. ***r. gamma*** in EEG, 50/second rhythm. ***r. idioventricular*** impulse originating from bundle of His or myocardium in consequence to complete A-V block. ***r. theta*** an EEG rhythm of 4 to 7 cycles/sec. r. tic-tac A rhythm where S1, and S2 are of same quality usually in cardiac distress or in fetus

rib one of the 12 pairs of narrow curved bones of chest wall connecting sternum to vertebra. ***r. cervical*** a super numerary rib arising from 7th cervical vertebra and often causing thoracic inlet syndrome by compression of lower cord of brachial plexus

riboflavin yellow-orange crystalline powder of B complex group functioning as coenzyme in cellular oxidation; Richly found in milk and milk products, green leafy vegetables, fish and meat; deficiency causes glossitis, seborrhea, cheilosis and corneal vascularization

ribonucleic acid (RNA) RNA differs from DNA in that its sugar is ribose and the pyrimidine compound it contains is uracil rather than thymine. RNA is principal constituent of cytoplasm and of certain viruses. Messenger RNA carries the transcription code for specific amino acid sequences from DNA to cytoplasmic reticulum for protein synthesis. Transfer RNA carries the amino acid groups to the ribosomes for incorporation into proteins

ribosome a constituent of cell cytoplasm that receives genetic information and translates them into synthesis of proteins

rickets a vitamin D deficiency disease in children where mineralization of newly formed osteoid tissue is defective. The child is restless with aches and pains, hepatosplenomegaly, delayed dentition, soft skull bones with proneness to skeletal deformities like kyphoscoliosis, bow leg, pigeon chest. ***r. renal*** rickets in chronic renal failure primarily due to inadequate formation of active vitamin D3 and accompanying acidosis causing bone dissolution. ***r. vitamin D resistant*** defects of renal tubular function causing excessive renal calcium and phosphorus loss so that the accompanying ricket responds poorly to vitamin D

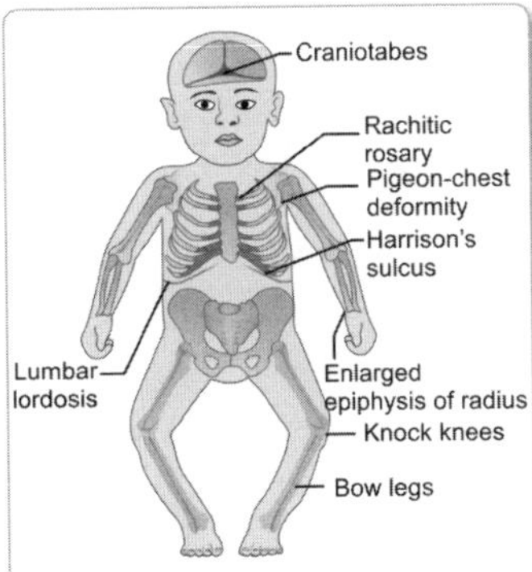

Rickets

rifampin an antibiotic from *Streptomyces*, used in treatment of mycobacterial diseases (leprosy, tuberculosis) and meningitis prophylaxis. Other congeners are rifabutin and rifapentia

rigor mortis the stiffening of body occurring soon after death

rigor paroxysmal chill

ripening 1. softening and dilatation of cervix during labor. 2. maturation of cataract

risk-benefit analysis in medicare, the analysis of risk and benefit from a procedure discussed between patient, doctor and relations

Ritgen's maneuver an obstetric procedure aimed to assist the delivery of the head of the fetus and protect the structure of perineum of the mother

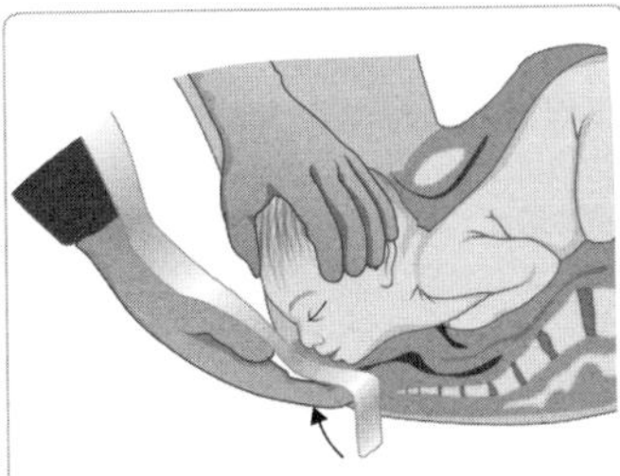

Ritgen's maneuver

R

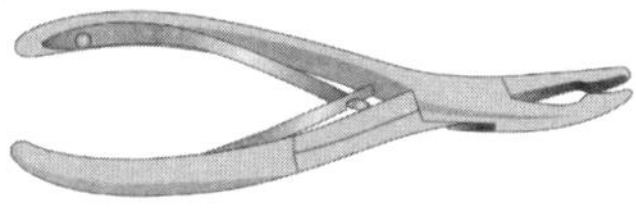

Rongeur

by applying an upward pressure from the coccygeal region to extend the head of the fetus

ritodrine Beta2 agonist for use in bronchial asthma

Roentgen German physicist who discovered Roentgen rays, (X-rays) and won noble prize in 1901

rongeur An instrument which is used to cut bone

rooming-in the baby remains by mothers bedside when she is in hospital, thus strengthening the bond between baby and mother

rooting-reflex a reflex in new born where stroking the cheek or side of mouth allows baby to turn towards side stimulated and open the month

Rose's position a position in which head and neck of the patient is extended and allowed to hang over the end of operating table so as to prevent aspiration of blood in the mouth and lips during surgery.

rotation the turning of the body along its long axis

rotavirus virus causing epidemic and sporadic enteritis

roth spots small white spot on retina close to optic disk in acute infective endocarditis

roughage fibers in cereals, fruits and vegetable, essential for patients of diabetes and those with constipation but inadvisable for patients of colitis

round ligament round cord-like structures passing from uterus in the broad ligament and then through the inguinal canal to end in soft tissues of labia majora

rubefacient agents causing redness of skin by vasodilatation, e.g. liniments of turpentine

rubella acute infectious disease of viral origin causing rash, cervical and post-auricular lymphadenopathy, in first trimester can cause fetal anomalies and in pubertal girls can cause oophoritis

Rubin test a test for potency of uterine tubes, also called tubal insufflation test

rugose, rugous having many wrinkles or creases

rule of nine formula for estimating percentage of body surface area, where head represents 9%, front and back of trunk 18% each, each lower extremity 18%, each upper extremity 9% and perineum 1%

rumination 1. regurgitation of previously swallowed food. 2. obsessional preoccupation with thoughts

rupture breaking apart of any organ or tissue e.g. of amniotic membrane, uterus, intestines, Fallopian tubes

Ryle's tube thin rubber tube with a weighted end introduced via nose to stomach for aspiration of gastric contents or administration of drugs and fluids

saber sin convex prominent anterior border of tibia in congenital syphilis

sabin vaccine oral polio vaccine containing inactivated poliovirus

saccharide a group of carbohydrates including mono-, di-, tri-, and polysaccharides

sacculation group of sacs or formed into group of sacs

sacculation of uterus a rare complication of incarceration of the retroverted gravid uterus in which the fundus remains under the sacral promontory and the anterior wall grows to accommodate the fetus

sacrococcygeus one of the two muscles, anterior and posterior extending from sacrum to coccyx

sacrovertebral angle angle formed between base of sacrum and fifth lumbar vertebra

sacrum the triangular bone of buttock lying in between the two iliac bones forming sacroiliac joints. Male sacrum is narrower and more curved

saddle nose a depressed nasal bridge, due to congenital absence of bony or cartilaginous support or destructive disease like leprosy and syphilis

sadism sexual pleasure from inflicting physical or mental torture on others

sagittal anteroposterior direction

sagittal plane the plane that divides body into left and right halves

sagittal suture suture between two parietal bones

salbutamol a beta sympathomimetic used to suppress premature labor; contraindicated in preeclampsia and antepartum hemorrhage

salicylate salt of salicylic acid. Methyl salicylate is a counter irritant whereas sodium salicylate is analgesic and antipyretic

saline enema 1 teaspoon of salt dissolved in a pint of water to which is added magnesium sulfate (epsum salt) to induce catharsis

saline solution of salt or salty; can be hypertonic >0.9% or hypotonic <0.85% concentration

saliva colorless, odorless, weakly alkaline secretion of salivary glands. Contains ptyalin, maltase and lysozymes. Daily secretion is up to 1500 mL

salk vaccine formalin inactivated poliomyelitis vaccine for intramuscular use

salmeterol beta2-adrenergic stimulant

salmonellosis infection with *Salmonella* group of organism producing typhoid fever, gastroenteritis and septicemia

salpingectomy surgical removal of fallopian tubes

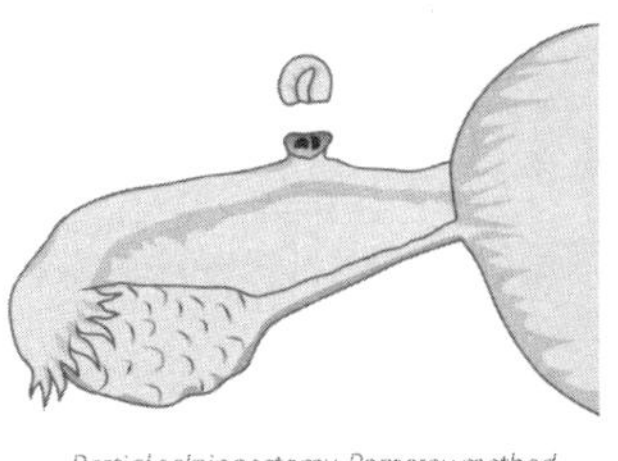

Partial salpingectomy, Pomeroy method

S

salpingitis inflammation of Fallopian tubes usually due to gonococci, tuberculosis, strepto and staphylococci

salpingo-oophorectomy excision of ovary and Fallopian tube

salpingo-oophoritis inflammation of Fallopian tube and ovary

salpingography imaging of Fallopian tubes by injection of radiopaque dye in investigation of infertility

salpingolysis surgical procedure to free the Fallopian tubes of adhesions

salpingopexy surgical fixation of Fallopian tube

salpingoplasty SYN: tuboplasty; plastic surgery of Fallopian tube to promote fertility

salpingorrhaphy ligation of Fallopian tube

salpingostomy surgical opening up of a Fallopian tube

salpingotomy incision on a Fallopian tube

salpinx the Fallopian or Eustachian tube

salt 1. sodium chloride. 2. a chemical compound formed from action of an acid with a base. ***s. bile*** salt of glycocolic and taurocolic acids present in bile, help in absorption of fat. ***s. iodized*** salt containing 1 part of sodium or potassium iodide per 10,000 parts of sodium chloride for iodine deficiency. ***s. smelling*** aromatized ammonium carbonate

sanguinous bloody

saphenous nerve a deep branch of femoral nerve supplying innerside of foot and leg

saphenous veins the long saphenous vein extends from foot to saphenous opening in upper thigh where as short saphenous vein runs up behind lateral malleolus to join popliteal vein

sarcoid 1. resembling flesh 2. small tubercle-like lesion characteristic of sarcoidosis

sarcoma cancer of connective tissue like muscle and bone. ***s. Ewing's*** a fusiform swelling of long bones containing round endothelial cells. ***s. Kaposi's*** a skin sarcoma in AIDS victims. ***s. osteogenic*** sarcoma in metaphysis of long bones containing variously shaped cells. ***s. reticulum cells*** a form of malignant lymphoma

satiety feeling satisfied with food

scab crust formed on a wound, pustule or ulcer

scald burn caused by moist heat or hot vapors

scalpel a straight surgical knife with a convex edge

scalp the hairy portion of head, consisting from out to inwards: skin, dense subcutaneous tissue, occipitofrontalis muscle with the galea aponeurotica, and periosteum

scan an image produced by moving detector or sweeping beam of radiation

scapula the flat triangular bone at the back of shoulder articulating with clavicle and humerus. ***s. winged*** paralysis of serratus anterior or trapezius causing prominence of medial border of scapula

Schilling test a test using radioactive B12 for assessment of vitamin B12 absorption and diagnosis of intrinsic factor deficiency as in pernicious anemia

schizoid personality disorder a personality cult with difficult interpersonal relationship, and a limited range of emotional experience and expression; the cold, lonely, aloof personality

schizophrenia a form of psychosis with disorder of thinking, affect and behavior. Patients have delusions and hallucinations with loss of self identity. **s. catatonic** patients have catatonic stupor or mutism, catatonic rigidity, catatonic posturing, etc. **s. paranoid** patient has delusions of persecution, jealousy

schultze expulsion of placenta at the end of third stage of labor; the placenta is expelled inverted, the fetal surface appearing first near vulva

sciatic pertains to hip or ischium

sciatica pain along the course of sciatic nerve from back of thigh along lateral border of leg to little toe usually due to disk prolapse at L5-S1

scissor gait crossing of the legs while walking as in cerebral diplegia

scissors a cutting instrument with two opposing blades with handles held together by a pin

sclera the outer tough white fibrous tissue of eyeball extending from optic nerve to corneal margin. ***s. blue*** abnormally thin sclera with visible choroid as in osteogenesis imperfecta

sclerema hardening of the skin

scleritis inflammation of sclera, can be anterior (adjacent to cornea), posterior or annular (in ring fashion around cornea)

sclerosis hardening or induration of a tissue due to excessive growth of fibrous tissue, a feature of degeneration. ***s. amyotrophic lateral*** a form of motor neurone disease which results in atrophy of anterior horn cells and the pyramidal tracts. ***s. multiple*** a slowly progressive disease of central nervous system marked by widespread demyelination producing visual disturbances, sensory motor deficit, and cerebellar symptoms

scoliosis lateral curvature of spine; the abnormal curve and the compen-

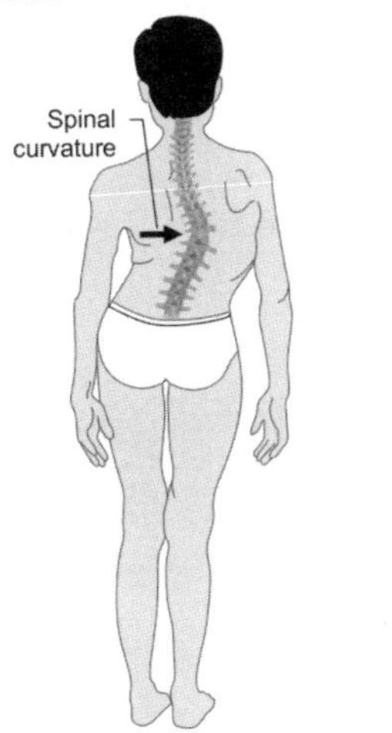

Scoliosis

satory curve in opposite direction; can be congenital, myopathic, ocular, paralytic, etc.

score a rating or grade as compared to standard. ***s. Apgar*** a scoring system for evaluation of neurological maturity of newborn from pulse, respiration, reflexes, skin color, grimace, etc.

Scriver test a biological test for diagnosing whole range of inborn errors of metabolism

scrotum the double cavity male pouch containing testicles and epididymis, composed of layers of skin, nonstriated dartos muscle, cremasteric, infundibular and spermatic fascia, cremasteric muscle and tunica vaginalis

scurvy vitamin C or ascorbic acid deficiency manifest with bleeding spongy gums, subperiosteal hemorrhage, muscle pain and induration, loosening of teeth and poor wound healing

sebaceous cyst sebum filled cyst of sebaceous gland with a black head, may need complete extirpation rather than drainage

sebaceous gland holocrine glands (secretion arising from complete disintegration of cells) in the skin that open into hair follicle and secrete oily substance, the sebum

sebum a fatty secretion from sebaceous gland, that from the ear is called cerumen and from pepuce is called smegma

secondary hemorrhage hemorrhage occurring after 48 hours of injury or operation commonly due to sepsis

secretin a hormone secreted from duodenum that stimulates secretion of pepsinogen and inhibits secretion of acid by stomach

secretion substances produced or the process of glandular secretion. ***s. apocrine*** a process by which the secreting cell breaks off to extrude the secretion, e.g. milk production. ***s. holocrine*** the process where the entire cell and its contents are extruded, e.g. sebum. ***s. merocrine*** the process where the cell remains intact and discharges its secretion through cell membrane

sedative agent that soothes, quietens or brings tranquility

sedimentation rate a test to determine the speed at which RBCs settle down when suspended in a test tube. The speed depends upon the size of RBC aggregate which is further dependent upon fibrinogen content of blood. Fibrinogen is an acute phase reactant and is increased in infection, inflammation of any etiology. ESR is reduced in polycythemia, congenital cyanotic heart disease and microcytic hypochromic anemia. Normal ESR is 10 to 15 mm/hr in male and slightly higher in female

segment a section or part ***s. upper uterine*** the upper three quarter of uterus that contracts and retracts during labor ***s. lower uterine*** the lowermost quarter of uterus that dilates during first stage of labor

segmentation division into similar parts; division of fertilized egg into many smaller cells

seizure a sudden attack of pain, disease or certain symptoms like convulsion, epilepsy

selenium sulfide drug used in treatment of tinea versiolor and dandruff

Sellick's maneuver the application of backward pressure on the cricoid cartilage in order to occlude esophagus to prevent aspiration of stomach content

semen thick viscid fishy odor discharge per male urethra during sexual climax. It contains the sperms 60 to 150 million/mL. The 80% are motile and normal in morphology. Semen is alkaline without any leukocytes, volume per ejaculation is 2 to 5 mL

seminal vesicle two sac-like structures close to prostate in the male giving rise to ductus deferens. Act to store semen and secrete a thick viscous fluid that forms part of semen

senna leaves of a plant, used as cathartic

sense 1. the general faculty responsible for perceiving the outside world. 2. to perceive. 3. normal power of understanding

sensitive 1. able to feel a sensation. 2. abnormal response to substances like drugs and foreign proteins

sensitivity 1. the term is employed in relation to accuracy of diagnostic tests/observations. It is the proportion of people who truely have a specific disease as identified by the test. 2. susceptibility of bacteria to antimicrobials

sensitization making a person susceptible to a substance by its repeated injection

sensorium the sensory apparatus of body or consciousness

sepsis a pathological state due to bacterial multiplication and toxin production. ***s. puerperal*** infection of genital passage resulting from childbirth. Common infecting agents are strepto, staphylo and *Escherichia coli*

septicemia multiplication of pathogenic bacteria in peripheral blood producing toxemia, disseminated cellulitis, lymphangitis, etc.

septum a partition wall dividing two cavities, e.g. interatrial, interventricular, atrioventricular, nasal septum, rectovaginal. ***s. pellucidum*** a thin triangular sheet of nervous tissue forming the medial wall of the lateral ventricles. s. primum The embryonic septum dividing the two atria in a developing heart

septuplet seven offsprings produced at one birth

sequela the final outcome of a disease with or without treatment

serology the scientific study of serum

seroma a localized collection of serum resembling a tumor, commonly after stitching of operational wounds

S

serosa a serous membrane like pleura, pericardium and peritoneum

serotonin 5 hydroxytryptamine present in platelets, mast cells, argentaffin cells of carcinoid tumors. A potent vasoconstrictor incriminated in migraine

serrate tooth-like, notched

serum the straw-colored fluid after blood coagulates

sex chromatin SYN: Barr body. It represents the inactivated 'X' chromosome in female somatic cells (Lyon hypothesis)

sex chromosome the X and Y chromosomes which determine the sex of an individual

sex the distinctive characteristics that separate living beings and plants into males and females

sextuplet six children in one pregnancy

sexual dysfunction sexual dissatisfaction due to defective arousal, orgasm, pain or penetration

sexually transmitted diseases (STD) diseases acquired during sexual intercourse with partner. They include syphilis, gonorrhea, lymphogranuloma venereum, granuloma inguinale, chancroid, acquired immunodeficiency syndrome, genital herpes and warts, viral hepatitis B, chlamydia urethritis, etc.

shaken baby syndrome presence of unexplained fractures in the long bones with subdural hematoma in child abuse

shake test Also called bubble test. A bedside test for amniotic fluid, formerly used for rapid estimation of fetal lung maturity and now largely replaced by more refined tests

sheath a connective tissue covering. ***s. carotid*** enclosure of carotid artery, vagus nerve and internal jugular vein by cervical fascia. ***s. myelin*** layers of lipid and protein forming a semifluid covering of nerves, an extension of plasma membrane of Schwann cells. ***s. synovial*** double walled tube like bursa enclosing the tendon of hands and feet

Sheehan's syndrome hypopituitarism secondary to pituitary infarction following postpartum hemorrhage and shock

shiatsu a form of alternate medicine based on principles similar to acupuncture

shingles SYN: Herpes zoster producing painful vesicles along course of a nerve

Shirodkar operation placement of purse-string suture around cervix to prevent premature delivery in incompetent cervix

shock a state of poor tissue perfusion due to deficient circulating blood volume, pump failure or sudden fear, anaphylaxis, overwhelming infection, drugs, toxins. ***s. anaphylactic*** shock following injection of foreign substances to a sensitized patient. ***s. cardiogenic*** shock due to pump failure following myocardial infarction or electrical disturbances.

s. endotoxic shock from endotoxins of gram-negative bacteria. ***s. spinal*** acute flaccid paralysis with loss of all sensations and reflexes following complete transection of spinal cord

shoulder the junction of upper arm with collar bone and scapula. ***s. dislocation*** slipping of humeral head from glenoid cavity of scapula

shoulder dystocia after delivery of head, the shoulder fails to rotate and descend due to large baby or contracted pelvis

shoulder presentation a state which develops when labor begins with the fetus lying obliquely and the position is not corrected so that on vaginal examination the presenting part feels high with palpable fetal ribs

show blood mixed thick mucoid discharge from vagina during first stage of labor

shunt diversion of flow. ***s. arteriovenous*** congenital abnormal arterio-venous communication or the one done for hemodialysis. ***s. left to right*** passage of blood from left side of heart to right side chambers as in VSD, ASD, PDA. ***s. right to left*** reverse of the above occurring in Fallot tetralogy, transposition of great vessels, single ventricle, DORV and Eisenmenger syndrome

Siamese twins (named after Chang and Eng joined Chinese twins born in Siam), cogenitally joined twins

sibling children of same parent

sickle cell anemia a form of congenital hemolytic anemia where there is abnormal hemoglobin (Hbs) resulting in sickling during splenic hypoxic conditioning

sickle cell crisis capillary plugging by sickle cells causing joint pain, abdominal pain, renal pain, etc. due to infarction

sickness illness. ***s. motion*** nausea and vomiting experienced during motion by road, air or water. ***s. morning*** nausea and vomiting of early pregnancy. ***s. mountain*** nausea, anorexia, insomnia and dyspnea of high altitude due to oxygen lack. ***s. sleeping*** 1. trypanosomiasis involving CNS (Chaga's disease), transmitted by tsetse fly. 2. encephalitis lethargica. ***s. serum*** joint pain, fever, lymphadenopathy following injection of serum

sigmoidoscopy examination of recto-sigmoid by sigmoidoscope

sign any objective evidence or manifestation of disease

sildenafil citrate specific inhibitor of cGMP, used in male erectile dysfunction

Silverman-Anderson score a system for evaluation of breathing performance of preterm infants based on chest retraction, retraction of lower intercostals muscles, xiphoid retraction, flaring of nares with inspiration, and expiratory grunt. Each of the five is graded as 0,1,2, with severe respiratory distress score can reach 10

silver nitrate a germicide and local astringent used for throat cauterization; causes grayish discoloration of mucous membranes

simian crease a single transverse crease on palm as in monkeys. Its presence may signify Down's syndrome, rubella syndrome, Turner's syndrome, Klinefelter's syndrome

Simmond's disease hypopituitarism due to pituitary atrophy

Simon's position an exaggerated lithotomy position with elevation of buttock and abduction of thighs, employed for operation of vagina

Sims position similar to left lateral position, right thigh and knee down up

Sims speculum a form of vaginal speculum

sinciput front and upper part of head

singer's test a test to distinguish fetal from maternal blood

sinoatrial node node at entry of superior vena cava into right atrium, the pacemaker of heart

sinus a cavity within bone, dilated venous channel, a cavity with small opening. ***s. cavernous*** the intracranial sinus extending from sphenoidal fissure to the apex of the petrous portion of temporal bone. ***s. circular*** a venous sinus around pituitary body communicating on each side with the cavernous sinus. ***s. coronary*** the vein in the atrioventricular groove of heart draining into right atrium. ***s. inferior petrosal*** a large venous sinus along lower margin of petrous part of temporal bone draining into cavernous sinus. ***s. maxillary*** cavity in the maxilla communicating with middle meatus of nose. Both maxillary sinuses are usually symmetrical. ***s. sigmoid*** continuation of transverse sinus along posterior border of petrous part of temporal bone to the jugular foramen to continue as jugular vein. ***s. superior sagittal*** a straight sinus along upper border of falx cerebri from the crista galli to the internal occipital protuberance where it joins transverse sinus, the left or right

Sjögren syndrome an autoimmune disorder marked by combination of rheumatoid arthritis with xerostomia

skeleton the bony framework supporting and protecting the viscera. It consists of 206 bones, 80 axial and 126 appendicular

Skene's glands paraurethral glands opening to the floor of terminal urethra. Constantly involved in gonococcal infection

skull the bony structure of head enclosing and protecting the brain divided into vault, base and face

slough a mass of necrotic tissue, to cast off a mass of necrotic tissue

small for gestational age a baby weighing less than expected for age of gestation, are vulnerable for birth asphyxia

smallpox a highly contagious and fatal disease caused by a poxvirus, variola

smear specimen of superficial cells from vagina or cervix, for histological and bacteriological examination

smegma the thick odorous secretion from Tyson's glands under prepuce and under labia minora

Smith-Hemli-Optiz syndrome Small stature, mental retardation, crypto-orchidism and failure to thrive

smoking in pregnancy can impair fetal growth and development from vasoconstriction

sneeze a sudden spasmodic expiration through nose

sniffing position proper position of the baby's head during bag and mask ventilation or endotracheal intubation. The baby's head and back are in straight alignment and the baby's chin is pulled as if sniffing. The neck is not hyperextended

snore the noise produced while breathing through mouth during sleep

snuffles noisy breathing and nasal catarrh of infants with syphilis

sodium chromoglycate mast cell stabilizer used in asthma as acrosol

sodium light, silvery white alkali metal which violently decomposes water forming sodium hydroxide and hydrogen. ***s. acetate*** systemic and urinary alkalizer. ***s. alginate*** a food additive. ***s. benzoate*** a food preservative. ***s. bicarbonate*** used IV to treat acidosis. ***s. carbonate*** washing soda. ***s. chloride*** table salt; 0.9% solution is osmotically compatible with blood. s. lactate In one-sixth or one- fourth molar solution used IV to correct acidosis. ***s. monofluorophosphate*** for topical application on teeth to prevent caries. ***s. morrhuate*** a sclerosing agent used to obliterate varices. ***s. nitrite*** antidote for cyanide poisoning. ***s. nitroprusside*** a powerful vasodilator. ***s. polystyrene sulonate*** cation exchange resin used to lower body potassium. ***s. propionate*** possesses antifungal action. ***s. salicylate*** analgesic and antipyretic. ***s. thiosulate*** antidote for cyanide poisoning

soft chancre/sore benereal ulcer of vulve due to Ducrey's bacillus

soft palate the posterior portion of roof of mouth

solute the substance that is dissolved in a solution

solution a homogeneous mixture of solid, liquid or gaseous substance in a liquid from which the dissolved substance can be recovered by crystallization or other physical process

solvent a liquid that has power to dissolve

soma the body as distinct from mind

somatic pertains to body, the nonreproductive cells, skeletal muscles

somatization expression of emotional conflicts as bodily ailment

S

somatoform disorder a group of disorders in which there are symptoms of a disease but no objective evidence to explain the symptoms

somatome an appliance for cutting body of the fetus

somatomedin insulin-like growth factors derived from liver (somatomedin C and A) that stimulate growth under influence of growth hormone

somatostatin a hypothalamic hormone that inhibits release of somatotropin, insulin, and gastrin

somatotrophin growth hormone

somnambulism sleep walking, the performance of any fairly complex act while in a sleep-like state or trance

sonar refers to ultrasound in medical diagnosis

sonogram ultrasonography record

sonolucent condition of not reflecting the ultrasound wave back to the source

soporific a drug producing sleep, narcotic

sorbitol a crystalline alcohol used as sweetening agent

sordes brown crusts that form on lips in unconscious

sore painful lesion of skin or mucous membrane

souffle a bruit, soft blowing sound. ***s. uterine*** blood flow within uterine arteries producing the sound

sound auditory sensation produced by vibrations, noise, measured in decibels. ***s. Korotkoff's*** sounds heard over an artery during blood pressure measurement. ***s. succussion*** splashing sound heard over a cavity filled with fluid. ***s. tubular*** breath sound heard over trachea and large bronchi

soyamilk a substitute for milk in lactose intolerance

spalding sign gross overlapping of fetal cranial bones in intrauterine fetal death

spasm sudden involuntary muscle contraction, can be clonic (alternate contraction and relaxation) or tonic (sustained contraction)

spasticity increased muscle tone with muscular stiffness as in upper motor neuron lesions

spatula flat instrument for mixing or spreading semisolids

specific gravity weight of a substance compared with equal volume of water. Specific gravity of water is taken as 1000

speculum instrument for examination of canals e.g. ear speculum, vaginal speculum

spermatic cord the cord suspending the testis and is composed of vas deferens, spermatic arteries, veins and lymphatics

spermatid a precursor cell of spermatozoon derived from secondary spermatocyte

spermatogenesis the process of formation of mature spermatozoa, i.e. spermatogonium–

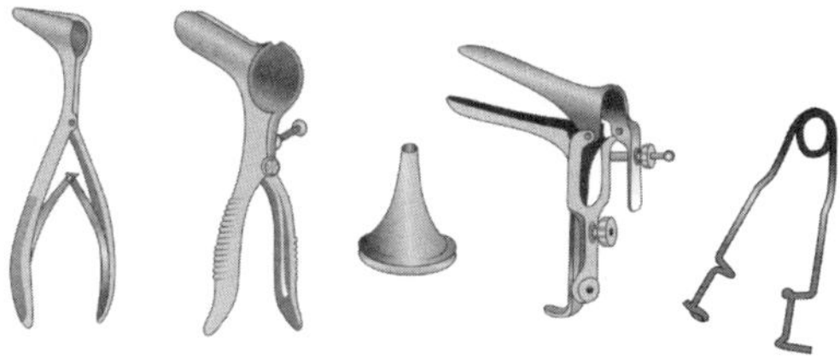

Speculum

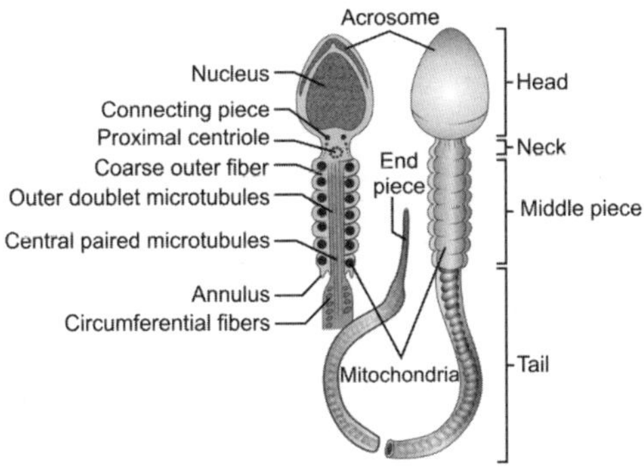

Spermatozoon

primary spermatocyte–secondary spermatocyte–spermatid–motile functional spermatozoa

spermatozoon the mature male germ cell formed within the seminiferous tubules of testis, freely mobile resembling a tadpole

spermicide agent that kills spermatozoa

sperm the male reproductive cell the spermatozoa

sphenoid bone large bone placed at base of skull between the parietal and temporal bones laterally, occipital bone behind and ethmoid in front

spherocyte erythrocyte assuming globular shape

spherocytosis a form of congenital hemolytic anemia characterized by hemolysis, anemia, splenomegaly and jaundice with increased red cell fragility

S

sphincter circular muscle fibers that close an orifice when contracted, e.g. anal sphincter, lower esophageal sphincter, pyloric sphincter and sphincter of Oddi

sphingomyelins phosphorus containing sphingolipids principally found in nervous tissue. They are derived from choline phosphate and a ceramide

sphygmomanometer instrument for indirect measurement of arterial blood pressure, can be aneroid or mercurial

spinal anesthesia anesthesia produced by injection of anesthetic agents into spinal canal

spinal column the vertebral column consisting of 33 vertebra: 7 cervical, 12 thoracic, 5 lumbar, 5 sacral and 4 in the coccyx

spinal cord the nervous tissue contained in spinal canal extending from medulla to lower border of first lumbar vertebra. The gray matter within spinal cord is in the form of H

spinal curvature curvature of spine which is often physiological like cervical and lumbar lordosis and thoracic kyphosis

spinal fluid cerebrospinal fluid lying in the central canal and around the spinal cord within the subarachnoid space

spinal nerves 31 pairs of nerves arising from spinal cord; 8 cervical, 12 thoracic, 5 lumbar, 5 sacral and coccygeal. Each nerve has a ventral efferent motor root and an afferent dorsal sensory root. Each nerve has white and gray rami communicant which pass to the ganglia of sympathetic trunk

spina the spine. ***s. bifida*** congenital nonunion between the laminae of vertebra

spin barkeit mucus on cervix, used to determine time of ovulation when the mucus can be drawn on a glass slide to maximum length

spirogram a record made by a spirograph depicting respiratory movements

spirometer an apparatus for measuring the air capacity of the lungs

spleen a lymphoid vascular organ in left hypocondrium at the tail of pancreas, consisting of red and white pulp, functions as erythropoietic organ in embryo, and filtrates bacteria, senescent red blood cells, inclusion bodies from the blood

splenic flexure junction of transverse colon with descending colon

splenomegaly enlargement of spleen

splint an appliance used for protection, fixation or union of injured part, can be movable or immovable. ***s. abutment*** adjacent tooth restorations that have been rigidly united at their proximal contact areas to form a single abutment with multiple roots. ***s. buccal*** a material such as plaster that can be placed on the buccal surfaces of assembled fixed partial denture units and onto which these components can be assembled and held in accurate relation after hardening. ***s. crib*** An appliance used for temporary tooth stabilization; constructed of gold, acrylic resin, chrome-cobalt alloys, or combinations thereof. It consists of a continuous crib clasp covering the facial and lingual surfaces of the teeth to be splinted. ***s. interdental*** an appliance made of plastic or metallic materials that is applied to the labial and lingual aspects of the teeth to provide points for applying mandibular and maxillofacial traction and fixation. ***s. labial*** an appliance of plastic, metal, or combinations of plastic and metal made to conform to the labial aspect of the dental arch. Used in the management of mandibular and maxillofacial injuries. ***s. Thomas*** a long wire splint with a proximal ring that fits into upper thigh, used for fracture femur

spondylitis inflammation of vertebra

spondylolisthesis forward subluxation of lower lumbar vertebra on sacral vertebra

spondylosis degenerative disease of vertebra and the intervertebral disk with new bone formation at vertebral margins and facet joint arthropathy

spondylos vertebra

sponge an absorbent pad made up of cotton and gauze to absorb fluids and blood, used in wound dressing. ***s. gelatin*** spongy substance of gelatin used to stop internal bleeding

spore an asexual reproductive unit of plants, some protozoa and bacteria

spotting appearance of blood-tinged discharge from vagina in between periods or at onset of labor

sprain trauma to the ligamentous capsular support of a joint with tearing of fibers and hemorrhage

spurious false, adulterated

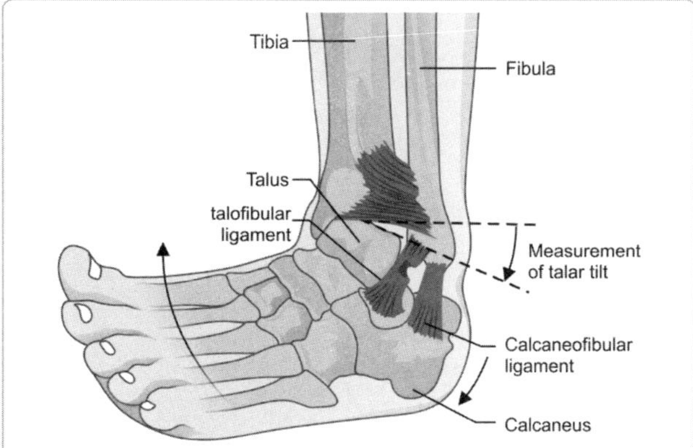

Sprain

sputum material expelled by coughing containing bronchial secretions, alveolar collections. ***s. nummular*** round coin-shaped flat forms of sputum sinking in water as seen in bronchiectasis

squatting sitting on ones haunches and heels

standard deviation in statistics, it is the square root of variance

standard error a measure of variability; the difference beween means of two samples

stanozolol anabolic steroid, used for muscle building

Staphylococcus gram-positive cocci appearing as bunch of grapes. Cause boils, carbuncles, internal abscess, food poisoning, toxic shock syndrome and scalded skin syndrome

stasis stagnation or stoppage

station the location of presenting part of fetus in the birth canal, designated as –5 to –1 according to number of centimeters, the part is above the imaginary plane passing through ilial spine. O when at the level of spine 1 to 5 according of number of centimeters the part is below the plane

statistics the systematic collection, organization and analysis of data and their interpretation

status a state or condition. ***s. asthmaticus*** persistent and intractable asthma. SYN: acute severe asthma. ***s. epilepticus*** recurrent convulsive episodes without regain of consciousness in between

Stein-Leventhal syndrome polycystic ovary syndrome with amenorrhea and infertility

stem cell the cell which is initial precursor of specific differentiated red blood cells

stenosis constriction or narrowing

stercobilin a brown pigment derived from bile that imparts the color to feces

sterile free from living microorganism; unable to procreate

sterility the state of being free from living microorganisms; state of being sterile

sterilization the process of destroying all microorganisms either by heat, chemical or ionizing radiation

sternum the narrow fat bone in the midline of thorax in front

steroid any organic compound containing cyclopentanoperhydrinophenanthrene ring

stethoscope instrument used to appreciate internal body sounds, i.e. respiratory, cardiovascular and intestinal

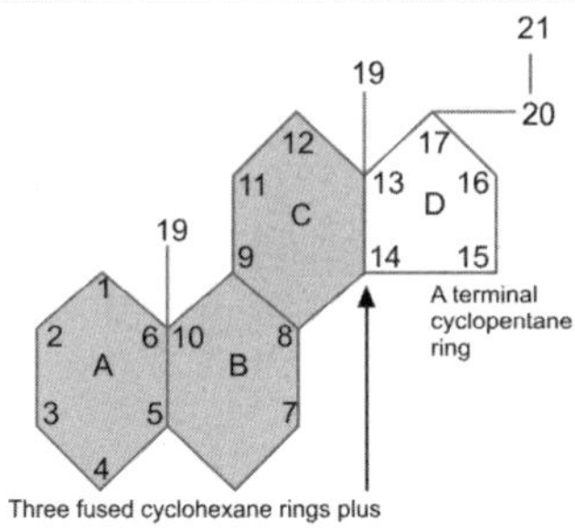

Steroid

stillbirth birth of dead fetus

stillette a wire for keeping clear the lumen of hollow structures like needles

stoma a mouth or opening

stomach the most dilated sac-like portion of alimentary tract in between esophagus and duodenum, secretes hydrochloric acid and pepsinogen, destroys the microorganisms and subserves as a reservoir

stomatitis inflammation of mouth. ***s. aphthous*** development of minute tiny painful ulcers on mucosa of mouth and tongue

stool the discharge from bowel through anus. The stool of newborn is first meconium then gradually changes to brown, and then to yellow

strabismus an abnormality of the eyes in which optic axes do not meet at the desired point due to incoordinate action of extraocular muscles

straight sinus the venous sinus at the junction of falx cerebri and tentorium cerebelli, prone to rupture with cerebral hemorrhage if there is excess molding of head during labor

strangury painful and interrupted urination

Streptococcus gram-positive cocci occurring in chains differentiated into alpha, beta and gamma types based on their reaction on agar plates. Those of alpha type (*S. viridans*) produce a greenish coloration about colonies and partially hemolyze the blood; those of beta type (*S. pyogenes*) form a clear zone about colonies and completely hemolyze the blood, gamma type (***S. faecalis***) are nonhemolytic and produce grayish discoloration about the colonies. ***S. pneumoniae*** gram-positive spherical capsulated cocci causing lobar pneumonia, otitis media. ***S. pyogenes*** hemolytic streptococci producing rheumatic fever, scarlet fever, puerperal sepsis. ***S. viridans*** organism producing endocarditis

streptokinase catalytic enzyme produced by hemolytic streptococci. It activates blood fibrinolytic system, used for dissolution of coronary thrombus

stress any stimulus that tends to disrupt body homeostasis to cause disease/disability

stress fracture hairline fracture often only visible 3 to 4 weeks after undue muscle stress as in runners

stress test method of evaluating cardiovascular fitness by exercise on treadmill or bicycle ergometer or after drugs (dipyridamole, dobutamine)

stress ulcer peptic ulcer caused by excessive stress as in burn, head trauma

stria a line or band differing in color and texture from surrounding tissue

striae gravidarum the bluish or pink streaks occurring on the abdomen, thighs and breasts during pregnancy due to the stretching of the abdomen as the uterus grows; the streaks turn silvertone in time

stroke 1. a sharp blow. 2. sudden neurological deficit with or without unconsciousness due to cerebral thrombosis, hemorrhage or embolism

stroma supporting framework of an organ including its connective tissue, vessels and nerves

stromatosis presence of mesenchyma like tissue throughout the endometrium of uterus

stupor a state of lessened responsiveness

stye inflammation of glands of Zeis and Moll at the edge of the lid. Internal stye involve Meiobomian or tarsal glands

stylet a thin probe

sub under, beneath, less in quantity

subarachnoid hemorrhage hemorrhage into subarachnoid space

subarachnoid space the space between arachnoid and pia containing CSF

subclavian below the clavicle

subcutaneous beneath the skin

subdural space space between dura and arachnoid

subinvolution incomplete or delayed return of uterus to nonpregnant size after childbirth

subluxation a partial or incomplete dislocation

submucosa connective tissue layer below the mucosa containing vessels and nerves

sudden infant death syndrome (SIDS) sudden death of apparently healthy infants between 3 weeks and 5 months

sugar sweet tasting carbohydrate either monosaccharose or disaccharose

sulbactam beta lactamase inhibitor

sulcus a furrow, groove, depression

sulfonamides a group of chemotherapeutic agents like sulfadiazine, sulfadoxine, sulfameraxine, sulfasalazine given orally for bacterial infections

sunscreen agents like PABA used for protection against solar dermatitis

superfecundation the fertilization of two or more ova ovulated more or less simultaneously by two or more coital acts, not necessarily involving the same male

superfetation fertilization of two ova in the same uterus at different menstrual periods within a short interval

superinfection a new infection caused by a different organism from the which caused initial infection

superovulation production of more than normal number of ova, which usually results from administration of gonadotropins

superoxide a highly reactive form of oxygen (oxygen with single electron) produced during phagocytosis and bacterial digestion by neutrophils, lipid metabolism

superscription the beginning of prescription marked by letter Rx meaning "you take"

supination turning the palm or foot upward; lying on the back

supine hypotension syndrome pressure of gravid uterus on inferior vena cava causing diminished venous return and hypotension

suppository a substance in the form of semisolid introduced into the vagina or rectum serving as vehicle for medicine

suppression of lactation prevention of lactation when breastfeeding is not desired or is contraindicated by giving bromocriptine that suppresses prolactin or by ethynil stilbestrol

suprarenal gland lying superior and medial to kidney secreting adrenaline and noradrenaline

surfactant an agent that lowers surface tension

surrogate mother mother who bears a child for another couple. She is impregnated with the fertilized ovum from that couple

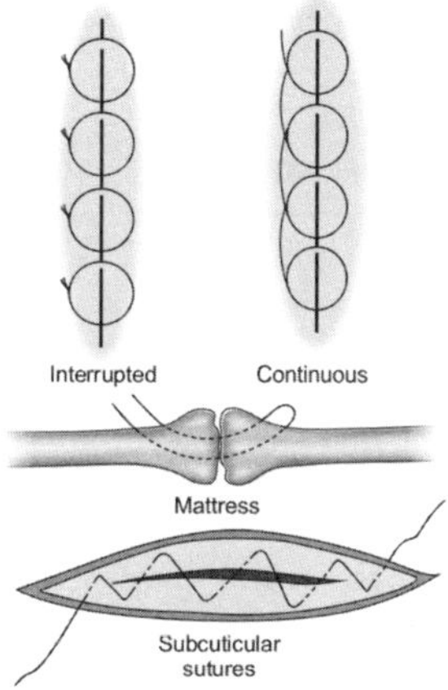

Suture

suture 1. the line of bony union as in skull bones. 2. to unite by stitching. 3. the thread, wire or other material used to stitch body parts together. ***s. absorbable*** sterile strand from mammalian collagen. ***s. catgut*** suture made from sheep's small intestine. ***s. coronal*** suture between the frontal and parietal bones. ***s. lamboid*** suture between parietal bones and superior border of occipital bones. ***s. nonabsorbable*** suture materials like silk, silkworm gut, horse hair, synthetic material and wire. ***s. purse string*** suture around the periphery of a circular opening which when drawn taught closes the opening. ***s. sagittal*** suture between the parietal bones. ***s. mattress*** an interrupted suture where the needle pierces both flaps of wound and then reenters to emerge at the same side of insertion and then tied. Particularly useful in holding together thick fragile tissues

swab a small piece of cotton or gauze wrapped around a slender stick for cleansing a wound, for applying medication, etc.

swelling an abnormal temporary enlargement on the surface of the body

symmetrical cortical necrosis a complication of abruptio placentae where cortical necrosis of both kidneys occurs due to renal vasospasm

sympathectomy surgical excision of part of sympathetic system; either nerve, ganglia or plexus

sympathomimetic producing effect similar to stimulation of sympathetic nerves

symphysiotomy section of symphysis pubis to increase capacity of contracted pelvis to facilitate child birth

symphysis fibrocartilaginous union of bones

symptom subjective description or manifestation of disease

synapse the point of junction between two adjacent neurons

synciotrophoblast outer layer of chorionic villi

synclitism a state of fetal hand when it enters pelvis with both parietal eminences at some level

syncope transient loss of consciousness due to inadequate blood supply to brain. ***s. cardiac*** syncope of cardiac origin as in Stokes-Adam's attack, tachycardia, tight aortic stenosis, HOCM. ***s. carotid sinus*** hypersensitive carotid sinus being stimulated by neck movement or tight collar producing bradycardia and syncope. ***s. vasovagal*** syncope occurring due to abrupt fall in blood pressure due to fall in peripheral resistance and hence reduced venous return

syncytium a mass of cytoplasm with numerous nuclei but no division into separate cells

syndactyly an abnormal fusion of the digits either partially or complete

syndrome a symptom complex indicating a particular disease

synthesis union of elements to produce new compounds

syphilis chronic venereal disease involving all tissues in body caused by Treponema pallidum, the spirochete

syphilitic macule small red nonitchy eruptions all over the body in secondary syphilis

syringe an instrument used for injecting or taking out fluids

syringomyelia a chronic progressive disorder with formation of cavities with surrounding gliosis in the spinal cord

syrinx Eustachian tube; pathological cavity within spinal cord, a fistula

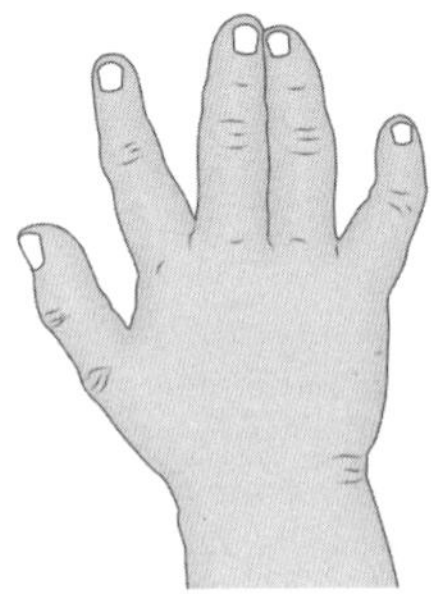

Syndactyly

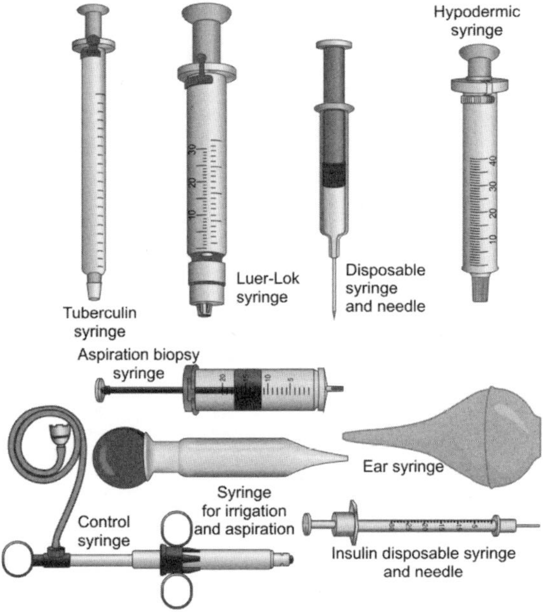

Syringe

systemic circulation blood flow from left ventricle to aorta and to arteries and return to heart via the superior and inferior vena cava

systemic lupus erythematosus (SLE) an autoimmune disease that can be life-threatening. Patients may have a distinctive pattern of facial redness and oral lesions. Endothelial damage to heart valves similar to those caused by rheumatic fever may occur

systole the period of myocardial contraction, usually of 0.3 seconds in a heart beat

T

tabes chronic progressive wasting disease. *t. dorsalis*. Degeneration of posterior column of spinal cord in syphilis

taboo setting apart of thing as sacred, thus forbidden for general use

tachycardia rapid heart rate; can be atrial, nodal, ectopic, ventricular or sinus depending upon the site of origin of the impulse

tachypnea abnormally rapid respiration

tactile perceptible to touch

Taenia a genus of parasitic, elongated ribbon like worms, the body being segmented. ***T. saginata*** tapeworm whose larvae live in flesh of cattle and adult worms (15 to 20 feet long) in human intestine. Men acquire the infestation by eating undercooked beef. ***T. solium*** tapeworm whose larval stage is in pigs and adult worms in human intestine. The disease is acquired by eating undercooked pork containing Cysticercus cellulosae

talipes congenital nontraumatic abnormal deviation of foot. ***t. calcaneus*** the heel alone touches the ground. ***t. equinus*** the person walks on the toes; can be varus or valgus depending on whether the heel is turned inward or outward

talus the ankle bone articulating with tibia fibula above and calcaneus and navicular bone below

tamoxifen antiestrogen drug used in adjuvant therapy of breast cancer

tampon a roll or pack made of various absorbent substances used to absorb body secretions or arrest hemorrhage, e.g. menstrual tampon

tapeworm parasitic worms belonging to class cestoda having a scolex with hooks and suckers and a series of proglottids. ***t. beef*** *Taenia saginata*. ***t. broad*** *Diphylobothrium latum*. **t. dog** *Dipylidium caninum*. **t. dwarf** *Hymenolepis nana*. ***t. pork*** *Taenia solium*

tarsus the ankle with its seven constituent bones, i.e. talus, calcans, cuboid, navicular and the three cuneiform bones

taurine an amino acid with high concentration in breast milk necessary for conjugation of bile acids in first week of life until glycine takes over the function

taxonomy laws and principles of classification of animals and plants

Tay-Sachs disease autosomal recessive form of gangliosidosis (lipid storage disease) manifesting with mental retardation, blindness, cherry red spot in macula, etc. due to deficiency of hexosaminidase. A leading to accumulation of sphingolipid in CNS

T cell a subset of lymphocytes responsible for cell-mediated immunity

tea tree oil essential oil having antibacterial, antifungal and antiviral property

teething eruption of teeth through the guns, the primary teeth 10 in number erupting between 6 to 30 months

telangiectasia dilatation of group of capillaries to form elevated dark red wart-like spots

telemetry transmission of data to a distant place by electronic means

temazepam benzodiazepine, sedative hypnotic produces central nervous system (CNS) depression at limbic, thalamic, hypothalamic levels of the CNS; used as sedative and hypnotic for insomnia

temperature the degree of intensity of heat. ***t. ambient*** temperature of surrounding. ***t. inverse*** a state where morning body temperature is higher than evening body temperature. ***t. normal*** oral temperature of 98.6°F (37°C). ***t. rectal*** more accurate than oral or axillary temperature. It is about 1°F higher than oral temperature, whereas axillary temperature is 1°F lower than oral temperature

temporal related to or limited in time

tenaculum a slender, sharp-pointed surgical instrument used mainly in surgery for seizing and holding parts

tendon fibrous connective tissue attaching a muscle to bone. ***t. Achilles*** the thickest and strongest tendon of gastrocnemius muscle attached to calcaneus

tension expansive force that stretches; a state of mental strain. ***t. premenstrual*** nervous instability, irritability, headache and depression occurring few days before menstruation

tentorium cerebelli the process of dura mater between cerebrum and cerebellum supporting the occipital lobes

tepid lukewarm

teratogen any substance capable of disrupting fetal growth and producing fetal malformation

teratogenic agent virus, irradiation or drugs, the exposure to which can damage the fetus in a pregnant woman

teratoma congenital tumor containing one or more of three embryonic germ layers

termination of pregnancy an abortion

term the end of pregnancy, 280 days or 40 weeks from LMP

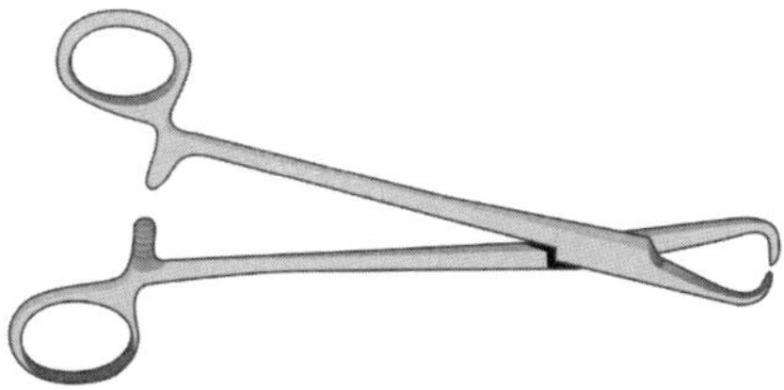

Tenaculum

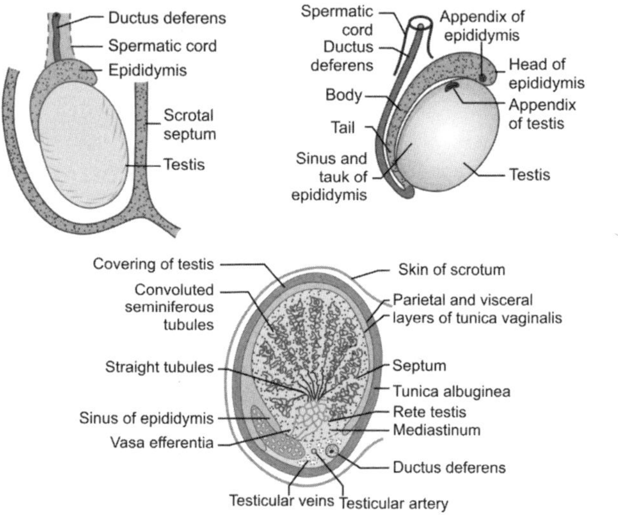

Testis

term infant a live born infant of between 38 and 42 weeks' completed gestation

tertiary care a level of medicare

tertiary third in order

testis the male reproductive gland located in scrotum about 4 cm long and 2 cm wide

testosterone an androgenic hormone secreted by Leydig cells of testes

tetanus an acute infectious disease caused by anaerobe *Clostridium tetani* manifesting with painful tonic clonic spasm of voluntary muscles

tetany a state of increased neuromuscular excitability caused by decreased serum ionized calcium or phosphorus and in alkalosis

tetracycline a broad-spectrum antibiotic

tetralogy a combination of four symptoms or elements. ***t. of Fallot*** Congenital heart disease with infundibular pulmonary stenosis, right ventricular hypertrophy, overriding aorta, and high ventricular septal defect

thalamus large ovoid masses of gray matter on either side of third ventricle, serving as gateway for all sensory projections to brain

thalassemia a group of congenital hemolytic anemia due to impaired synthesis of hemoglobin polypeptide chains, alpha or beta. ***t. major*** the homozygous form of deficient beta chain synthesis manifesting with severe microcytic anemia, splenomegaly, jaundice, gallstones, leg ulcers and thickened cranial bones. ***t. minor*** heterozygous state for alpha or beta chain production with mild microcytic hypochromic anemia and raised HbA2

thalidomide alfa glutarimide previously used as sedative but now only used in lepra reaction; causes severe birth defects if given to pregnant mothers

theophylline a plant product and bronchodilator. ***t. ethylenediamine*** aminophylline

therapeutic a curative. ***t. abortion*** termination of pregnancy that disrupts mother's physical or mental health (as a sequence of rape) or is likely to produce a physically or mentally handicapped child. ***t. index*** the ratio of toxic dose of a substance to its therapeutic dose; an index of safety of the drug

therapy the means employed to effect a cure or manage a disease. ***t. collapse*** production of pneumothorax to effect pulmonary collapse as a method of treatment of nonhealing cavitary pulmonary tuberculosis. ***t. electroconvulsive*** passing of electric current in the convulsive dose to treat psychosis or suicidal depression. ***t. photodynamic*** method of treating cancer by using light absorbing chemicals that are selectively retained by malignant cells. ***t. physical*** use of physical agents such as massage, heat, hydration, electricity, exercise in the treatment of disease. ***t. replacement*** therapeutic use of medicine as a substitute for natural body substances, e.g. thyroid hormone, insulin

thermometer instrument for recording temperature

thiamine vitamin B1 present in wheat germ, rice water, animal and plant foods. Acts as a coenzyme in carboxylation of pyruvic acid. Deficiency produces beriberi

thiopental sodium an ultrashort acting barbiturate used for inducing surgical anesthesia

third degree perineal tear the tear extending into rectum with damage to perineal body and anal sphincter

third stage of labor the time period from birth of baby to complete expulsion of placenta and membranes; it is on average 20 to 30 minutes but ranges from 5 minutes to 2 hours

thoracic duct the main lymphatic duct of body arising at cisterna chyli, ascending up to join left subclavian vein near its junction with left internal jugular vein

T

thorax the part of the body between diaphragm below and base of the neck above. ***t. barrel-shaped*** Rounded chest as in emphysema

threatened abortion vaginal spotting with abdominal pain but dilatation of cervix

threshold 1. point at which physiological response is produced. 2. a measure of sensitivity of an organ or function

thrill a palpable murmur

thrombin an enzyme derived from prothrombin by action of thromboplastin

thromboangiitis inflammation of blood vessel with thrombus formation. ***t. obliterans*** chronic occlusive vascular disease common to cigarette smokers commonly affecting the feet with propensity for gangrene formation. SYN: Buerger's disease

thrombocytopenia decrease below normal in number of platelets (>50,000 cmm)

thrombocytopenic purpura a hematological disorder in the newborn in which the bleeding time is prolonged, platelets are greatly decreased and there is cell fragility

thrombocytosis increase in number of platelets (>400,000 cmm)

thromboembolism a detached thrombus causing occlusion of a vessel

thromboembolus a blood clot in a vein

thrombokinase factor 'X' or Stuart factor

thrombophlebitis inflammation of vein with thrombus formation

thromboplastin the coagulation factor III present in most tissues which accelerates clot formation by converting prothrombin to thrombin

thrombosis the formation or existence of thrombus or clot within the vessel

thrombus a blood clot

thrus infection caused by *Candida albicans* in mouth and throat with formation of white patches and ulcers

thymus the capsulated bilobed organ in anterior mediastinum which is essential for immune function of body

thyroid gland the bilobed gland joined by isthmus located at the base of the neck, secreting T3 and T4

thyromegaly abnormally enlarged thyroid gland

thyrotoxicosis hyperfunctioning of thyroid gland with tachycardia, fine tremor, anxiety, nervousness, diarrhea, etc.

thyroxine tetraiodothyronine, the principal hormone of thyroid gland

tidal periodically rising and falling

tinea fungus infection. ***t. capitis*** fungal infection of head. ***t. corporis*** fungal infections of body with scaly eruptions and clearing center. ***t. cruris*** fungal infection of genital area. ***t. nigra*** superficial fungal infection of palm with pigmented nonitchy nonscaly macules. ***t. pedis*** fungal infection of foot (SYN:

athlete's foot). ***t. versicolor*** yellow or fawn colored skin patches due to *Malassezia furfur*

tissue a group or collection of similar cells performing a particular function

tissue fluid interstitial fluid or extracellular fluid whose excess causes edema

tissue macrophage a large wandering branched cell with single nucleus capable of ingesting particulate matter

tissue plasminogen activator (TPA) a thrombolytic agent that is dot specific, acting on plasminogen causing breakdown of fibrin

titer the amount or concentration

toco childbirth or labor

tocograph device for recording force of uterine contraction

tocology science of parturition

tocolysis suppression of uterine contraction

tocopherol compounds with vitamin E activity

tomography a method of X-ray that shows details of image of structures at a particular plane of tissue by blurring images of structures in all other planes

tone 1. a state of partial contraction of muscle. 2. normal tension in arterial wall

tongue a fleshy leafy organ lying in the floor of mouth. Helps in mastication, deglutition, speech production and taste. ***t. smooth*** a tongue with atrophy of papillae as in anemia and malnutrition. ***t. strawberry*** a bright red tongue with prominent papillae as in scarlet fever

tongue tie congenital shortness of frenum linguae with poor protrusion, difficulty in articulation and sucking

tonic uterine contraction powerful continuous contractile state of uterus leading to anaxia of fetus due to reduced placenta fetal blood flow

TORCH syndrome an acronym for a group of infections, which are particularly damaging to the fetus or newborn; includes toxoplasmosis, rubella, cytomegalovirus and herpes virus type 2

torsion twisting as occurs in pedicle of ovarian cyst or myoma with gangrene

torticollis spasmodic contraction of neck muscles causing head to tilt to one side and chin pointing to other side

tourniquet any item used to exert pressure over an artery to stop bleeding. ***t. rotating*** a technique of applying tourniquets to three extremities in rotation to reduce venous return to heart as in pulmonary edema

tourniquet test test for determining capillary fragility from their ability to withstand pressure

toxemia circulation of toxins throughout the body producing symptoms like fever, diarrhea, vomiting, hypotension, flushing tachycardia, etc. ***t. of pregnancy*** a series of changes occurring in pregnancy leading to hypertension, proteinuria, convulsion and intrauterine growth retardation

toxin a poisonous substance of animal or plant origin

T

toxoid a toxin without toxicity but with intact antigenicity so that when injected can produce antibodies

Toxoplasma a form of protozoa, e.g. *T. gondii* causing toxoplasmosis

toxoplasmosis a disease due to infection with *Toxoplasma gondii* manifest with pneumonitis, hepatitis, encephalitis (in the severe form) or mild fever and malaise in mild form. In congenital form, the newborn may have encephalopathy, jaundice, anemia, hepatosplenomegaly and generalized lymphadenopathy

trachea the round cartilaginous air tube extending from larynx to bronchi (6th cervical to 5th dorsal vertebra)

tracheoesophageal fistula a congenital anomaly in which there is an abnormal tube like passage between the trachea and the esophagus

tracheomalacia softening of cartilaginous framework of trachea

tracheostomy surgical opening up of trachea to put an airway to facilitate respiration in laryngeal obstruction or a condition requiring prolonged respiratory assistance

trait a characteristic or property of an individual

tranquilizer a drug reducing mental tension and anxiety without interfering with normal mental activity

transcutaneous nerve stimulation a method of pain relief by application of mild electrical current over painful area by electrodes, can be applied pain relief of labor by placing 4 electrodes at T10, T11 and S2, S4 on the spine

transducer device that converts one form of energy into another e.g., ultrasonic transducers that convert sound energy to electrical energy

transferrin iron-transporting globulin in plasma

transfusion injection of blood, blood products or IV solutions into vein. ***t. exchange*** transfusion of blood and withdrawal of blood at same time until blood volume is entirely replaced as in hemolytic disease of newborn

transient ischemic attack (TIA) symptoms of neurological deficit lasting for few hours without residual damage due to transient interference with blood supply to brain

transillumination inspection of a cavity or organ by passing a light through its wall, e.g. examination of paranasal sinus by means of a light placed across mouth; examination of hydrocele contents in scrotum and examination of brain in hydrocephalus in infants

translocation the displacement of part or whole of chromosome to another

transplantation the operation of transplanting an organ or tissue from one person to another, e.g. heart, lung, kidney, liver and bone marrow. ***t. heteroplastic*** transplantation of a part from one individual to another of the same or closely related species. ***t. heterotopic*** transplantation in which transplant is placed in a different location in host than it had in donor

transport movement of materials in biological systems particularly across cell membrane

transposition a change in position of an organ or viscera usually to opposite side

transsexual an individual who has overwhelming desire or feels psychically to be of opposite sex or has got his external sex changed by surgery

transudate a fluid that passes through the capillary wall

transverse arrest in obstetrics, arrest of transverse axis of descending fetal head in maternal pelvis

transverse lie a state where longitudinal axis of fetus lies across the uterus can cause shoulder presentation with obstructed labor if not corrected before labor

transverse sinus a sinus of dura mater running from internal occipital protuberance along attached margin of tentorium cerebelli to reach jugular foramen

transvestism dressing or masquerading in the clothing of opposite sex to be accepted as a member of opposite sex

trauma a physical injury or wound caused by external force or violence. ***t. psychic*** a painful emotional experience

travel in pregnancy travel in first and last trimester be restricted

treatment any specific procedure employed for amelioration of a disease or pathological condition. **t. empiric** treatment based on observation and experience rather than having a scientific basis. ***t. expectant*** relief of symptoms that arise during an illness but treatment not directed at specific cause of illness. ***t. palliative*** symptomatic treatment rather than a cure

Trendelenburg position position in which patient's head is low and the legs are on an elevated and inclined position

trial labor it is attempted when cephalopelvic disproportion is very mild and head is not engaged. If head fails to descend and cervix fails to dilate, it should be quickly terminated

Trichinella a genus of nematode. *Trichinella spiralis* of this genus causes trichinosis from ingestion of undercooked pork containing the cyst

Trichomonas genus of flagellated protozoa. ***T. hominis*** intestinal flagellate causing diarrhea and bacillary dysentery-like disease. ***T. vaginalis*** flagellate inhabiting vagina causing profuse white watery often blood-stained discharge and intense itching

triglyceride combination of glycerol with three different fatty acids

trigone a triangular area at the base of bladder, i.e. between the two openings of ureter and internal urinary meatus

trimester a block of 3 months

trimethoprim antibacterial agent used for urinary tract infection; when combined with sulfamethoxazole causes sequential block in enzyme synthesis within a wide range of bacteria

tripartite placenta a placenta divided into three lobes, each lobe with a cord that join to form one cord

triple test blood test alfa-fetoprotein unconjugated estriol and LCG at 16 to 18 week gestation to exclude Down syndrome

triplet three children in one pregnancy

triple vaccine combination of tetanus, diphtheria and whooping cough vaccines

trisomy having three homologous chromosomes instead of two

trocar the instrument which is contained within the cannula for removal of fluid from body cavity

trochanter bony processes. **t. greater** outward projection at upper end of femur below its neck. **t. lesser** conical tuberosity at the inner and posterior surface of upper end of femur at the junction of shaft and neck

trophoblast the outermost layer of developing embryo consisting of inner cytotrophoblast and outer syntrophoblast that comes in contact with uterine endometrium

trypsin proteolytic enzyme formed by action of enterokinase on pancreatic trypsinogen

tubal insufflation assessment of tubal patency by insufflation with carbon dioxide

tubal ligation ligation of Fallopian tubes for sterilization

tubal mole a mass of blood clot retained in Fallopian tube after tubal pregnancy

tube a long hollow cylindrical structure. ***t. endotracheal*** a tube usually with an inflatable cuff put into trachea for airway during anesthesia. ***t. nasogastric*** rubber tube passed into stomach for aspiration/decompression of stomach. ***t. stomach*** a wide bore tube for stomach wash in poisoning

tubectomy surgical removal of a part or whole of fallopian tube

tuberculosis an infectious disease caused by *Mycobacterium tuberculosis* having propensity to infect lungs, bone, GU tract, meninges and the GI tract

tuberosity an elevated bony process, e.g. ischial tuberosity

tubular necrosis (acute) death of renal tubules, usually a consequence of prolonged renal ischemia or following incompatible blood transfusion or sepsis

tubule a small tube. ***t. collecting*** tubules having transport function in renal medulla. ***t. convoluted*** the constituent parts of a nephron of kidney. ***t. seminiferous*** very small tubules in testis in which the spermatozoa develop and leave the testis to enter the epididymis

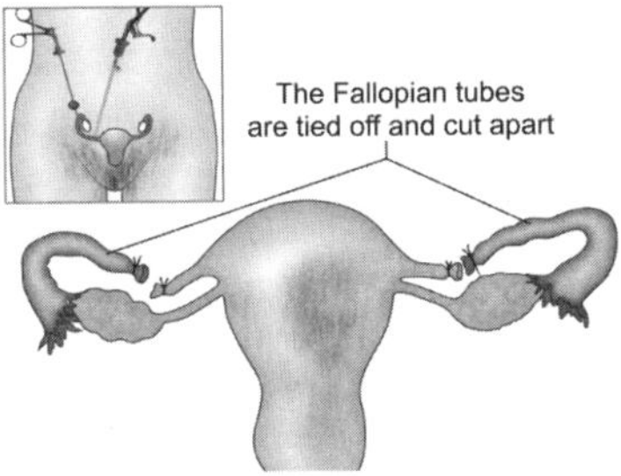

Tubectomy

tumescence swelling

tunica a covering. ***t. adventia*** the outer fibrous coat of blood vessels. ***t. intima*** the innermost layer of endothelial cells and the basement membrane including the internal elastic lamina of blood vessels. ***t. media*** the middle layer in the wall of a blood vessel containing circular smooth muscle and elastic fibers. ***t. serosa*** the mesothelial lining of the pleura, peritoneum and pericardium. ***t. vaginalis*** the serous membrane surrounding the testes

tunnel a narrow channel. ***t. carpal*** the fibro-osseous canal in the wrist through which pass the flexor tendons and the median nerve. ***t. tarsal*** the osteofibrous canal bounded by flexor retinaculum and tarsal bones giving way to posterior tibial vessels, tibial nerve and flexor tendons

Turner's syndrome 45(XO) chromosomal pattern in girls manifested with amenorrhea, infertility, short stature and poor sexual maturation

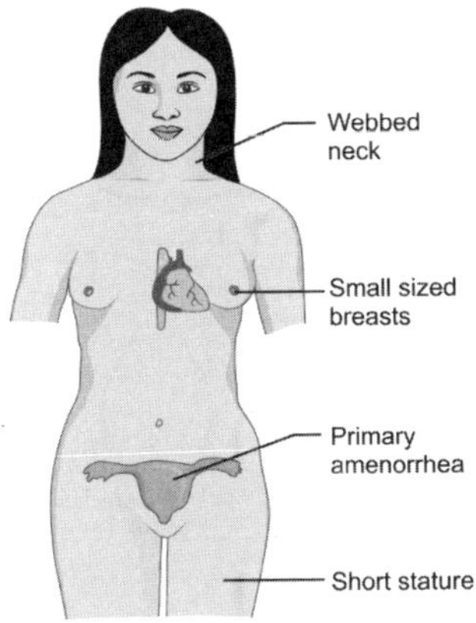

Turner's syndrome

twin two fetuses developing within uterus in one pregnancy. ***t. dizygotic*** twins developed from two separate ova. ***t. monozygotic*** twins developing from a single fertilized ovum; hence have identical genetic makeup, are of same sex, have common placenta and one chorion sac. ***t. siamese*** symmetrically united twins

twin-to-twin transfusion transfer of blood from one fetus to other leading to former being anemic and latter plethoric

tympanic membrane membrane at the junction middle ear and external ear

typing identification of types, e.g. 1. Bacteriophage typing, i.e. determination of bacterial species by bacteriophages. 2. tissue typing, i.e. testing for histocompatibility of tissues to be used in transplant or graft

tyramine an intermediate product during conversion of tyrosine to epinephrine, found in cheese, beer, yeast, beans, wine and chicken liver

tyrosine an amino acid serving as precursor for epinephrine, thyroxine and melanin

ulcer discontinuity in the skin or mucous membrane with sloughing. ***u. curling*** stress-induced peptic ulcer as in postburn or cerebrovascular accident patient. ***u. decubitus*** ischemic necrosis and tissue ulceration over bony prominence in bedridden patients. ***u. Hunner's*** painful slowly healing ulcer in urinary bladder. ***u. rodent*** deeply infiltrating ulcer with undermined edges as in basal cell carcinoma

ulna the inner and larger bone of forearm

ultrasonic sound frequency above 20,000 cycles per second, not audible to human ear

ultrasonography use of ultrasound to image body organs

ultrasound sound frequency in the range of 20,000 to 109 cycles per second, employed to image body organs and for therapeutic purposes (ultrasonic ablation/stone dissolution)

umbilical relating to the navel

umbilical catheterization insertion of catheter into umbilical vein or artery in neonates for giving fluids or drugs, monitoring of blood, gases, etc.

umbilical cord the cord consisting two arteries and one vein embedded in Wharton's jelly attaching fetus to placenta

umbilical hernia hernia in which part of the intestine protrudes through the umbilical ring

umbilicus the navel or depression in the center of abdomen

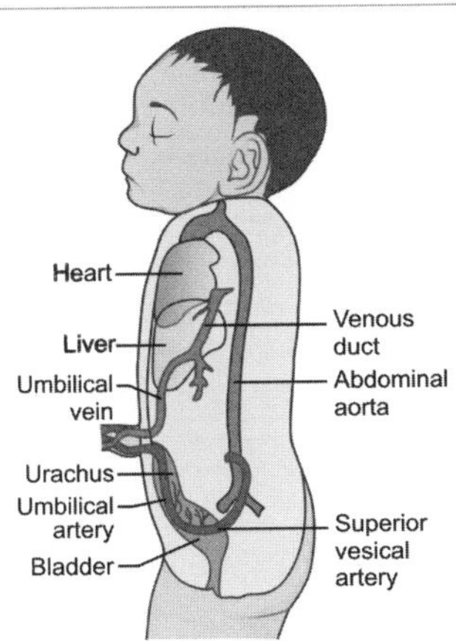

Umbilical vessels

unconscious lacking awareness of surrounding

unicellular consisting of single cell

unilateral affecting or occurring at one side

universal antidote two parts of activated charcoal, one part magnesium oxide and one part tannic acid used in poisoning by unknown agents by oral route

universal donor a person of blood group 'O', Rh-negative

universal recipient a person of blood group AB, Rh-positive

unstable lie a condition when fetus changes its lie from one examination to another after 36 weeks of gestation

urachus a fibrous cord extending from apex of bladder to umbilicus. Often

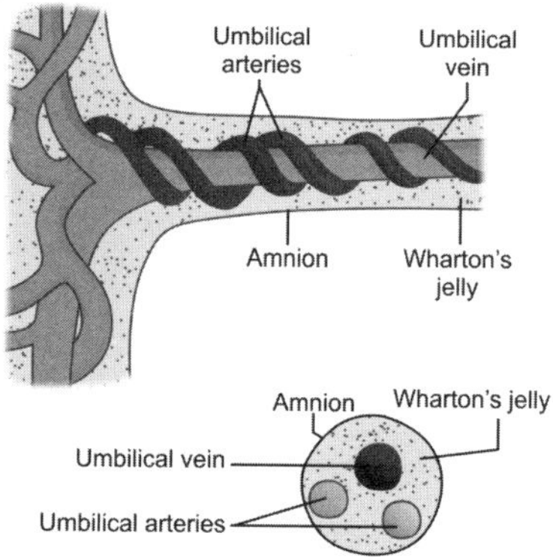

Umbilical cord

urachus remains patent resulting in an umbilical urinary fistula

urea the diamide of carbonic acid derived from ammonia by deamination representing 80–90% of total urinary nitrogen

uremia a complex biochemical abnormality in kidney failure, characterized by azotemia, acidosis, anemia and many systemic symptoms. ***u. prerenal*** uremia occurring not primarily due to kidney disease but due to fluid loss

ureter 28–34 cm fibromuscular tubes conveying urine from kidney to urinary bladder

urethra the canal extending from bladder neck to exterior for discharge of urine

urethritis inflammation of urethra. ***u. anterior*** inflammation of anterior portion of urethra (portion anterior to triangular ligament)

urethrocele prolapse urethral wall in female consequent to birth trauma

uric acid an end product of purine metabolism responsible for clinical manifestations of gout

urine the fluid excreted by kidneys with a specific gravity of 1005 to 1030, acidic in reaction and amber colored; 24 hour urine contains nearly 75 grams of solids, i.e. 25% as urea, 25% as chloride 25% as sulfates

urinometer device for measuring specific gravity of urine

urodynamics study of bladder function both neural and muscular

urogenital diaphragm the sheet of tissue stretching across the pubic arch, formed by deep transverse perineal and sphincter urethrae muscles. SYN: triangular ligament

urography X-ray study of urinary tract after introduction of radiopaque dye. Can be ascending type: dye is injected into bladder or descending type: the dye is given IV and is excreted by the kidneys

urticaria eruption of itchy wheals on skin. ***u. pigmentosa*** brown itchy eruptions of mastocytosis. ***u. solaris*** urticaria on exposure to sunlight

uterine souffle the sound of blood flow in uterine vessels in gravid uterus

uterine subinvolution failure of uterus to return to its normal size after child birth

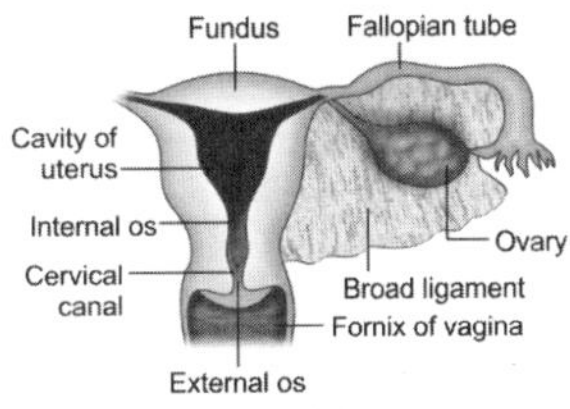

Uterus and adnexa

uterosacral ligament two ligaments extending from back of cervix to sacrum encircling the rectum, thus maintaining uterus in anteversion

uterus the womb, the seat of embryo's imbedment and growth; a hollow muscular pelvic organ

uvulectomy removal of uvula by surgery

uvula a small fleshy structure hanging from soft palate

vaccination inoculation with a vaccine to achieve resistance against an infectious disease

vaccine a suspension of live attenuated/killed infectious agent or its products/parts for achieving immunity against that infectious agent. ***v. BCG*** bacille Calmette-Guérin, a preparation of dried live-culture of *Mycobacterium tuberculosis* whose virulence has been reduced by repeated cultures on glycerinated ox bile. ***v. DPT*** a preparation of diphtheria and tetanus toxoid and killed pertussis organisms given intramuscularly. ***v. hepatitis B*** vaccine containing recombinant viral capsular antigen of hepatitis B virus. ***v. human diploid cell*** an inactivated rabies virus vaccine prepared in human diploid cell tissue culture. ***v. influenza*** a polyvalent vaccine containing inactivated antigenic variants of the virus for rendering immunity in chronically ill and aged. ***v. measles*** a live attenuated virus vaccine. ***v. mumps*** a live attenuated virus vaccine. ***v. pneumococcal*** a polyvalent vaccine effective against 23 strains of pneumococci, given to children under 2 years of age and to those who have undergone splenectomy. ***v. polio*** oral poliovaccine containing 3 types of live attenuated (v. Sabin) or inactivated viruses (v. Salk)

vacuum aspiration a method to perform abortion during first 3 months of pregnancy and remove hydatidiform mole

vacuum extractor a device with a suction cup which is placed on fetal head for applying traction during delivery

vagina the musculomembranous passage between the cervix and vulva

vaginal birth after cesarean (VBAC) permits patients the opportunity of a trial of labor and possibly a vaginal delivery after previously delivering by cesarean section

vaginal hysterectomy surgical removal of uterus through vagina

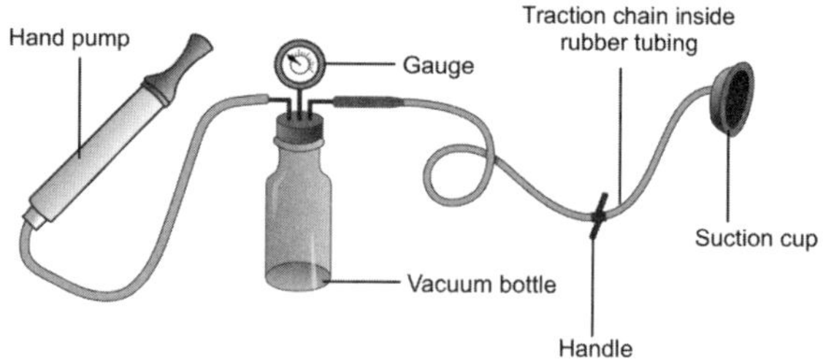

Vacuum extractor or ventouse

vaginal vibrator a vibrator placed in vagina for erotic stimulation

vaginismus painful spasm of vagina often preventing coitus; may be idiopathic, following trauma, vaginitis or psychological aversion to coitus

vaginitis inflammation of vagina causing purulent malodorous discharge, itching, pain in perineum, and during coitus and painful micturition. ***v. atrophic*** atrophy of vagina in postmeno-pausal women with reduced introitus and dryness. ***v. trichomonial*** vaginitis due to Trichomonas causing red frothy discharge with fishy odor

vagus the tenth cranial nerve, a parasympathetic nerve supplying heart, liver, lungs and part of alimentary tract

Valsalva maneuver forcible expiration against closed glottis, nose, and mouth; used to increase pressure within middle ear to correct retracted ear drum

valve membranous structures that allow flow of fluid in one direction

valvoplasty dilatation of valve

valvotomy incision into a valve to dilate it

vanilylmandelic acid (VMA) metabolite of epinephrine and norepinephrine in urine, amount increased in pheochromocytoma

variability the change in the baseline fetal heart rate caused by the interplay of the sympathetic and parasympathetic nervous systems; may vary from 5 to 10 beats/minute with contractions and fetal or maternal movements

variable deceleration a periodic slowing of the fetal heart rate either with a contraction or between contractions, due to umbilical cord compression; variable in duration, intensity and timing of the deceleration

variance in statistics, the square of standard deviation

varicella chickenpox, the viral disease with polymorphic maculovesico-pustular eruptions

varicose means distended, tortuous and knotted

varicose veins dilated tortuous veins as developing in legs due to venous incompetence or the development of esophageal varices in portal hypertension

variola SYN: smallpox, the vesicopustular generalized eruptive viral disease that has disappeared from the globe for past two decades

varix dilatation of a vein, artery or lymphatic channel

varus turned inward

vas a duct. ***v. deferens*** the 18″ long excretory duct of testis transporting sperm to urethra

vasa pleural of vas. ***v. recta*** 1. straight collecting tubules of kidney. 2. tubules that become straight prior to entering the mediastinum testis. ***v. vasorum***

V

the tiny blood vessels supplying the fibromuscular coats of arteries and larger veins

vasa previa the presentation infront of the fetal head during labor of blood vessels of umbilical cord

vasectomy removal of a segment of vas deferens bilaterally to induce male sterility

vasoconstriction spasm or temporary narrowing of blood vessels

vasodepressor an agent that depresses circulation, i.e. lowers blood pressure by dilating blood vessels

vasodilator agent causing relaxation of blood vessels

vasomotor pertains to or regulating the contraction and relaxation of blood vessels

vasopressin a posterior pituitary hormone having antidiuretic, and vasopressor effect (causes coronary spasm, hence not used to raise blood pressure)

vasopressor agent bringing about contraction of blood vessels

vasovagal syncope sudden fainting due to hypotension caused by emotional stress, pain or trauma

vault the part of fetal skull excluding the base and face

v. cap a contraceptive device which attaches to vaginal vault by suction preventing sperm entry uterus

vegan a strict vegetarian who even abstains from milk and milk products

vegetation wart-like luxuriant growth from heart valves; consisting of fibrin mesh with enmeshed blood cells

vein vessel carrying unsaturated blood towards the heart except for pulmonary veins that carry saturated oxygenated blood to left atrium

velamentous expanding like a veil or sheet

vena cava one of the two main venous trunks, superior and inferior draining upper and lower portions of body and entering right atrium

veneral wart moist reddish elevations on genitals and anus

venereal disease disease acquired by sexual intercourse. It includes gonorrhea, syphilis, AIDS, viral hepatitis B, trichomoniasis, chlamydia infection, granuloma inguinale and lymphogranuloma venereum (LGV)

venesection surgical incision into a vein for draining out blood or introducing blood/colloids

venipuncture puncture of a vein for drawing out blood or introducing any substance

ventilation circulation of fresh air in lung alveoli. ***v. continuous*** positive pressure Mechanical method of artificial ventilation where the respirator delivers air to the lungs under a continuous positive pressure. ***v. intermittent positive pressure*** the respirator delivers air under positive pressure to initiate inspiration but expiration is passive

ventilator an apparatus to give artificial ventilation

ventricle a small cavity or pouch, e.g. in the heart and in the brain. ***v. third*** the median cavity of brain bounded by thalamus and hypothalamus on either side, anteriorly by optic chiasm; communicating with lateral ventricles and fourth ventricle. ***v. fourth*** the CSF containing cavity at base of brain extending between upper end of spinal canal and cerebral aqueduct. Its roof is formed by cerebellum and floor by rhomboid fossa. ***v. lateral*** the ventricle in each cerebral hemisphere with triangular-shaped body, inferior and posterior horns; communicating with third ventricle by interventricular foramen

ventricular septal defect a congenital defect in the interventricular septum of heart leading to passage of blood from left ventricle into right ventricle

ventrosuspension fixation of displaced uterus to anterior abdominal wall

vernix caseosa a sebaceous deposit covering the fetus, abundant on creases and flexor surfaces, consisting of sebaceous secretion, lanugo and exfoliated skin

version change in position of fetus within uterus. ***v. bipolar*** a combination of both external and internal manipulation to bring a change in fetal position. ***v. cephalic*** turning of the fetus so that head becomes the presenting part. ***v. external*** version of fetus with both hands placed on abdomen. ***v. internal*** version of fetus with one hand placed inside vagina. ***v. podalic*** version by holding feet of the fetus to make the presenting part breech

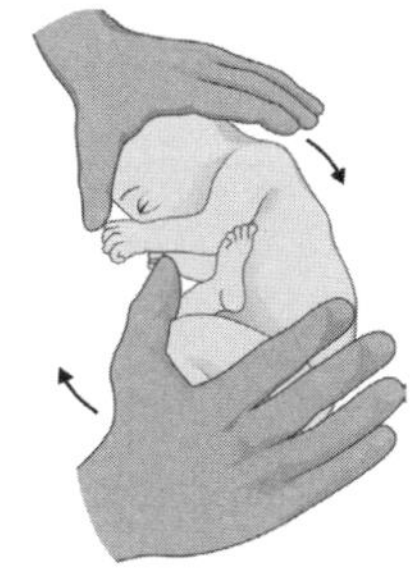

External version

vertebra one of the 33 bony segments making up the spinal column, consisting of 7 cervical, 12 thoracic (dorsal), 5 lumbar, 5 sacral and 4 coccygeal

vertex presentation The fetal head or cranium is the presenting part with the head flexed on the chest and the chin in contact with the thorax; also called cephalic presentation

vertex the top portion of head

vertical perpendicular to the horizontal plane, upright

vertigo the sensation of moving around in space (subjective vertigo) or experiencing the surrounding objects moving around oneself (objective vertigo)

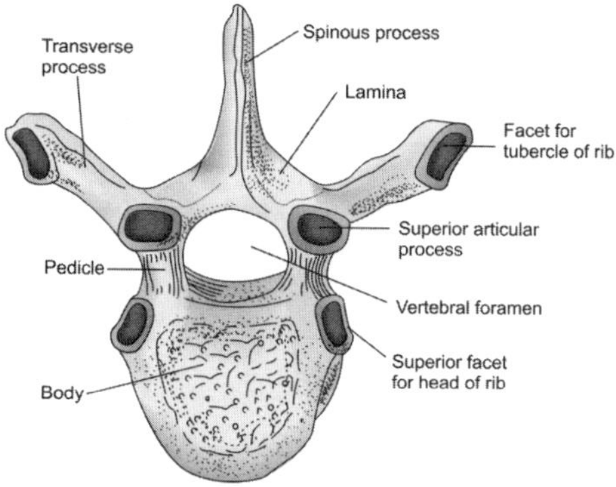

Vertebra

very low birth weight (VLBW) infant when an infant weighs less than 1,500 grams

vesica a bladder

vesical shaped like a bladder

vesicle elevated skin lesions containing serous fluid. **v. seminal** membranous sacculated tubes at the base of bladder acting as reservoir of semen

vesicovaginal concerning urinary bladder and vagina

vesiculitis inflammation of seminal vesicle

vestibule an entrance, the part of the vulva lying between labia minora

vestige a small incompletely developed structure

viability ability to live or capable of living, e.g. a fetus reaching 24 weeks gestation or 500 grams of weight can live outside uterus

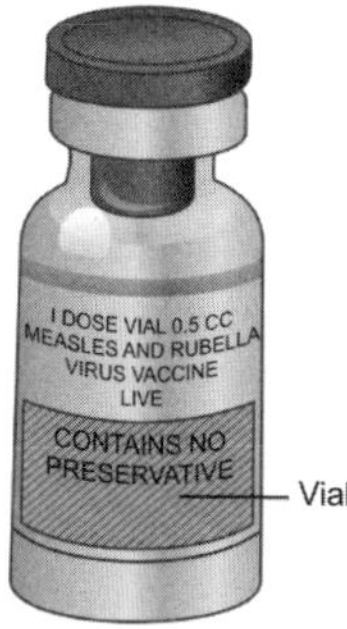

Vial

viagra sildenafil citrate, used in treatment of erectile dysfunction in male

vial a small glass bottle for storing medicines, chemicals, perfumes, etc.

Vibrio a genus of comma-shaped motile gram-negative bacilli, e.g.

V. cholerae, the organism causing cholera

vicarious acting as alternative or substitute

villus short slender filamentous processes found on some membranous surfaces. ***v. arachnoid*** protrusion of arachnoid into dural venous sinus. ***v. chorionic*** tiny branching processes on surface of chorion that become vascular and form placenta. ***v. intestinal*** the projecting structures into lumen of small intestine that help to absorb fluid and nutrients

virgin woman who has had no sexual intercourse; uncontaminated, fresh

virilism appearance of male secondary sexual characteristics in female

virion a complete virus particle

virulence degree of pathogenicity

virus minute submicroscopic organisms with a central core of DNA or RNA and a capsid but no cell wall. They utilize the cell metabolic processes for their nutrition and replication. ***v. cytomegalic (CMV)*** a member of the herpes virus group transmitted transplacentally from mother to fetus with mental retardation and hepatosplenomegaly in the newborn. ***v. enterocytopathogenic human orphan (ECHO)*** virus responsible for epidemic pleurodynia, menin-goencephalitis, myocarditis, etc. ***v. immunodeficiency*** the RNA virus containing reverse transcriptase that confers it capacity to change the antigenicity indefinitely and hence the difficulty in producing a successful vaccine. It causes the dreaded disease AIDS for which there is no cure. ***v. respiratory syncytial*** the virus causing lower respiratory infection in infancy and childhood and that produces large syncytial masses in cell cultures

viscera internal body organs

visceroptosis downward displacement of a viscus

viscid sticky, adhering, gummy

viscosity 1. the state of being sticky or gummy. 2. resistance of a fluid medium to changeability due to existing intermolecular force

vision act of seeing external objects; sense by which light and color are perceived

visual acuity a measure of the resolving power of eye. A normal person is able to read letters at a distance of 20 feet that subtend angle of 5°

vital capacity the quantity of air that can be expelled following deep inspiration

vital signs the traditional signs of life: like pulse, blood pressure, respiration, urination

vital statistics statistics relating to birth, death, marriage, sickness, etc.

vitamin micronutrients essential for metabolism, growth and development

vitamin A fat-soluble vitamin derived from carotenes (alpha, beta and gamma) in food, responsible for growth, development and integrity of epithe-

V

lial tissues, and functioning of Rods, the visual sensory cells that contain visual purple for dim vision

vitamin B12 cyanocobalamin, essential for cytoplasmic maturation of red cells and intactness of neurons

vitamin B1 thiamine, an essential coenzyme for decarboxylation of pyruvate to acetyl coenzyme

vitamin B2 riboflavin; constituent of flavoproteins responsible for tissue oxidation

vitamin B6 pyridoxine, a coenzyme for over 60 different enzyme systems, required for heme synthesis and neuroexcitability

vitamin C ascorbic acid, a factor essential for integrity of intercellular cement in many tissues, especially capillaries

vitamin D one of several vitamins (D2, D3, D4 and D5) that have antirachitic property. Vitamin D2 (calciferol) D3 (irradiated 7 dihydrocholesterol), D4 (irradiated 22 dihydro ergosterol), D5 (irradiated dehydrositosterol), all are essential for calcium and phosphorus metabolism

vitamin E tachysterol (alpha tocopherol), which prevents oxidation of polyunsaturated fatty acids in cell membranes

vitamin K naphthoquinone derivative that helps in synthesis of prothrombin in liver

viviparous giving birth to young alive offspring rather than larvae or embryo

v liability a situation in which the employer is vicariously liable for torts of employee during course of his/her employment

vocal cord two thin mucous folds in larynx enclosing vocal ligaments responsible for production of sound

v of newborn bile-stained vomit without passage of meconium indicates intestinal obstruction, V in pregnancy normal feature in first 3 months of pregnancy but can be disabling with electrolyte disturbance in hyperemesis gravidarum

volvulus twisting of bowel upon itself causing obstruction to lumen and even blood supply of the segment leading to necrosis

vomiting the act of ejection of gastric contents through mouth

vomitus material ejected by vomiting

vulsellum a forcep with hook on each blade

vulva the external genital organ in female consisting of labia majora, labia minora, clitoris, vestibule and vaginal opening

vulvectomy excision of vulva

vulvitis inflammation of vulva

vulvovaginitis inflammation of vulva and vagina; most commonly in diabetes

vulvovaginoplasty surgical reconstruction of vulva and vagina

v vaginal the roof of vagina to which cervix protrudes

warfarin a synthetic coumarin anticoagulant

wart a small, hard outgrowth on the skin caused by a virus

water birth a form of parturition in water to achieve pain relief and relaxation

wean to discontinue breastfeeding and substitute with other food

web a tissue or membrane, w laryngeal the most common congenital malformation of larynx causing obstruction of airways

wedge a piece of material thick at one end and thin at other end

Weil's disease spirochetal disease with jaundice and hemolysis

Wernicke's encephalopathy hemorrhagic encephalitis occurring due to vit B deficiency in alcoholics and in hyperemesis gravidarum

wet nurse a woman who breastfeeds infants other than her own

Wharton's jelly connective tissue of umbilical cord

wheal localized area of edema, often with itching

wheeze a whistling sound of small bronchiole spasm as in asthma

whipworm the nematode *Trichuris trichiura*

white matter the protion of cerebrum containing myelinated nerve fibers

whit low herpetic infection of terminal finger

whoop the sonorous and loud inhalation of whooping cough

widal test blood test for diagnosis of typhoid and paratyphoid

Wilson-Mikity syndrome bronchopulmonary dysplasia, a condition occurring in babies ventilated for long with oxygen

Wolffian bodies the primitive kidneys in developing embryo

world health organization (WHO) public health arm of United Nations

wound discontinuity in any structure or organ by injury causing tissue loss, can be penetrating lacerated perforating

Wrigley's forceps obstetric forceps used for low forcep delivery

xanthelasma deposition of a yellow lipid-rich plaque on the eyelids

xanthoma a tumor of skin tendon composed of lipid-laden foam cells. ***x. eruptive*** associated with raised triglycerides, usually in diabetics

xanthopsia yellow vision

xenograft a graft received from animal

xenon the chemical element whose radioactive isotope 133 Xe is used in assessment of pulmonary function, lung imaging and cerebral blood flow studies

xenophobia irrational fear of animals/ strangers

xeroderma a dry rough discolored state of skin

xerophthalmia dryness and thickening of conjunctiva in vit A deficiency

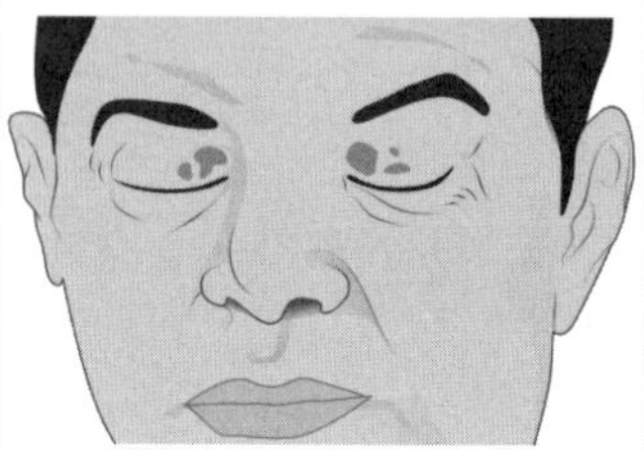

Xanthelasma of the eyelids

xeroradiography a photoelectric process of making radiographs using semiconductor-coated metal plates, specially useful for breasts

xerostomia dryness of mouth due to salivary gland dysfunction

X-linked transmitted by gene present on x- chromosome

XO a symbol for turner syndrome where females contain only one X-chromosome

X-ray Powerful electromagnetic radiations of extremely short wavelength.

x tuberous yellowish orange nodules on skin over joints in hyperlipoproteinemia, biliary cirrhosis and myxedema

XXY syndrome Klinefelter's syndrome where a male has two X chromosomes and one Y chromosome

xylitol a sweetener used as sugar substitute in diabetics

xylocaine lignocaine, a local anesthetic

xylometazoline adrenergic agent used as topical nasal decongestant

xylose a pentose sugar used in diagnosis of intestinal malabsorption

XYY syndrome a supermale with 2Y chromosomes tend to be all and may exhibit aggressive and antisocial behavior

yaws nonvenereal treponemal disease of skin often involving bone and joint

Y chromosome the complimentary male sex chromosome

yeast unicellular fungi fermenting carbohydrate, e.g. Baker's yeast also a source of B complex vitamins and protein

Yersinia a genus of gram-negative nonencapsulated bacteria causing gastroenteritis and mesenteric lymphadenitis (*Y. enterocolitica*, *Y. pseudotuberculosis*) and plague (*Y. pestis*)

yin-yang the feminine and masculine energies in human being whose balance is crucial to good health as believed by Chinese

yoga a set of exercises of disciplined body and mind

yogurt a semisolid fermented food made by adding bacterial strains of *Lactobacillus* and *Streptococcus* to raw milk

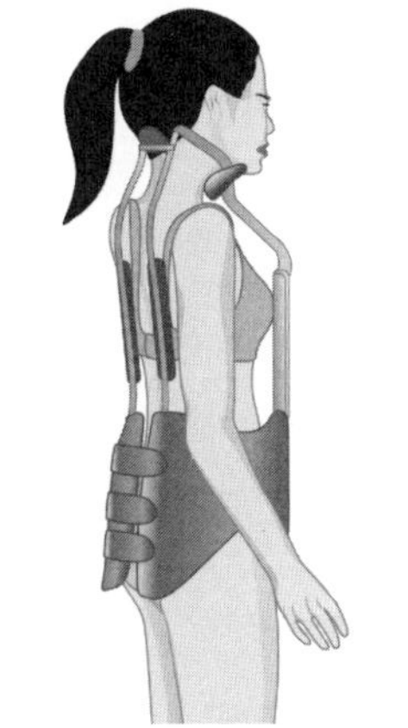

Yale brace

yolk sac the cavity in the developing embryo surrounded by entodermal cells

yttrium beta-emitting isotope used in radiotherapy

yale brace a device used for the stabilization of cervical spine

zafirlukast a leukotriene receptor antagonist used in bronchial asthma

zalcitabine a reverse transcriptase inhibitor used in treatment of HIV patients

Ziehl-Neelsen method a method of staining acid-fast organisms like tubercle bacillus with boiled carbol fuschin followed by rinsing alcohol

zileuton a leukotriene synthesis inhibitor used in bronchial asthma

zinc an essential micronutrient vital for enzyme function. ***z. acetate*** an astringent and hemostyptic, ***z. chloride*** used as nutritional supplement in total parenteral nutrition and applied topically as an astringent and a desensitizer for dentin. ***z. oxide*** a topical astringent. ***z. sulfate*** a topical astringent for eyes. ***z. undecylenate*** a topical antifungal

zolmitriptan a selective serotonin reuptake inhibitor used in migraine

zolpidem a nonbenzodiazepine used for insomnia

zona pellucida the cellular transparent membrane surrounding ovum which is to be penetrated by sperm for fertilization

zoology the biology of animals

zoonosis disease of animals transmissible to man

zoophilia abnormal fondness for animals

zoophobia irrational fear for animals

zydovudine a reverse transcriptase inhibitor used in treatment of HIV patients

zygoma zygomatic process of temporal bone

zygote intrafallopian transfer (ZIFT) a method of infertility treatment where the zygote is placed into midampullary portion of Fallopian tube

zygote the fertilized ovum prior to segmentation

zymoprotein any protein which also possesses enzymatic activity

Appendices

Appendix 1

Abbreviations used in prescriptions

Abbreviation	*Latin*	*English*
a.c.	ante cibum	before food
ad lib.	ad libitum	to the desired amount
b.d. or b.i.d.	bis in die	twice a day
c.	cum	with
o.m.	omni mane	every morning
o.n.	omni nocte	every night
p.c.	post cibum	after food
p.r.n.	pro re nata	whenever necessary
q.d.	quaque die	everyday
q.d.s.	quaque die sumendum	four times daily
q.i.d.	quater in die	four times a day
q.q.h.	quater quaque hora	every four hours
R	recipe	take
s.o.s.	si opus sit	if necessary
stat.	statim	at once
t.d.s	ter die sumendum	three times a day
t.i.d.	ter in die	three times a day

Appendix 2

Abbreviations for diseases, investigations and procedures

AC	Air conduction
AFB	Acid-fast *Bacillus*
ALT	Alanine aminotransferase
ANA	Antinuclear antibodies
ANF	Antinuclear factor
APB	Atrial premature beat
AR	Aortic regurgitation
ARF	Acute rheumatic fever
AS	Aortic stenosis
ASD	Atrial septal defect
ASO	Antistreptococcal `O' titer
AST	Antistreptozyme titer Aspartate transaminase
ATT	Antitubercular treatment
AVM	Arteriovenous malformation
BC	Bone conduction
BPH	Benign hypertrophy of prostate
CABG	Coronary artery bypass grafting
CAD	Coronary artery disease
CHF	Congestive heart failure
CMV	Closed mitral valvotomy, cytomegalovirus
CNS	Central nervous system
COPD	Chronic obstructive lung disease
CP	Creative protein
CPK	Creatine phosphokinase
CT	Computerized tomography
Cx	Circumflex
DAT	Differential agglutination test
DCM	Dilated cardiomyopathy
DIC	Disseminated intravascular coagulation
DLC	Differential leukocyte count
ECE	Extracapsular cataract extraction
EF	Ejection fraction
ELISA	Enzyme-linked immunosorbent assay

Contd...

Contd...

ERCP	Endoscopic retrograde cholangiopancreatography
FEV	Forced expiratory volume
FVC	Forced vital capacity
G6PD	Glucose-6-phosphate dehydrogenase
HAV	Hepatitis A virus
HBcAg	Hepatitis B core antigen
HBsAg	Hepatitis B surface antigen
HBV	Hepatitis B virus
HIV	Human immunodeficiency virus
HOCM	Hypertrophic obstructive cardiomyopathy
HSV	Herpes simplex virus
ICCE	Intracapsular cataract extraction
ICCU	Intensive coronary care unit
ICT	Intracranial tension
ICU	Intensive care unit
IHD	Ischemic heart disease
INO	Internuclear ophthalmoplegia
ITP	Idiopathic thrombocytopenic purpura
JVP	Jugular venous pressure
LA	Left atrium
LAD	Left anterior descending artery
LDH	Lactate dehydrogenase
LIMA	Left internal mammary artery
LMN	Lower motor neuron
LP	Lumbar puncture
LV	Left ventricle
LVEDP	Left ventricular end-diastolic pressure
LVEDV	Left ventricular end-diastolic volume
LVH	Left ventricular hypertrophy
MCP	Metacarpophallangeal joint
MDM	Mid-diastolic murmur
MND	Motor neuron disease
MR	Mitral regurgitation, mental retardation
MRCP	Magnetic resonance cholangiopancreatography
MS	Mitral stenosis
MTP	Metatarsophallangeal joint, medical termination of pregnancy

Contd...

Contd...

MVI	Multivitamin infusion
MVP	Mitral valvoplasty, mitral valve prolapse
NMR	Nuclear magnetic resonance
NSAID	Nonsteroidal anti-inflammatory drugs
OS	Opening snap
PaO_2	Partial pressure of oxygen
PCWP	Pulmonary capillary wedge pressure
PDA	Patent ductus arteriosus
PIP	Proximal interphallangeal joint
PKP	Penetrating keratoplasty
PNH	Paroxysmal nocturnal hemoglobinuria
PS	Pulmonary stenosis
RA	Right atrium
RIND	Reversible ischemic neurologic deficit
RK	Radial keratotomy
RV	Right ventricle
SAH	Subarachnoid hemorrhage
SBE	Subacute bacterial endocarditis
SCAT	Sheep cell agglutination test
SGOT	Serum glutamic oxaloacetic transaminase
SGPT	Serum glutamic pyruvic transaminase
TB	Tuberculosis
TCA	Transient ischemic attack
TGV	Transposition great vessels
TIPS	Transjugular intrahepatic portohepatic shunting
TLC	Total leukocyte count
TOF	Tetralogy of Fallot
TR	Tricuspid regurgitation
TS	Tricuspid stenosis
TTP	Thrombotic thrombocytopenic purpura
UMN	Upper motor neuron
VPB	Ventricular premature beat
VSD	Ventricular septal defect

Appendix 3

Child and infant resuscitation

Infant younger than 1 year		*Child older than 1 year*
Shake, pinch gently Shout for help	Check conscious level ↓	Shake, pinch gently Shout for help
Head tilt. Chin tilt (jaw thrust)	Open airway	Head tilt. Chin tilt (jaw thrust)
Look, listen, feel	↓	Look, listen, feel
Five breaths (mouth to mouth and nose)	Check breathing ↓	Five breaths (mouth to mouth)
Feel brachial pulse. Start compression if <60/min	Breathe ↓	Feel carotid pulse. If no pulse start chest compressions
Two fingers, over sternum Rate 100/min, depth 2 cm. Five compressions: One	Check pulse ↓ Chest compressions	Heel of one hand, over sternum Rate 100/min, depth 3 cm. breath. Five compressions: One breath

Appendix 4

A. Food sources of water-soluble vitamins

Vitamin	*Food sources*
C (ascorbic acid)	Fruit—especially citrus fruit, blackcurrants Green vegetabls—especially frozen peas, tomoatoes, capsicums New potatoes
B_1 (thiamin)	Meat—especially pork, duck Cereal products—especially brown and wholemeal bread, breakfast cereals, wheatgerm Yeast, yeast extract Pulses, nuts
B_2 (riboflavin)	Dairy products, eggs Bread, fortified breakfast cereals Wheatgerm, wheatbran Mushrooms, yeast extract Liver, kidney Pulses
B_6 (pyridoxine)	Meat, fish, milk, eggs, liver Wholegrain cereals Peanuts, walnuts Bananas, avocados
B_{12} (cobalamin)	Meat—especially liver, kidney, rabbit Sardines, oysters Dairy produce, eggs
Niacin (nicotinic acid)	Meat—especially offal Fish Brewer's yeast, yeast extract Wholemeal wheat, bran Peanuts, pulses, coffee
Folate (folic acid)	Liver, kidney Dark green leafy vegetables (easily destroyed by cooking) Beetroot, bran, peanuts Avocados, bananas, oranges Wholemeal bread Eggs, chocolate Some fish

B. Food sources of fat-soluble vitamins

Vitamin	*Food sources*
A	β-carotene—orange and green vegetables, apricots, melon, egg yolk Preformed vitamin A—offal, dairy produce, fortified margarine, oily fish, fish liver oils
D	Fish liver oils, oily fish Fortified margarine Liver, egg yolk Full cream milk, cheese, butter
E	Vegetable oils—especially wheatgerm oil Margarine Eggs, butter Wholemeal cereals Broccoli
K	Green vegetables Liver oils Potatoes

C. Food sources of minerals

Mineral	*Food sources*
Calcium	Dairy products Green leafy vegetables Cereal products, especially wheat flour products Pulses
Iron*	Red meat, egg yolk Green vegetables Wholemeal, cereal products Pulses
Sodium	Milk, table salt and in all food products except oil and sugar. Tends to be high in readymade and tinned foods
Potassium	Oranges, bananas, dried fruit Vegetables and most other foods High in instant coffee, chocolate
Iodine	Drinking water, iodized salt Seafish and shellfish Bread, spinach
Fluoride	Tea, seafish, drinking water (depending on the area)

*Absorption enhanced in the presence of vitamin C.

Appendix 5

Psychomotor development

Birth through	Ability to suck, swallow, gag, cry, and maintain eye contact with a person
1st Month	The head needs to be supported. Loud noises may cause a startle reflex
2nd Month	May turn to either side when on their backs; will follow moving objects, able to lift head but not for a sustained period; begin to smile, frown, and turn away
3rd Month	Greater movement and vocal response to stimuli; notice own hands and suck on them; head will be steady while in a supported position
4th and 5th Months	Able to lift head higher when lying on stomach; will reach for objects and may be able to encircle a bottle with both hands; may drool a lot; attempt to put all kinds of objects in mouth
6th–9th Months	Develop ability to grasp and pick up food; are able to pull themselves up to a sitting position and eventually will crawl; they begin to make noises that sound like words and to recognize certain words; will play peek-a-boo
9th–11th Months	Develop ability to handle food and to drink from a cup; may imitate sounds and say certain words; crawl by pulling body along with arms, and pull themselves to a standing position; they will point at objects and throw things; they want to feed themselves and to help with dressing and undressing; they will walk while holding a person's hand
12th Month	Can eat food alone and drink from a cup with assistance; able to move around easily, and crawl upstairs, and out of crib

Appendix 6

A. Nutrition ready reckoner for international foods

	Calories (Kcal)	*Proteins (g)*	*Fats (g)*	*Carbo-hydrates (g)*	*Fiber (g)*	*Calcium (mg)*	*Iron (mg)*	*Carotene (mcg)*	*Retinol (mcg)*	*Vit B_1 (mg)*	*Vit B_2 (mg)*	*Niacin (mg)*	*Vit C (mg)*	*Serving portion*
BEVERAGES														
Hot tea	34	0.6	1.0	5.7	0.0	31.0	0.0	0.0	7.00	0.01	0.01	0.0	0	1 Tea cup
Instant coffee	149	1.0	13.3	6.3	0.0	31.0	0.0	0.0	7.00	0.01	0.01	0.0	0	1 Tea cup
Cold coffee (with cream)	279	3.9	17.0	27.7	0.0	144.0	0.3	487.0	183.00	0.06	0.23	0.1	2	1 Tall glass
Banana milkshake	228	6.2	7.5	33.8	0.0	223.0	0.5	40.0	101.00	0.11	0.37	0.4	7	1 Tall glass
Mango milkshake	237	6.2	7.7	35.6	0.8	227.0	1.3	2067.0	608.00	0.15	0.41	9.0	16	1 Tall glass
Lemonade	107	0.3	0.3	25.7	0.5	21.0	0.1	0.0	0.00	0.01	0.00	0.0	12	1 Glass
BREAKFAST CEREALS														
Cracked wheat porridge	292	10.0	10.4	39.7	2.5	296.0	1.5	152.0	39.00	1.29	0.49	1.3	5	1 Bowl
Oat meal porridge	217	6.6	6.6	32.8	2.0	154.0	1.0	70.0	18.00	0.80	0.26	0.3	2	1 Bowl
Cornflakes with milk	291	9.8	10.8	38.7	1.2	290.0	0.9	157.0	41.00	1.28	0.48	0.6	5	1 Bowl
EGGS														
Boiled egg	87	6.7	6.7	0.0	0.0	25.0	0.7	300.0	180.00	0.05	0.20	0.1	0	1 Egg
Poached egg	87	6.7	6.7	0.0	0.0	25.0	0.7	300.0	180.00	0.05	0.20	0.1	0	1 Egg
Fried egg	160	6.7	14.8	0.0	0.0	25.0	0.7	620.0	260.00	0.05	0.20	0.1	0	1 Egg
Scrambled egg	172	6.7	15.8	0.8	0.0	57.0	0.7	620.0	267.00	0.06	0.22	0.1	0	1 Egg
Baked egg	124	6.7	10.8	0.0	0.0	25.0	0.7	460.0	220.0	0.05	0.20	0.1	0	1 Egg
Fluffy omelette	160	6.7	14.8	0.0	0.0	25.0	0.7	620.0	260.00	0.05	0.20	0.1	0	1 Egg
Cheese and mushroom omelette	308	12.9	27.1	3.0	0.0	182.0	1.3	780.0	373.00	0.09	0.42	1.5	1	1 Egg

Contd...

Contd...

	Calories (Kcal)	Proteins (g)	Fats (g)	Carbo-hydrates (g)	Fiber (g)	Calcium (mg)	Iron (mg)	Carotene (mcg)	Retinol (mcg)	Vit B_1 (mg)	Vit B_2 (mg)	Niacin (mg)	Vit C (mg)	Serving portion
SOUPS														
Minestrone soup	90	1.4	5.2	9.4	1.2	43.0	0.7	491.0	123.00	0.07	0.03	0.5	17	1 Bowl
Chicken sweet corn soup	322	25.5	13.5	24.6	6.0	23.0	2.6	107.0	93.00	0.21	0.34	8.6	6	1 Bowl
French onion soup	208	4.8	11.6	21.1	2.4	102.0	0.8	321.0	110.00	0.08	0.05	0.6	8	1 Bowl
Tomato soup	82	2.1	4.5	8.3	2.3	101.0	1.3	862.0	216.00	0.25	0.21	0.8	55	1 Bowl
Green pea soup	186	9.0	6.4	23.1	2.2	70.0	1.9	375.0	109.00	0.28	0.08	1.1	11	1 Bowl
Spinach soup	561	3.9	8.9	116.2	5.9	81.0	1.5	5902.0	1475.00	0.06	0.27	0.08	29	1 Bowl
Mixed vegetable soup	146	3.3	9.2	12.5	1.4	124.0	0.9	779.0	225.0	0.11	0.16	0.6	23	1 Bowl
Cream with tomato soup	245	5.4	16.6	18.5	2.3	180.0	1.5	984.0	287.00	0.32	0.25	1.0	45	1 Bowl
Cream with spinach soup	307	8.5	23.2	16.0	5.1	200.0	2.2	6214.0	1644.0	0.20	0.52	0.9	32	1 Bowl
Cream with carrot soup	250	4.6	16.2	21.5	2.0	172.0	1.4	1935.0	531.00	0.17	0.17	0.9	6	1 Bowl
Cream with mixed vegetable soup	263	7.5	13.4	28.0	3.2	179.0	2.0	1160.0	331.00	0.33	0.24	1.5	45	1 Bowl
Cream with mushroom soup	308	6.6	22.4	19.9	0.7	136.0	1.5	554.0	189.00	0.13	0.41	2.9	6	1 Bowl
Hot and sour soup	181	11.2	9.3	13.2	1.6	65.0	2.8	86.0	22.00	0.22	0.25	23	6	1 Bowl
CEREALS														
Boiled rice	277	6.0	0.8	61.4	3.6	8.00	2.6	2.0	0.40	0.17	0.13	3.1	0	1
Beans and macaroni	352	12.1	16.8	38.0	3.7	243.0	2.2	673.0	242.00	0.20	0.20	1.5	40	1 Plate
Spaghetti shallow dish bolognese	346	14.6	14.9	38.3	33.0	174.0	3.2	867.0	236.00	0.28	0.21	4.8	30	1
Chicken shallow dish chowmein	542	31.4	24.2	49.6	3.9	104.0	5.6	9.8	333.00	0.39	0.36	8.1	59	1

Contd...

Contd...

	Calories (Kcal)	Proteins (g)	Fats (g)	Carbo-hydrates (g)	Fiber (g)	Calcium (mg)	Iron (mg)	Carotene (mcg)	Retinol (mcg)	Vit B_1 (mg)	Vit B_2 (mg)	Niacin (mg)	Vit C (mg)	Serving Portion
MEATS														
Shepherd's pie	486	23.8	34.5	20.0	2.2	206.0	3.5	339.0	98.00	0.31	0.18	9.2	15	1 Bowl
Roast chicken	297	25.3	21.8	0.0	0.0	18.0	2.0	334.0	166.0	0.13	0.20	10.0	0	1 Bowl
Chilli chicken	464	27.3	35.5	8.8	1.9	46.0	3.1	222.0	135.0	0.35	0.31	10.9	50	1 Bowl
Chicken sweet and sour	420	27.0	33.3	3.1	0.8	39.0	2.7	270.0	181.0	0.28	0.35	10.6	30	1 Bowl
Fried fish with chips	443	26.3	26.2	25.4	2.2	307.0	3.3	165.0	94.00	0.09	0.11	0.9	9	1 Bowl
Fish in coconut milk	371	27.0	17.1	27.2	3.2	150.0	3.2	4.0	1.00	0.06	0.03	0.5	7	1 Bowl
Prawn curry	342	30.1	19.9	10.5	2.7	509.0	9.3	3.0	0.80	0.05	0.18	7.5	4	1 Bowl
Crispy baked fish	390	32.3	15.1	31.2	4.1	461.0	4.1	496.0	153.00	0.13	0.13	1.3	16	1 Bowl
VEGETABLES														
Egg curry	314	15.5	17.6	23.3	2.8	85.0	2.8	483.0	237.00	0.38	0.25	1.2	21	1 Bowl
Stuffed tomatoes	233	6.0	15.6	17.1	2.8	138.0	1.5	829.0	228.00	0.27	0.08	1.1	41	2 Tomatoes
Stuffed okra	132	2.3	10.2	7.7	5.9	79.0	0.5	62.0	16.00	0.08	0.12	0.7	16	1 Bowl
Roast potatoes	191	2.4	5.0	34.0	3.8	15.0	0.8	228.0	57.00	0.15	0.01	1.8	26	1–2 Potatoes
Stuffed baked potato	334	7.1	18.8	34.0	3.8	33.0	1.3	698.0	248.00	0.19	0.16	1.8	26	1–2 Potatoes
Creamed bowl	429	21.4	29.8	18.8	9.3	458.0	3.5	11812.0	3195.00	0.25	1.00	1.4	58	1 Small spinach
Creamed spinach and mushrooms	363	13.4	25.8	19.2	7.1	366.0	2.9	8692.0	2284.00	0.23	0.90	3.5	45	1 Bowl

Contd...

Contd...

	Calories (Kcal)	*Proteins (g)*	*Fats (g)*	*Carbo-hydrates (g)*	*Fiber (g)*	*Calcium (mg)*	*Iron (mg)*	*Carotene (mcg)*	*Retinol (mcg)*	*Vit B_1 (mg)*	*Vit B_2 (mg)*	*Niacin (mg)*	*Vit C (mg)*	*Serving portion*
SALADS														
Russian salad	959	19.7	85.6	27.5	3.3	100.0	3.8	879.0	333.00	0.38	0.33	5.4	39	1 Small bowl
Beetroot and egg salad	366	8.9	30.8	13.4	3.6	62.0	2.1	300.0	180.00	0.12	0.29	0.6	15	1 Small bowl
Tossed green salad	153	1.5	12.2	9.2	2.0	50.0	0.9	225.0	57.00	0.18	0.04	0.5	43	1 Small bowl
Cucumber and yogurt salad	29	1.3	1.3	2.9	1.0	53.0	0.5	10.0	4.00	0.04	0.05	0.2	6	1 Small bowl
French dressing	722	0.0	80.0	0.4	0.0	1.0	0.0	0.0	0.00	0.00	0.00	0.01	1	3/4 Cup
Mayonnaise	1220	7.1	131.8	1.3	0.0	56.0	1.4	380.0	229.00	0.08	0.26	0.0	4	1 Cup
Mayonnaise without eggs	886	7.7	90.1	11.0	0.0	288.0	0.5	139.0	36.00	1.20	0.46	0.3	6	1 Cup
DESSERTS														
Vanilla ice cream	288	2.3	22.9	18.2	0.0	90.0	0.2	415.0	139.00	0.03	0.14	0.1	0	1 Ice cream cup
Strawberry ice cream	288	2.3	22.9	18.2	0.0	90.0	0.2	415.0	139.00	0.03	0.14	0.1	0	1 Ice cream cup
Chocolate ice cream	288	2.3	22.9	18.2	0.0	90.0	0.2	415.0	139.00	0.03	0.14	0.1	0	1 Ice cream cup
Fruit ice cream	323	2.6	23.0	26.5	0.3	95.0	0.4	832.0	246.00	0.05	0.16	0.3	5	1 Sundae glass
Cold lemon	534	6.9	41.9	32.3	0.4	41.0	0.8	1000.0	355.00	0.05	0.20	0.1	8.8	1 Souffle dish

Contd...

Contd...

	Calories (Kcal)	*Proteins (g)*	*Fats (g)*	*Carbo-hydrates (g)*	*Fiber (g)*	*Calcium (mg)*	*Iron (mg)*	*Carotene (mcg)*	*Retinol (mcg)*	*Vit B_1 (mg)*	*Vit B_2 (mg)*	*Niacin (mg)*	*Vit C (mg)*	*Serving portion*
Souffle cold orange	594	7.8	42.0	46.2	1.5	64.0	1.2	2656.0	769.00	0.05	0.20	0.1	45	1 Souffle dish
Souffle cold pineappple	525	6.7	42.0	30.00	0.0	25.0	0.7	1000.0	355.00	0.00	0.20	0.1	0	1 Souffle dish
Souffle cold vanilla	536	7.3	42.7	30.6	0.0	57.0	0.7	1000.0	362.00	0.06	0.20	0.1	0.2	1 Souffle dish
Souffle cold chocolate	536	7.3	42.7	30.6	0.0	57.0	0.7	1000.0	362.00	0.06	0.20	0.1	0.2	1 Souffle dish
Souffle bread and butter pudding	222	7.4	11.3	22.7	1.0	124.0	0.7	316.0	177.00	0.08	0.27	0.2	2	1 Small plate
SANDWICHES														
Tomato and cheese	268	7.2	11.8	33.3	4.6	88.0	0.9	460.0	145.00	0.09	0.06	0.6	11	2 Pcs
Tomato and cucumber	231	5.2	8.6	33.1	4.9	28.0	1.0	460.0	115.00	0.10	0.02	0.6	12	2 Pcs
Tomato grilled	313	9.6	15.0	34.8	5.0	160.0	1.2	530.0	192.00	0.12	0.12	0.6	16	4 Pcs
French toast	443	14.6	27.6	34.0	4.6	144.0	1.7	1088.0	407.00	0.15	0.20	0.6	11	2 Pcs
Cheese open	340	11.7	18.6	31.5	7.4	196.0	1.1	328.0	168.00	0.14	0.11	1.5	0	2 Pcs
Danish luncheon	350	16.2	17.5	31.9	4.6	42.0	2.1	620.0	260.00	0.24	0.22	1.2	3	2 Pcs
Chicken and corn open	340	15.6	15.0	35.6	5.5	18.0	1.8	362.0	124.0	0.12	0.11	4.6	3	2 Pcs
CAKES														
Sponge cake	177	6.2	4.6	27.8	0.5	20.2	0.9	202.0	120.00	0.05	0.14	0.4	0	1 Pc
Sponge chocolate cake	156	5.5	4.5	23.3	0.3	18.8	0.7	201.0	120.00	0.05	0.14	0.3	0	1 Pc
Pineapple pastry	279	7.1	13.2	32.9	0.6	23.1	1.0	390.0	176.00	0.06	0.16	0.5	0	1 Pastry
Chocolate pastry	228	5.5	12.5	23.3	0.3	19.0	0.7	361.0	160.00	0.05	0.14	0.3	0	1 Pastry
Chocolate cream cake	223	3.1	13.1	23.2	0.4	9.0	0.5	526.0	158.00	0.03	0.06	0.3	0	1 Pc

B. Fishes and sea food

Food	*Protein (g)*	*Fat (g)*	*Carbohydrate*	*Calories*	*Calcium (mg)*	*Iron (mg)*
Anchovy	19.4	9.5	0.2	165	142	1.5
Cat fish	21.2	—	—	88	550	0.4
Blue mussel	9.9	2.0	3.6	70	1130	8.0
Crab small	11.2	5.8	3.3	59	1370	20.4
Crab mussel	8.9	1.1	3.7	109	590	—
Lobster	20.5	0.9	—	90	16	—
Shrimp small dried	68.1	8.5	—	349	4380	—
Silver belly	19.2	1.6	—	91	715	2.2

C. Animal food

Food	*Protein*	*Fat*	*Carbohydrate*	*Calories*	*Calcium (mg)*	*Iron (mg)*
Beef meat	79.2	10.3	0.2	410	6	18.8
Beaf mussel	22.8	2.5	—	114	10	0.8
Duck	21.6	4.8	0.1	130	4	—
Buffalo meat	19.4	0.9	—	86	3	—
Fowl	21.8	0.6	—	109	24	—
Goat meat	21.4	3.6	—	118	12	—
Liver goat	2.0	3.0	—	107	17	—
Liver sheep	19.5	7.5	1.3	150	10	6.3
Mutton	18.5	13.3	—	195	148	2.3
Pigeon	23.3	4.9	—	114	3	2.2
Snail small	12.6	1.0	3.7	75	1320	—
Snail big	10.5	0.5	12.4	98	870	—
Turtles meat	16.5	1.5	1.5	88	7	
Finch	26.6	3.0	—	133	90	—

Appendix 7

Normal hematological values

Test	*Normal values*
Total WBC count (TLC)	0–1 year: 10,000–25,000/cmm 1–3 years: 6,000–18,000/cmm 4–7 years: 6,000–15,000/cmm 8–12 years: 4,500–13,500/cmm Adults: 4,000–11,000/cmm
Differential WBC count (DLC)	Polymorphonuclear cells: 50–70% Lymphocytes: 20–40% Monocytes: 4–8% Eosinophils: 0–2% Basophils: 0–1%
RBC count	4.5–5.5 million/cmm
Hemoglobin	At birth: 18 g% Adults Men: 13–16 g% Women: 12–15 g%
Erythrocyte sedimentation rate (ESR)	Men: 0–9 mm/hour Women: 0–20 mm/hour
Bleeding time (BT)	1–6 minutes
Coagulation time (CT)	5–18 minutes
Blood urea	20–40 mg/dL
Blood glucose	Fasting: <110 mg/dL Post-prandial: <140 mg/dL Random: 80–120 mg/dL (after waking up) 100–140 mg/dL (at bedtime)
Total bilirubin	0.1–1.0 mg/dL
Thyroxine	4.5–11.5 µg/dL
Uric acid	2.5–8 mg/dL
Aspartate transaminase (AST) or serum glutamic oxaloacetic transaminase (SGOT)	5–40 IU/L
Alanine transaminase (ALT) or serum glutamic pyruvic transaminase (SGPT)	7–56 IU/L
Alkaline phosphatase	25–100 IU/L
Total cholesterol	<200 mg/dL
Triglycerides	<150 mg/dL
Serum creatinine	1–2 mg/dL

Appendix 8

Normal values in urinalysis

Test	*Normal values*
Color	Pale yellow to deep amber color
Specific gravity	1.015–1.025
pH	4.5–8
Protein (albumin)	Negative
Sugar	Negative
Bilirubin	Negative
RBCs	Nil
WBCs	Nil
Creatinine	0.8–8 g/24 hours
Urobilinogen	Random: <25 mg/dL 24-hour urine: 4 mg/24 hours
Uric acid	250–750 mg/24 hours

Appendix 9

Abbreviations used regarding the route of administration of medicine

Abbreviation	*Meaning*
AD	Right ear
AS	Left ear
AU	Each ear
H	Hypodermic
IM	Intramuscular
INJ	Injection
IV	Intravenous
IVP	Intravenous push
Rx	Take, prescription
OD	Right eye
Sc	Subcutaneously
SQ	Subcutaneous
OS	Left eye
OU	Both eyes
p or P	After, per
PO, per os	By mouth
EC	Enteric-coated
Elix	Elixir
Ext	External, extract
Os	Mouth

Appendix 10

Differential diagnosis of abdominal pain

Region	*Possible causes*
Generalized or diffuse abdominal pain	• Perforation • Aortic aneurysm • Diabetic ketoacidosis • Bilateral pleurisy • Acute pancreatitis • Peritonitis • Severe pelvic inflammatory disease • Gastroenteritis
Central abdominal pain	• Early appendicitis • Acute gastritis • Ruptured aortic aneurysm • Small bowel obstruction • Mesenteric thrombosis • Acute pancreatitis
Epigastric pain	• Aortic aneurysm • Esophagitis • Acute pancreatitis • Gastric and duodenal ulcer
Right upper quadrant pain	• Appendicitis • Hepatic and gallbladder diseases • Duodenal ulcers, myocardial infarction • Acute pancreatitis • Duodenal ulcers • Acute pancreatitis • Basal pneumonia • Subphrenic abscess
Left upper quadrant pain	• Gastric ulcer • Diaphragmatic pleurisy • Acute pancreatitis • Acute perinephritis • Spontaneous splenic rupture • Aortic dissection • Ischemic colitis • Subphrenic abscess

Contd...

Contd...

Region	*Possible causes*
Right lower quadrant pain	• Acute appendicitis • Mesenteric adenitis • Ruptured ectopic pregnancy • Perforated duodenal ulcer • Diverticulitis • Pelvic inflammatory disease • Salpingitis • Ureteric and biliary colic • Crohn's disease • Torsion of ovarian cyst or tumor
Left lower quadrant pain	• Diverticulitis • Constipation • Irritable bowel syndrome • Pelvic inflammatory disease • Rectal carcinoma • Ulcerative colitis • Ruptured ectopic pregnancy • Torsion of ovarian cyst or tumor • Salpingitis
Suprapubic pain	• Acute urinary retention • Urinary tract infection • Cystitis • Pelvic inflammatory disease • Ectopic pregnancy • Diverticulitis
Loin pain	• Muscle strain • Urinary tract infection • Renal stones • Pyelonephritis

Appendix 11

Conditions leading to systemic or localized edema

Systemic edema	• Congestive cardiac failure • Cirrhosis • Nephrotic syndrome or other conditions leading to hypoalbuminemia • Drug-induced • Idiopathic
Localized edema	• Inflammation • Venous or lymphatic obstruction • Chronic lymphangitis • Resection of regional lymph nodes • Filariasis

Appendix 12

Common forms of drug preparation

Drug preparation	*Description*
Capsule	Powder or gel form of drug encased in a relatively stable and soluble shell, usually made of gelatin, to make it easily palatable
Elixir	A solution containing varying amounts of alcohol, a sweetening agent or flavor, and water and may or may not contain active medicine
Emulsion	Drug which is a mixture of 2 or more immiscible liquids
Enteric-coated tablet	Tablet coated with a substance that does not allow the absorption of drug anywhere in gastrointestinal tract, but small intestine
Lotion	A medicated liquid for external application on skin
Lozenge	Sweetened medicated candy that is intended to dissolve slowly in mouth to soothe the irritated tissues of throat
Ointment	Semisolid preparation of a drug that has a base of fatty or greasy material
Plaster	Medicated solid dressing used as an adhesive or a counterirritant
Poultice	Soft, moist mass often heated and medicated and used to treat painful and inflamed part of the body
Suppository	Solid base of drug(s) inserted into the body cavities, other than mouth like rectum and vagina, that melts slowly at body temperature to release the drug
Syrup	Drug dissolved in a thick, sweet, and sticky liquid intended to soothe the irritated membranes
Tablet	Small, flat pellet of drug to be taken orally
Transdermal patch	Medicated adhesive patch, placed on skin, to release a specific dose of medicine

Appendix 13

Australia Vaccine Schedule: 2010

Vaccine	*Birth*	*2 mo.*	*4 mo.*	*6 mo.*	*12 mo.*	*18 mo.*	*4 yrs*	*10–13 yrs*	*15–17 yrs*	*≥65 yrs*
Hepatitis B	HepB	HepB	HepB	HepB						
Rotavirus		RV	RV	RV						
Diphtheria, pertussis, and tetanus		DTPa	DTPa	DTPa			DTPa		dTpa	
Haemophilus influenzae type b		Hib	Hib	Hib	Hib					
Pneumococcal		7vPCV	7vPCV	7vPCV						23vPPV
Poliovaccine (inactivated)		IPV	IPV	IPV			IPV			
Measles, mumps, and rubella					MMR		MMR			
Varicella						Vari-cella				
Meningococcus					Men CCV					
Human papillomavirus vaccine								HPV[1]		
Influenza										Yearly

(Shaded) Range of recommended ages except certain high-risk groups. See references for more details including "catch-up" immunizations, and recommendations for high-risk groups

1. 12–13 years, females only

Source: "National Immunisation Program Schedule". Australian Government. Retrieved 2010-05-05.

United kingdom vaccine schedule: 2013

Vaccine	*2 mo.*	*3 mo.*	*4 mo.*	*12 mo.*	*3–4 yrs*	*12–13 yrs*	*13–18 yrs*
Diphtheria, pertussis and tetanus	DTaP + IPV + Hib	DTaP + IPV + Hib	DTaP + IPV + Hib		DTaP + IPV		Td + IPV
Poliovaccine (inactivated)							
Haemophilus influenzae type b				Hib + MenC			
Meningococcus		MenC					MenC (13–15 yrs)
Rotavirus (from July 2013)	Rotavirus	Rotavirus					
Pneumococcal	PCV		PCV	PCV			
Measles, mumps, and rubella				MMR	MMR		
Human papillomavirus vaccine						HPV x 3[1]	

1. Females only 3 vaccinations over 12 months

Source: Department of Health and National Health Service. "Vaccination schedule". National Health Service. Retrieved 2013-06-04.

United states vaccine schedule: 2012

Vaccine	*Birth*	*1 mo.*	*2 mo.*	*4 mo.*	*6 mo.*	*9 mo.*	*12 mo.*	*15 mo.*	*18 mo.*	*19–23 mo*	*2–3 yrs*	*4–6 yrs*	*7–10 yrs*	*11–12 yrs*	*13–18 yrs*	*19–26 yrs*	*27–59 yrs*		*60–64 yrs*	*≥65 yrs*
Hepatitis B	HepB	HepB			HepB					Complete 3-dose series						3 doses				
Rotavirus			RV	RV	RV															
Diphtheria, pertussis, and tetanus			DTaP	DTaP	DTaP			DTaP				DTaP	DTaP, 1 dose	DTaP	DTaP, 1 dose	Td (every 10 years)				Td or Tdap
Haemophilus influenzae type b			Hib	Hib	Hib		Hib													
Pneumococcal			PCV	PCV	PCV		PCV				PPSV									PPSV
Poliovaccine (inactivated)			IPV	IPV	IPV							IPV	IPV, complete 3-dose series							
Influenza					Influenza (yearly)															
Measles, mumps, and rubella							MMR					MMR	Complete 2-dose series			1 or 2 doses	1 dose			
Varicella (chickenpox)							Varicella					Vari-cella	Complete 2-dose series						Addition of shingles vaccine	
Hepatitis A							HepA, dose 1				HepA Series		Complete 2-dose series							
Meningococcus						MCV								Dose 1	Booster at 16	1 or more doses				
Human papillomavirus vaccine														3 doses	Complete 3 dose series [note]					

▯ Range of recommended ages for everyone.
▮ Range of recommended ages for certain high-risk groups.
▮ Range of recommended ages for catch-up immunization or for people who lack evidence of immunity (e.g., lack documentation of vaccination or have no evidence of prior infection). CDC provides more detailed information in catch-up immunizations.

1. Note on HPV vaccine: Males who have not yet received 3 doses of HPV4 are generally recommended to have done so through age 21. HPV4 is recommended for men who have sex with men through age 26 years who did not get any or all doses when they were younger.

Source:

1. Available from http://www.cdc.gov/vaccines/schedules/hcp/child-adolescent.html.
2. "Recommended Adult Immunization Schedule—United States, 2012". CDC. Retrieved 2012-06-29.